The Holistic Rx
for Kids

The Holistic Rx
for Kids

Parenting Healthy Brains and Bodies
in a Changing World

Madiha Saeed, MD

ROWMAN & LITTLEFIELD
Lanham • Boulder • New York • London

Published by Rowman & Littlefield
An imprint of The Rowman & Littlefield Publishing Group, Inc.
4501 Forbes Boulevard, Suite 200, Lanham, Maryland 20706
www.rowman.com

86-90 Paul Street, London EC2A 4NE, United Kingdom

British Library Cataloguing in Publication Information Available

Library of Congress Cataloging-in-Publication Data

Names: Saeed, Madiha M., author.
Title: The holistic Rx for kids : parenting healthy brains and bodies in a
   changing world / Madiha Saeed.
Description: Lanham : Rowman & Littlefield, [2021] | Includes
   bibliographical references and index. | Summary: "As physical and mental
   health conditions and destructive behaviors skyrocket, Dr. Saeed
   uncovers how our children's brains, bodies, and behaviors are being
   hijacked and presents evidence-based actionable steps parents can take
   to help their children make better decisions, build resilience, and heal
   and prevent acute/chronic conditions at any age"—Provided by
   publisher.
Identifiers: LCCN 2021019625 (print) | LCCN 2021019626 (ebook) | ISBN
   9781538152157 (cloth) | ISBN 9781538152164 (ebook)
Subjects: LCSH: Children—Diseases—Alternative treatment. | Child mental
   health. | Holistic medicine. | Integrative medicine. | Parenting.
Classification: LCC RJ53.A48 S24 2021 (print) | LCC RJ53.A48 (ebook) |
   DDC 618.92/89—dc23
LC record available at https://lccn.loc.gov/2021019625
LC ebook record available at https://lccn.loc.gov/2021019626

To my loving parents and my children,
Abdullah, Zain, Emaad, and Qasim,
who work alongside me
to create a worldwide healing revolution!

Contents

Contents

Disclaimer

This book represents reference material only. It is not intended as a medical manual, and the data presented here are meant to assist the reader in making informed choices regarding wellness. This book is not a replacement for treatment that the reader's personal physician may have suggested. If the reader believes he or she is experiencing a medical issue, professional medical help is recommended. Mention of particular products, companies, or authorities in this book does not entail endorsement by the publisher or author.

Foreword

$\mathcal{I}$'m often asked, "How on earth do you do it all?" And Dr. Madiha Saeed is the person I ask that same question all the time. I'm in awe of her ability to seamlessly balance being a present mom to her four incredible sons, managing an active family-physician practice as a board-certified doctor, and prolifically writing and educating millions of people through her online work.

I first met Madiha at a health event and was immediately struck by her presence and knowledge. Her energy was infectious, and her passion for helping families was immediately noticeable. We spent hours talking about health research, parenting, and dozens of other topics, and I left that weekend knowing that she would be a growing force for good.

Since then, she has become a good friend and a core member of my medical review board, and it has been a pleasure to continue to work with her. She has an unmatched skill for making complex topics actionable and easy to understand and inspiring life-changing action in her patients and readers.

Madiha has a burning desire to help improve health and wellness for families and shares the mission of changing the myriad statistics pointing to the rising problems our children's generation will face. As a practicing board-certified family physician, she works hands on each day with her patients and spends much of her free time (after caring for her family) researching and writing to help others worldwide.

Her first bestselling book, *The Holistic Rx: Your Guide to Healing Chronic Inflammation and Disease*, provided a practical blueprint for families to move toward healing and vibrant health. Dr. Madiha walks the walk, building on her own experience overcoming autoimmune disease, joint pain, fatigue, weight struggles, skin issues, and more, and pulling from the best of current research and clinical expertise to shorten the learning curve for everyone she helps.

The best part?

As a busy mom, she understands just how hectic family life can be and how moms have limited free time and extra bandwidth.

In her timely new book, Dr. Saeed focuses specifically on children, offering specific holistic parenting and health guidelines for raising healthy children: brain, body, and soul.

This volume is a much-needed solution as chronic physical and mental health conditions are drastically on the rise . . . in children. Madiha fearlessly takes on the threats hijacking our children's bodies and brains and gives parents a road map to creating resilient and healthy children in a world working against us.

If you ever feel overwhelmed, are dealing with health struggles, or have children who have been affected by any health condition, read this book and then reread it! Take notes, highlight, underline, and implement these simple steps. Dr. Madiha has done the research and real-world work to provide the most straightforward path for your children and your family to follow. You'll feel like you are getting wisdom and advice from one of your closest and most trusted friends . . . because you are! She will show you the steps without adding extra steps or stress to your life.

I'm grateful to Madiha for her work, and you will be, too!

Warmly,
Katie Wells
Founder, WellnessMama.com

Acknowledgments

I CAN'T THANK GOD ENOUGH!

I am so thankful for all the blessings in my life—especially my children, Abdullah, Zain, Emaad, and Qasim—for opening my eyes and heart to this mission. I am also thankful for my parents, Muhammad and Nusrat Saeed, and my family. My parents sacrificed everything, literally everything, for my siblings and me to be where we are today. They sold our home; left loved ones, family, and friends; and moved multiple times only because they wanted us to live our lives without debt. They opened my heart to the power of unconditional love and what it truly means to trust your heart when the world is telling you something different.

I am grateful for my husband, Omer; my siblings/best friends (Athar, Fasiha, Sophia, and Atif); and my in-laws (Mumtaz, Tahira, Usman bhi, Sadaf, Sadia, and Shazia), who supported me through every hurdle, took on my "out-of-the-box" ideas, respected me, and loved me through everything I learned. I've had to change our entire lifestyle, change foods, change restaurants, change outings, and change dietary habits, and my family supported me through thick and thin. I couldn't have asked for a better and more supportive family.

I wouldn't have developed a passion for parenting if it weren't for Dr. Dominic Vachon, who guided me to a world of compassionate care. I extend my heartfelt thanks to Uthman Cavallo, Susan Hart-Cavallo, Shelly, Krista, Becky, Nancy, Deanne, and everyone at Physicians HolisticHealth Alliance for believing in me, taking me under their wing, and helping me bloom into who I am today.

I am grateful for my friends and family—Zaina, Yvonne, Huma, Samia, Lobna, Aliya and Tayibba Baji, Laura, Noor, Adina, Fatima, Sr. Jill, Dr. Ahmad,

Aunty Ayesha, my aunts and uncles—and so many more who supported me, edited my books, listened to my ideas on educating the world, and encouraged me every step of the way. I owe a debt of gratitude to Rowman & Littlefield; my editor, Suzanne, and her team; and my agent, Jeff Herman, for helping me make my dreams a reality. I am so very thankful for all the leaders in functional, integrative, and holistic medicine—Dr. Mark Hyman, Dr. Jeffery Bland, Dr. Amy Myers, Dr. Deanna Minich, Dr. Terry Wahls, Dr. Tom O'Bryan, Dr. Izabella Wentz, Dr. Maya Shetreat, Dr. David Perlmutter, Beth Lambert, Margot Sunderland, Erik Goldman, Kimberly Whittle, Katie Wells (Wellness Mama), Kaya and Dhru Purohit, JJ Virgin, Dr. Steven Masley, Jason and Colleen Wachob, and so many more—who have educated and opened my eyes to the holistic system of healing and the importance of a healthy lifestyle. I also thank Mary Agnes and the late Tommy Antonopoulos for believing in me and blessing me with their guidance, love, and support. Thank you all for changing my life forever!

The power of unconditional love and sacrifice opened doors that I never could have imagined. Love has brought me here today. Love has brought me to you. Love can save our future. Together we can raise each other up to create a healing revolution. Our children depend on it.

Introduction

From Medical Doctor to HolisticMom, MD

$\mathcal{O}$ur children are our treasures, our eternal loves, and our little miracles; wrapped in a receiving blanket, they are beautiful gifts to hold in our arms forever. As you stare into your bright new child's eyes, your heart skips a beat, your heart grows, and each cell in your body leaps with happiness; immediately, your thoughts turn to concern. You are now responsible for a little human being. How can we keep these little miracles safe from the world? Do we really have what it takes to allow these children to thrive and be healthy, or do we leave it all up to chance and fate?

The overall health of the family is critical to our society. If our families are healthy, society is healthy. If our families are sick, and if our brains and bodies are not working appropriately, it trickles down to our society and our world. This is today's sad reality. Despite the advances in modern medicine, our families, our society, and our world are getting sicker and sicker.

According to the Centers for Disease Control, about 60 percent of all adults in the United States have at least one noncommunicable chronic health condition, while 40 percent have two or more, and the numbers continue to grow at an alarming rate. Worldwide obesity has nearly tripled since 1975.[1] Obesity affects one in every three adults; almost two billion adults are overweight, and one in every five children is obese. One out of every two children has a chronic health condition, and this statistic is estimated to increase to eight out of every ten by 2025. Johns Hopkins Bloomberg School of Public Health reports that the prevalence of autism has nearly tripled since 2000.[2] If we continue on the current trajectory, one in every four children will have a form of autism by 2033.[3]

Health aside, in the next twenty-four hours, 1,439 teens will commit suicide, 3,506 teens will run away, and 15,006 teens will use drugs for the first time. Every seven minutes a youth is arrested for a drug crime, and destructive

1

behavior overall is on the rise.[4] During the COVID-19 pandemic, the Children's Hospital Association and the American Association of Pediatrics found a nearly 20 percent spike in the number of young people attempting suicide and more than a 40 percent increase in behavioral issues.[5] That is a lot of children! With chronic disease on the rise, what will happen to humanity if our children are all sick and continue to get sicker and more destructive?

What is going on with our children? Are our children's futures just left to chance? Did you know our children's brains, body, and behaviors are being hijacked, making parenting these children ten times harder? It's time for a parenting revolution. It's time to start parenting a child's brain, body, and behavior so our children are ready and prepped to make better decisions, develop resilience, build deeper relationships, and heal and prevent acute and chronic conditions at any age, no matter what life throws at them.

WHERE TO START? PARENTING IS OVERWHELMING!

Wake up. Feed the kids. School. Work. Home. Feed the family. Homework. Work. Sleep. Repeat. I get it. As a mom of four boys, I completely get it! Life is very overwhelming! There's all the feeding, the chores, the whining, and the arguing on top of meeting the emotional, physical, and psychological needs of every person in your household.

The craziness doesn't end! And when it's quiet, you know someone is creating a pool in a sink somewhere! Now if I have to tell you that you have to learn a totally different way to parent and change your family's lifestyle . . . *forget it!*

As a family physician, mother, international speaker, author, cook, butt wiper, referee, grocery shopper, accountant, cleaner, teacher, and so much more . . . let me tell you a secret . . .

Healthy children with healthy bodies and brains
are soooo much easier to parent!
Better brain, body, and behavior are keys to parenting success.

You are probably asking, "Dr. Saeed, you are a medical doctor. What does medicine have to do with parenting?" When children are healthy, their brains function better, their bodies function better, they make better decisions, they behave better, and you can talk to them like real human beings. Depending on the age, they will have less destructive behaviors or temper tantrums and fewer anger outbursts; they will be more empathetic and mindful; and they will have better relationships. But most important, they are satiated (meaning *less* time in the kitchen for you! Yay!). When your child's brain and body function the way they are supposed to, your child is so much easier to parent. But with more and more children getting sicker, parenting sick children is different and more challenging for the whole family on so many different levels compared to parenting healthy children.

Let me tell you another secret . . . .this is crazy! This blew my mind in residency. . . ready for it?

Your pediatrician or family physician has most likely
never taken a parenting class!

Crazy, right? That is what I thought as I was seeing one child after another for well-child checkups. We would check for their physical developmental milestones but skipped over the child's emotional, spiritual, and mental needs. Doctors are almost never taught nutrition and little stress management, so we have no idea how to feed and help your child thrive in a stressful, changing world. I learned this harsh reality in my final year of residency and was so passionate about it that I even started to educate our family medicine residents about parenting. I had found my calling.

Seeing child after child for the last thirteen years, I have been meticulously studying parenting and functional medicine. I have combined what I have learned over thirteen years in both fields and applied what I learned in my home and in my practice with thousands of patients. I have seen everything from families with healthy children to families with sick children, from families with peaceful children to families with oppositional defiant children with juvenile delinquencies. This world is not the same as our grandparents' world. I am honored to share what I have learned and my real-life experiences with you in this book.

ONCE UPON A TIME

Before becoming a board-certified integrative holistic family physician, I was—like most Americans—unhealthy and overweight. I had many of the same bad habits that have led 60 percent of all Americans down the road toward chronic disease. I was suffering from thyroid disease, acne, seborrheic dermatitis, weight and hormonal problems, digestive issues, severe fatigue, joint and muscle aches, and even lupus (SLE), a disease that literally attacks every cell and organ of the body, eventually killing you. My husband and I were both residents working eighty-hour work weeks, and I was a new mother and wife living far away from family, just trying to keep my head above water. I continued on that hamster wheel, like it was my new normal, until one day when the wheel that I was on came to an abrupt and screeching *halt*!

At noon, my husband had a gut inclination. He asked me, "Can you go and check up on Abdullah? I feel like something is wrong." Almost laughing it off, I walked across to the hospital's day care. I was not prepared for what would unfold next—I walked into every parent's worst nightmare.

When I walked into the day care's infant room, immediately I felt something was off. The lights were dimmed. The day care provider was rocking back and forth, back and forth. As I approached her, she immediately started to stare. Trying to break the awkward silence in the room, I started to talk. Then I heard a barely audible murmuring in the back of the room. I ran back to find my first-born son; his arms and legs had been strapped down with a receiving blanket and a pacifier had been stuck in his mouth. His plush green Winnie the Pooh blanket was wrapped tightly around his mouth and nose. His eyes were bloodshot, he was red in the face, and his swollen cheeks were shiny with tears. He was almost suffocating to death. I quickly picked him up, and as I cradled him in my arms, I unwrapped his face. "You could have killed my child!" I screamed at the day care provider and ran out.

That day, God saved my child. That day, I made a heartfelt solemn promise to take care of these blessings, the best I know how. But how could I take care of these gifts if I couldn't even take care of myself? I, a family physician, was falling apart!

Despite being a physician, I went to one doctor after another to find out how I could stop these diseases from progressing and slowly killing me from the inside out.

No one could answer my question or even had time to listen to my concerns. They simply brushed me off like I was overreacting and offered me medications with side effects like "possible death"! That is what I was trying to prevent . . . something didn't make sense to me. Now bombarded with so much extra stress, my last straw was shingles! Seventy-year-olds have shingles. How did I get this disease?! Why was my body falling apart at such a young age? And what answer did the doctors give me? "It's just stress . . ."

"I know I'm freakin' stressed! How am I supposed to manage this stress?" When I asked what I could do to make sure this problem didn't progress, I was told, "Just sit back and let the disease take its course; there is nothing you can do." Nothing I could do . . . that didn't sit right with me. I was not satisfied with that answer; I took matters into my own hands. Nothing was going to stop me from being there for my children. I continued to research, learn, and look for answers.

What could I do to take back control of my life? I refused to sit back and watch this disease kill me; there had to be another way. As both medical doctor and patient, I was tired of a methodology that covered up symptoms and didn't answer my question: Why did I get sick in the first place? I knew I had the potential to fly but was tired of being weighed down by my chronic symptoms. Hopeless, I was guided to holistic, integrative, and functional medicine, and I was blessed to have joined a holistic medical practice. Working with board-certified physicians, mental health professionals, nutritionists, exercise physiologists, chiropractors, homeopaths, acupuncturists, and so many more, I quickly realized that medical school and residency hadn't taught me what I really needed to know about how to keep people, especially our children, healthy and happy. I was not taught one class on nutrition and almost no stress management, and, surprisingly, my colleagues and siblings in pediatrics, internal medicine, gynecology, and psychiatry were all in the same boat. With all the children we saw, we were taught zero parenting classes!

I promised I would take care of these children—mind, body, and soul—the best I knew how; it's a vow I take seriously with every breath I take. What I learned in the science of parenting and functional, holistic, and integrative medicine research blew my mind! I not only learned how to take care of myself and my family but also learned to combine both for the most effective parenting I have ever come across! It is all about balance and raising mindful children who can immediately feel when they are starting to go off balance.

Our lifestyles are the key to optimal brain and body function.
Balanced Lives + Healthy Brains + Healthy Body = Easy Parenting
Win for You and Win for Them!

Let me explain: On my quest for optimal brain and body health, I came to understand that our imbalanced immune system is one of the primary processes behind most chronic health conditions, and it occurs when our bodies are out of balance, which is one of the consequences of our changing world. Putting the body (including our immune system) back into balance can optimize the mitochondria (powerhouse of the cell) and brain function. That is the key to healthy children who are easier to parent because their brains work better; however, the importance of balancing the immune system is often overlooked. I discovered that the solution lies in the fields of holistic and functional medicine, which gets to the fundamental reasons of why you're feeling the way you're feeling. It uses all the effective tools available—complementary, alternative, and integrative medicine, combined with conventional treatments and unconditional love—to help get the body back into balance. Years of study in holistic, integrative, and functional medicine (as well as parenting)—and applying everything I learned with my family and my patients' families—have transformed my life as a medical doctor and a parent. I now know how to help my families live and parent their children easily and, as a bonus, optimize their immune system and mitochondrial function and help their brains work better. Most important, I walk the talk, so I will be able to provide real-life experiences.

PARENTING DILEMMAS TO PARENTING SUCCESS

Which child do you think would be easier to parent? Is it the child who loves life, is able to get out of bed without a problem, has no aches or pains, and eats a variety of foods? Or is it the child who is depressed, wants to commit suicide, is angry all the time, is destructive, cries without reason, is a picky eater, or is always complaining? It's a no-brainer, right?

Children do better when they feel better. With years of seeing patients and families—especially children with chronic health conditions like depression, suicidal tendencies, bipolar disorder, anxiety, attention-deficit/hyperactivity disorder (ADHD), acne, fatigue, sinus issues, and so much more—I have noticed that if we can help the child's and parents' brains and bodies work better, then everything else in the house improves. Let's take the example of two teens.

The first, a fourteen-year-old boy, had been dealing with depression for nine years. Over the course of the last two years, he had tried nine different antipsychotic medications with no relief from his depression, oppositional defiant disorder, anxiety, ADHD, digestive issues, acne, fatigue, and anger. After extensive blood work and studying his deficiencies, we found he was also dealing with severe insulin resistance and vitamin D deficiency. In two weeks after the initial appointment, by addressing his root causes, he claimed, crying, "I am finally happy that I am finally happy again!" Gradually, as his body continued to heal, with the help of his physician, he was able to wean off of all medications! He is now able to recognize when his mood, mind, and body are imbalanced and then immediately reflect on his lifestyle, recognize what is out of balance, and fix it. He is now excelling in all that he puts his mind to—loving life. He has the power to get his body and mind back into balance and is living a more mindful life.

Now let's take a look at another teen's story. She was a thirteen-year-old female with a history of anger issues, oppositional defiance, ADHD, depression, anxiety, hypercholesterolemia, fatigue, and irritability, who even tried to commit suicide. She was on so many medications, but nothing seemed to help. After we went through a full history, including lab work, and changed her lifestyle, we found out that she also had Hashimoto's disease, insulin resistance, and vitamin deficiencies! Once we gave her body what it needed to work well, she began to thrive off her medications!

If we give our body exactly what it needs to heal, healing is possible at any age. I have twelve years of stories of patients—adults and children—who have reclaimed their lives. These families are now living more fulfilling lives when they put their bodies and brains back into balance. These stories are among thousands of examples that add fuel to my fire to help spread the word of true healing and real living. Patients like you and your child are improving the quality of their lives and are preventing (or recovering from) autoimmune diseases, skin problems, mood disorders, digestive issues, cancer, allergies, asthma, autism, chronic pain, and weight problems (along with a very wide range of nonspecific symptoms) simply by implementing evidence-based, cost-effective lifestyle changes. Even more amazing is that once you target the root cause, you can improve not just one chronic condition or behavior but all of them simultaneously—*and* help make your parenting so much easier!

All these stories are meant to inspire and empower you—that at any age or background, you and your family can have a healthier and more peaceful life. If they could do it, and I could do it, you can do it!

HOW TO NAVIGATE THIS BOOK

The Holistic Rx for Kids targets parenting healthy brains and bodies in a changing world in three simple parts. A child's behavior is the tip of the iceberg. In the first part of the book, we will dive into why our children's brains, bodies, and behavior have been hijacked; why parenting is more challenging today; and why the previous parenting books will not work for today's sicker generation. We will explore the crisis of today's world situation; why our children's brains and bodies are sicker now than ever before; and how our imbalanced lives are leading to inflammation, resulting in a dysfunctional brain and body that doesn't work well. We will then briefly explain the science of holistic parenting and how what we do as parents can affect our children's brain and body chemistry, optimize the immune system, lower overall chronic inflammation in our children's bodies, and build mindful children. With all that in mind, we will discuss the foundations of holistic parenting to raise mindful, resilient children: digestive health, detoxification, and the four S's (stress management, sleep, social health, and spiritual health).

In the second part, we will dive into the foundations of holistic parenting and give real-life parenting solutions to common parenting dilemmas. Children do better when they are able to, so by restoring digestive health, nourishing the body, detoxifying the body, reducing stress, getting quality sleep, building social support, and cultivating spirituality, we can help balance the child from the inside out. This section will examine daily parenting struggles and dilemmas like discipline, optimizing self-esteem, sleep training, and weaning; offer solutions on dealing with chronic stress, acute childhood events/trauma, and bullying; provide suggestions on what to do when you eat out at restaurants or go to parties; and give kid-friendly meal ideas and other practical tips.

Part III highlights what to do when your child does get sick with acute or chronic conditions. This section will delve deeper into a physician-designed, HolisticMom-approved functional medicine approach to managing chronic diseases and highlight integrative modalities (such as supplements, homeopathics, acupressure, and aromatherapy) that can complement your child's conventional care to optimize health and healing.

The Holistic Rx for Kids gives parents and their children everything they need to know without overwhelming them. As a physician mom of four young boys, I offer evidence-based, easy, time-saving, and cost-effective recommendations. Along with my clinical and personal experience, this book features easy action plans based on age, weaning guides, shopping lists, and kid brain- and body-friendly recipes for any busy parent's lifestyle. *The Holistic Rx for Kids* is the missing key parents needed to help their children truly thrive from the inside out, with an added bonus of easing our parenting struggles.

We as parents need to cultivate and help our children grow physically, mentally, and spiritually to the best of our ability. When we provide their little bodies with what they need and allow their brains and bodies to function appropriately, we optimize their potential to truly thrive and, most important, make our parenting so much easier! Families now can have peace of mind that they are doing everything they can to help their children thrive naturally— body, mind, and spirit. Our children are the key to creating a healthier and happier world.

Let's dive into how our children's brains, bodies, and behavior have been hijacked by this changing world—leading to sicker, difficult children—and how we can change the current paradigm.

Part I

PARENTING TODAY'S CHILD

• 1 •

Today's Dilemma

Is Our Changing World Threatening Our Future?

OUR PRESENT, OUR FUTURE, AND OUR WORLD ARE CHANGING

Rapidly changing technology, immediate online deliveries, growing social media platforms, advancements in medical innovations, 5G, food engineering, agriculture . . . we are no longer living in the world of our ancestors. We are living in a vastly changing world that comes with its consequences—good and bad. With all the benefits, the changing world is contributing to imbalances in how we are supposed to be living our lives, contributing to a silent suffering. This suffering is affecting our present, the future of humanity, and our world.

Our Suffering Present

Despite the United States spending more on health care than any other country, we rate forty-sixth in life expectancy worldwide. Chronic disease is on the rise, as six in every ten adults have a chronic health condition and four in every ten have two or more chronic health conditions; these numbers are growing at an alarming rate, affecting about 133 million Americans. It is projected that in ten years, eighty-three million Americans will have three or more chronic conditions, as compared to thirty million in 2015. Every forty seconds someone is dying from a heart attack[1] or suicide.[2] Eighty-eight percent of Americans are metabolically unhealthy. Heart disease, cancer, and stroke account for more than half of all deaths each year. The Centers for Disease Control (CDC) states that chronic diseases are the leading causes of death and disability in the United States and are responsible for seven out of ten deaths every year.[3]

Even scarier, NPR reported that it found an overall 52.4 percent decline in sperm concentration and a 59.3 percent decline in the total sperm count

11

over a thirty-nine-year period.[4] That is a lot of unhealthy people—and a lot less sperm.

Our Suffering Future

If you thought that was scary, let's look at the statistics with regard to our children: Chronic diseases have quadrupled among children since the 1960s. In 1994, one in eight children had a chronic condition; now, 54 percent of all American children have been diagnosed with a chronic health condition, with numbers estimated to increase to 80 percent by 2025.[5]

Our children are not just getting sicker; they are also getting bigger, as childhood obesity continues to climb. Obesity rates have doubled in more than seventy countries since 1980 and tripled in children.[6] Seventy percent of obese children have at least one cardiovascular disease risk factor, and 39 percent have two or more risk factors. One in every six kids has type 2 diabetes,[7] and given current trends, one in every three children born in 2000 will develop diabetes over the course of a lifetime.[8] In 2021, CNN reported that cases of childhood type 2 diabetes have more than doubled during the coronavirus pandemic! And one in five US adolescents are prediabetic. This will be the first generation of kids to not outlive their parents, as our children are living shorter and sicker lives!

Unfortunately, our children's brains are also getting sicker. Our children's mental health has continued to decline with increasing rates of attention-deficit/hyperactivity disorder (ADHD), neurodevelopmental disorders, depression, suicide, and behavior problems, much of which is related to our children's diet.[9]

One in six American children has at least one neurodevelopmental disorder like autism, ADHD, dyslexia, specific learning disorders, communication disorders, sensory processing disorders, and more. ADHD has increased 167 percent! The CDC reports one in six American children aged two to eight has a diagnosed mental, behavioral, or developmental disorder. A study published in the *Journal of American Academy of Child & Adolescent Psychiatry* looked at 301,311 antipsychotic prescriptions filled by privately insured children ages two to seven in the United States from 2007 to 2017. Antipsychotics were more often prescribed to boys, especially between the ages of six and seven. Children who took antipsychotic medication were at increased risk of weight gain, diabetes, high cholesterol, cardiovascular disease, and unexpected death. In very young children, antipsychotics might cause developmental and other long-term adverse effects.[10] Serious depression is worsening, with the pandemic making the situation even worse. Worldwide, suicide is the third leading cause of death in older adolescents and the second leading cause of death in both young adults ages fifteen to nineteen and children ages ten to fourteen in the United States. Suicidal thoughts and self-harm are increasing in young kids (aged six to twelve), and, as reported by the Children's Hospital Association, this trend began even before the pandemic. The suicide rate among teen girls reached a forty-year high, and it has increased for thirteen years in a row, hitting those who live in less populated and rural areas the hardest.[11] Suicide risks soared to 56 percent between 2007 and 2016[12] despite the 400 percent increase of antidepressant prescriptions in the United States since the 1990s.[13] The number of teenage girls out of a hundred thousand who were admitted to a hospital every year because they were cutting or harming themselves was stable until 2011; then it started to climb to about 62 percent for older teen girls and 189 percent for preteen girls, which is nearly triple! We are also seeing the same patterns for suicides. The suicide rate for older teen girls (aged fifteen to nineteen) is up 70 percent compared to the first decade of the century. The rate for preteen girls, who normally have low rates to begin with, is also up 151 percent! *JAMA Network Open* reported that the prevalence of suicide ideations, attempts, and self-injury in children between the ages of nine and ten "was higher than previously estimated," after they analyzed more than eleven thousand children and their caregivers, associated mostly with family factors.[14]

If that wasn't enough, autism is also on the rise. Autism prevalence rates have nearly tripled since 2000. In 2020, the CDC reported that autism spectrum disorder affects one in fifty-four children and one in thirty-four boys, with boys being four to five times more likely to be identified with autism than girls. If we continue at the current trajectory, one in every four will have autism by 2033![15]

Many kids have overlapping comorbid diagnoses, as there is a rise in inflammatory conditions like allergy and autoimmune conditions linked to poor diet.[16] Cancer is one of the leading causes of death for children aged five to fourteen. One in five kids has eczema, one in thirteen children (under the age of eighteen) has asthma,[17] and one in thirteen children has food allergies.

There is also a rise in misbehavior and behavior issues. The CDC reports that 7.4 percent of children aged three to seventeen have a diagnosed behavior problem, which is around 4.5 million children in the United States. Sixty-two percent of teachers wish they could spend less time disciplining students, not limited to any particular demographic group. According to a recent survey, juvenile crime and drug abuse are rated first and third as the biggest worries among Americans. In all, 25 percent of all serious violent crimes involved a juvenile offender. Every four minutes a youth is arrested for an alcohol-related crime, and every seven minutes a youth is arrested for a drug crime. In the next twenty-four hours, 2,795 teenage girls will become pregnant, 1,439 teens will attempt suicide, and 3,506 teens will run away.[18]

The CDC reports that by grade 12 roughly two-thirds of students have tried alcohol; about half of kids between grade 9 and grade 12 have tried marijuana, and 40 percent in this age group have tried cigarettes; and 20 percent of twelfth-graders reported using a prescription medicine without a prescription. One-tenth of all alcohol consumed in the United States is consumed by adolescents between the ages of twelve and nineteen! The frequency with which teenagers use marijuana and alcohol has risen during the pandemic. Studies in *JAMA Pediatrics* have shown that teens between twelve and seventeen who use alcohol, cannabis, illegal drugs, and/or tobacco are more likely to develop lifelong substance abuse disorder than those who start at a later age.[19] Because a teen's brain is still developing, unfortunately, teen drug abuse can have long-term behavioral and cognitive effects.

What is going on with our children? Are we not seeing these statistics? This is crazy! Some may think that this is just "better diagnosis," but one thing is for sure: I know very few autistic adults, and I know way too many autistic children. There is a problem, as a whole generation of kids are more anxious, more depressed, and more fragile. They are much less comfortable taking risks, and even the rate at which they are getting driver's licenses is dropping. Our changing world is threatening our future. These are not the same children of our ancestors.

Our Suffering World

Unfortunately, suffering puts not only the health of our families but also the health our planet at risk. Our world that we will be leaving for our children is also suffering. Climate change (changes that are happening to our planet, which are leading to droughts, rising sea levels, unpredictable weather, and global warming causing temperature extremes) has with it lingering effects on our food, plants, and animals.

With about 200 million tons per year of fertilizer used globally[20] on our land, we are losing not only wildlife but also the plants and the soil that nourish our families. We are losing 1 percent of consumable food calories of the ten top world crops and about 2 billion tons of topsoil per year. We have lost about one-third of the soil in the last 150 years and are left with lifeless dirt with limited nutrients to feed the plants. This has led to a loss of biodiversity, to desertification, and to a loss of marine life, and it has pushed forty million people a year off their land because their soil is no longer adequate. By 2050, one billion people will be refugees of soil desertification. All these chemicals and toxins we are dumping into the land and water have led to marine death and decreased biodiversity of the planet. The United Nations estimates we only have sixty years of topsoil left![21]

Studies have shown that one-third of all animal and plant species on the planet could face extinction by 2070,[22] and we have already lost 90 percent of the plant varieties and half of the livestock.[23] We have lost 75 percent of the pollinator species, which are disappearing at the rate of mass extension. The oceans feed more than 500 million people, but now there are at least five hundred marine dead zones around the world (the size of Europe if all combined), up from fewer than fifty in 1950. A dead zone refers to a reduced level of oxygen in the water, leading to marine life death and biological deserts. The second-largest dead zone in the world is located in the United States in the northern Gulf of Mexico, and the largest is in the Arabian Sea covering almost the entire 63,700-square-mile Gulf of Oman.[24]

What happens when we don't have soil, don't have plants, and don't have food? That means no humans—and that is something to think about! We are at a critical moment in human history. Processed food and the consequences of how we eat and live our lives are the biggest threats to our economy and our border security. This changing world has also brought cheap-engineered food, lack of in-person social interaction, lack of nature, and decreased movement, which are all costing us more than we bargained for. We are literally destroying our future and present with the decisions we and our children are making every day.

HOPELESSNESS TO HOPE

What comes to mind when you read these statistics? Like most, you are likely stunned and feeling hopeless, wondering what will happen to our children. We can't fix what we don't know is broken, so these statistics were only meant to shed light on the grave situation. The question is: Are we going to stick our heads in the ground and pretend everything is okay? This problem will not go away if we continue to ignore it. Will we finally do what we can to make sure that our children don't become part of those statistics?

I know what you are thinking . . . your child's primary care doctor isn't worried, so why should you be? Well, conventional medicine is great for acute care, but when it comes to healing/preventing chronic disease and changing behaviors, we need to dig a little deeper. We need to look past drug treatments, as they alone will not keep us healthy and happy and will not help us make the right decisions. Remember, conventionally trained medical doctors are taught to address the problem and to band-aid with quick approaches; they are not taught to answer the question *why?*

Why are our children sick?
Why are they misbehaving?
Why are they making the wrong decisions?
Why are they difficult to parent?
Why are our children suffering?

Understanding the *why* . . . therein lies the hope. If we can understand what the root cause of this suffering is, we can help put our children's brains and bodies back into balance. If we can put our children in an environment, internally and externally, that allows their brains to work better, they will start to make better decisions, take steps to improve the immune system, and actually have the energy and overall health to take care of the world, fix our food system, improve our economy, and even save the planet.

Lots of hope! It all starts with you and how you choose to parent your child. But let's face it, parenting is so difficult! Why does it seem that kids today are more difficult to parent than the kids of yesteryears?

WHY IS PARENTING SO HARD?

What Parenting Books Got Right, and What They Are Missing

Kids Who Make the Right Decision = Easy Parenting

Kids Who Constantly Make the Wrong Decision = Difficult Parenting

Our kids' decisions—what they wear and what they choose to eat—and how they feel are all dictated by the brain. If your child is constantly making the wrong decision, it makes your parenting harder. If your child is frequently making the right decision, it makes your parenting so much easier. For decades, parenting books have talked about the two main critical players in your child's brain that are involved in decision making (neuroeconomics): the prefrontal cortex and the amygdala.

The prefrontal cortex—the more developed part of the brain—is responsible for rational decision-making skills; it examines the pros and cons and helps our children think through their actions after taking a look at the whole picture. The amygdala—the reactive part of the brain—is responsible for primitive, impulsive, fight or flight types of reactions and decisions. To make a thought-out rational decision and form healthy habits, we need to have both working together. That is what parenting books got right. But with today's children, these parenting books are not taking into consideration the health and lifestyle of the child—which play a large role in influencing how these parts of the brain interact with each other and affect our children's decision-making skills.

Today our children's lifestyles are completely out of balance, which leads to an imbalanced population. Despite warnings about unhealthy diets and obesity, American kids and adolescents are eating more fast food than ever before.[25] Increased artificial/junk food consumption, limited diet variety, lack of sleep, lack of nature, lack of exercise/play, and negative social environment, along with increased exposures to toxins inside and outside the home, contribute to an imbalanced child, an imbalanced immune system, and chronic inflammation, one of the underlying reasons for chronic disease.

Inflammation is disconnecting our children's connections between the prefrontal cortex and the amygdala. This imbalanced lifestyle is now creating children who are out of control, who are unable to use the whole brain to make logical decisions, and who have decreased empathy, poor relationships, and more anger, which fosters an "everyone hates me" mentality. Anything that heightens the inflammatory response leads to chronic inflammation that can compromise the access of the prefrontal cortex, which threatens our children's ability to use it effectively and, in turn, impedes our every parenting move.

OUR CHILDREN'S BRAINS AND BODIES HAVE BEEN HIJACKED!

The first step of our children's better brain, body, and behavior journey is to understand what's fueling their symptoms—that is . . .

Why are your children feeling the way they do?

When a child goes to the doctor, let's say for a headache, the doctor prescribes an anti-inflammatory. What about for eczema? An anti-inflammatory. For pain? An anti-inflammatory. Allergies? An anti-inflammatory. Autoimmune condition like juvenile arthritis? An anti-inflammatory. Cancer? Anti-inflammatory. Get the picture?

No matter what the chronic conditions or symptoms your child is dealing with—depression/mood disorders, thyroid disease, autoimmune disorders, digestive issues, skin disorders, cancer, autism, or more general symptoms like chronic pain, fatigue, sinus issues, allergies, constipation, ear infections, or even simply constant misbehavior[26]—one of the key underlying processes is an imbalanced immune system leading to chronic inflammation. Doctors know that the underlying mechanism is inflammation, but doctors are rarely taught to address why the person is getting sick in the first place and what is leading to the imbalance. Let me help you understand what chronic inflammation actually is.

What Is Inflammation?

If I told you that your child was on fire, what would you do? Would you try to do everything in your power to put out the fire to save your child, even if it meant risking your own life? When your child is dealing with a chronic condition, he literally has a fire within him—a fire that is destroying him from the inside out. If you want to save his future, that fire burning inside needs to be put out.

Inflammation actually means "fire inside," and it is the body's natural defense response to the immune system trying to keep the bad guys out and the good guys in and even trying to heal wounds. Inflammation can cause redness, swelling, heat, and pain. Without inflammation, we would be in danger, with no way to fight microbial invaders or repair the damage constantly inflicted on us.

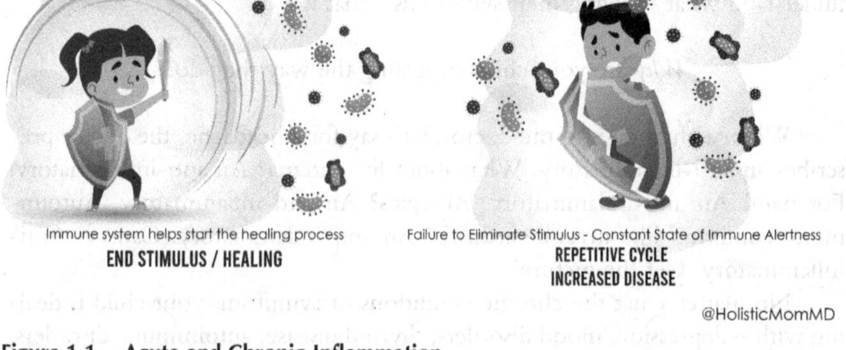

INFLAMMATION

ACUTE INFLAMMATION
Innate Immunity

STIMULUS
Trauma & Infection

Immune system helps start the healing process
END STIMULUS / HEALING

CHRONIC INFLAMMATION
Adaptive Immunity

ONGOING STIMULUS
Environment Triggers, Stress, Chronic Infection

Failure to Eliminate Stimulus - Constant State of Immune Alertness
REPETITIVE CYCLE
INCREASED DISEASE

@HolisticMomMD

Figure 1.1. Acute and Chronic Inflammation

There are two forms of inflammation: acute and chronic.[27] A healthy inflammation response, or acute inflammation, lasts for a short time and is a good sign that your child's body and its defenses are working properly. For a baby, this kind of reaction can be caused by hearing a sudden loud sound or noticing the absence of a parent or caregiver.

If the switch to our immune system gets stuck in the "on" position, it can be too much of a good thing. Modern life's constant daily exposures to triggers like chronic stress, toxins, toxic food, allergens, low-grade infections, or even ongoing abuse, deep poverty, and racism can all start to drive disease, destroying our miracle of a body. This takes a little longer to kick in and takes time to develop.

A properly functioning immune system can keep this fire under control, but constant exposures to triggers causes the inflammatory molecules (like cytokines) to go out of control, destroying everything in their path, which damages tissues and organs and leads to chronic disease of every stripe.[28] Chronic inflammation can lead to or worsen conditions (e.g., mood disorders, cardiovascular disease, asthma, cancer, and diabetes) that hijack our children's little brains and bodies. Even before their diseases become noticeable, inflammation starts brewing in their bodies, so when symptoms are actually felt, damage has already started.

Inflammation Hijacks Our Children's Brains and Behavior

Chronic inflammation hijacks your child's brain. Studies have shown that inflammation decreases the strength of the connection between the prefrontal cortex and amygdala,[29] leads to a heightened response when the brain is presented with something that may be threatening,[30] impairs cognitive function,[31] and contributes to brain aging.

Behavior and inflammation are intimately connected. Studies have shown that children who suffer from chronic conditions were at an increased risk for developing depression, anxiety, and emotional problems that persisted beyond childhood and adolescence into adult life.[32] When looking at a group of four thousand children, researchers even determined that children with behavioral problems may be at increased risk for many chronic diseases in adulthood, including heart disease, obesity, and even diabetes. Studies have found that signs of behavioral and emotional functioning problems in children at the age of seven were associated with inflammation in adulthood, showing a potential childhood origin of adult inflammatory risk, and those children who experienced cognitive problems like poor memory, low attention, or lack of inhibition may suffer from mental health issues later in life.[33] Studies have also shown that depressed children and teenagers have increased risk of suffering from premature death and a wide range of illnesses later in life.[34] In 2021, in the *Journal of American Academy of Child & Adolescent Psychiatry*, a twenty-year study linked childhood depression (ages ten to twenty-four) to disrupted adult health, social functioning issues, substance abuse, lower financial and educational achievement, and increased criminality.

Inflammation not only influences the amygdala and prefrontal cortex but also disrupts brain chemistry; leads to the production of inflammatory precursors like kynurenic acid, quinolinic acid, and picolinate; and antagonizes an important neurotransmitter called serotonin, which in turn leads to further inflammation and mood disorders.[35] In addition, serotonin has been linked to neurodevelopment.[36]

Prenatal inflammation can also lead to behavioral problems. Researchers have shown that brain networks in babies can reflect the degree of inflammation their mothers have experienced even in pregnancy. When the child was assessed for working memory at the age of two, researchers found that the higher the interleukin-6 levels (which are important in stimulating immune responses, such as inflammation) were during pregnancy, the lower the child scored.[37] In another study, researchers found that a mother's inflammation during pregnancy was associated with cognitive problems and a decrease in impulse control in the child at the age of two;[38] additionally, prenatal maternal depression (PMD) can alter the amygdala-prefrontal circuits in infants,[39] putting them at risk for developing a range of neuropsychiatric disorders. This study has shown that the maturation and coordination of the central and peripheral physiology are altered by prenatal exposure to depression, and that PMD-associated variations in the development of the amygdala-prefrontal cortex circuits are relevant for future neurobehavioral maturation. Childhood psychiatric symptoms are strongly linked to adverse environmental exposures during pregnancy. Researchers studied more than nine thousand children between the ages of nine to ten living in twenty-one communities in the United States and found that children subjected during pregnancy to two or more adverse exposures (like maternal use of tobacco, alcohol, or marijuana; unplanned pregnancy; complications during pregnancy like gestational diabetes and high blood pressure; and complications during labor and delivery) were more likely to have clinically significant scores on the Child Behavior Checklist, indicating a higher level of problems like depression, anxiety, and attention deficits.[40] This is especially worrisome now, as studies have shown that new mothers are twice as likely to have postnatal depression in this pandemic lockdown.[41] Even with the most resources in the world, the United States still ranks thirty-seventh out of seventy-nine countries in math proficiency. So what will happen to our children's brains and bodies as a consequence of this pandemic?

It is undeniable that our children's brains are being shaped by changes in media, technology, lifestyles, and other conditions of our modern society.

Inflammation Hijacks Our Children's Bodies

Chronic inflammation will eventually start to damage healthy tissues, cells, organs, and DNA. Inflammation also damages your child's mitochondria (key energy source for our bodies, or the powerhouse of the cell), which are important for a child's overall health and well-being. Mitochondria are little factories in our cells (each cell holds hundreds to thousands) that take the food we eat and convert it to energy (adenosine triphosphate, or ATP); this energy is used to support our bodily functions. Our mitochondria are able to perceive signals of inflammation and can be damaged through uncontrolled oxidative stress that can degrade membranes and the DNA of the mitochondria. Dysfunctional mitochondria have been shown in children with autism[42] and even in children with behavioral issues.[43]

Inflammation and Our Children's Genes

Every thought, every action, and every bite we take can influence everything down to our genetic code, altering the activity of our DNA through a science called epigenetics. Epigenetics is the study of change in our gene function without physical mutations to the DNA structure—meaning we can control our genes. Adults and children all have around 25,000 genes that control the production of proteins in the body. The human genome is made up of about 1 percent that codes for genes; the other 99 percent, also known as "junk DNA," does not code for genes. Science has proven that this is where the information resides that tells the genes how they are going to be expressed—determining when and where genes are turned on and off,[44] depending on our lifestyles and experiences.

Some conditions have a genetic component, but many researchers have determined that less than 10 percent of those with the genes for an autoimmune disease will actually develop it. Genes may load the gun, but the environment pulls the trigger—our children can turn their genes on and off with the decisions they make each day and the experiences they have. Those control mechanisms, above our genes, are controlling factors that regulate how we look, act, and feel in direct communication with our environment and lifestyle. Factors such as family lifestyle; medications; internal and external environment; digestive health, including our microbiome (our gut's bacteria); nutrition, toxins, stressors, and trauma; and exercise, sleep, optimism, spiritual health, or any other life experiences can turn these genes on and off, and all alter how these genes are expressed. Genes can actually shape the behavior of the individual, which is all determined through a person's lifestyle.

Is Your Child Inflamed?

We know that inflammation impedes a child's brain, body, and behavior. How do you know whether your child is inflamed? First, let's examine the criteria of a healthy child.

A healthy child really has no chronic symptoms. The child wakes without difficulty; is filled with energy; has no rashes, food sensitivities, or allergies; is able to focus on the task at hand; and loves life. The healthy child's eyes are without swelling or dark circles. He eats a wide range of foods, does not have digestive issues, and goes to the bathroom without difficulty, forming nice "snakes" in the toilet. At bedtime, a healthy child is able to fall asleep in less than thirty minutes. A healthy child is able to control her emotions; has empathy; makes sound decisions; is able to maintain good, fulfilling relationships; experiences deep calm; has the will and motivation to follow her dreams; and is mindful. A healthy child has normal wanted behaviors of being polite, doing chores, and doing homework. A healthy child can get sick with occasional viral illnesses but then recovers fairly quickly with no remaining symptoms. The healthy child does not exhibit violent behaviors.

An imbalanced child is one where you see the smoke coming from her little chimney; the "smoke" is her symptoms. The unhealthy child is dealing with general symptoms like fever, congestion, stiffness, dry eyes, irritability, fatigue, mood disorders, and concentration issues, as well as more specific

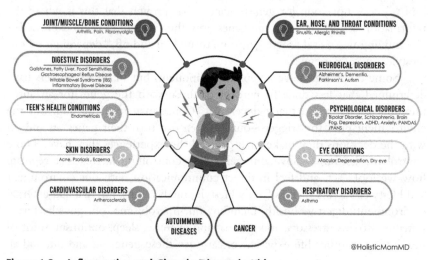

Figure 1.2.   Inflammation and Chronic Disease in Kids

symptoms like allergies, depression, anxiety, headaches, weight issues, behavioral issues, and so much more. It is when the child starts to fall off the healthy child train and experiences more frequent infections and chronic symptoms that she shows signs of becoming an inflamed, imbalanced child with an increased toxin load.

Everyone is different; a child's symptoms are dependent on the body part affected by the inflammation. The body can't literally speak to us, but it can speak to us through symptoms and signs. So think of symptoms like the body calling out for help—help from an external or internal world that is out of balance.

CHANGING WORLD; IMBALANCED LIFESTYLES

Child's Lifestyle Out of Balance = Bad Decisions =
Unhealthy Brain, Body, and Behavior

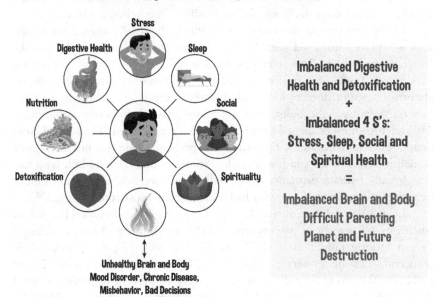

Problems with an Imbalanced Life
Factors Leading to an Unhealthy Brain and Body

Stress
Digestive Health
Sleep
Nutrition
Social
Detoxification
Spirituality

Unhealthy Brain and Body
Mood Disorder, Chronic Disease,
Misbehavior, Bad Decisions

Imbalanced Digestive
Health and Detoxification
+
Imbalanced 4 S's:
Stress, Sleep, Social and
Spiritual Health
=
Imbalanced Brain and Body
Difficult Parenting
Planet and Future
Destruction

@HolisticMomMD

Figure 1.3.

As we discussed, our children's decisions are largely determined by their lifestyle and experiences. The main components of their lifestyles can include the following:

- Digestive health and nutrition
- Detoxification and toxic environments
- Stress
- Sleep
- Social health
- Spiritual health

Digestive Health and Detoxification Out of Balance

Altered Digestive Health and Nutrition

Children's brains and bodies are made from food. Our children are eating the wrong food, are not eating enough of the right foods, and are overeating. What is the difference between a child with a chronic condition and a child without a chronic condition? The environment. The biggest connection between our children's insides and outsides is their gut/digestive tract. Science shows that the gut encompasses our total health. The majority of our children's immune system (70–80 percent) and one hundred trillion microbes (that dictate their health, influence their decisions, and even affect their genes) are in the gut.

In the first part of the twentieth century, chemically altered food substances replaced real food with fake food. Our children's diets lack diversity and lack real food. The overconsumption of fake food—and not eating enough real foods—has caused an epidemic of hormonal/metabolic/immune abnormalities, gut disturbances, and changes in mood and behavior, making kids act violently, fight, bully, show aggression, have feelings of worthlessness, and suffer from other mental health issues. In a report titled "Health and Academic Achievement," the CDC stated that poor nutrition was linked to poor academic performance and lower grades. Studies found that children who had a high carbohydrate/protein-ratio breakfast had increased social punishment behavior compared to those who had a low carbohydrate/protein meal.[45]

In a 2016 poll conducted by the C. S. Mott Children's Hospital in Michigan, 97 percent of parents reported that eating habits during childhood have a lifelong impact on a child's health, but only 17 percent rated their own children's diet as very healthy. Only 21 percent of parents limited their children's fast food and junk food intake; only 16 percent of parents limited their children's sugar drinks.[46] Children are overeating a diet filled with "fake food"—that is, food filled with sugar (the average child in America consumes 34 teaspoons of sugar a day!), additives, and artificial colors and packed with chemicals. Today there are an estimated ten thousand chemicals we commonly use in our food, whereas in 1958 there were around eight hundred chemicals. At least one thousand of these current food additives have never been reviewed for their safety by the Food and Drug Administration (FDA). It's not just what our kids are eating; it's also what they aren't eating. When looking at the diets of children in the United States between 2007 and 2010, the CDC reported that nine out of ten children didn't eat enough vegetables.[47]

A study published in the *Lancet* estimated there were eleven million children between the ages of five and nineteen suffering from obesity in 1975, and the number increased to 124 million in 2016! The number of obese or overweight children aged five and younger went from thirty-two million in 1990 to forty-one million in 2016, and if we continue on the current trajectory, that number could grow to seventy million by 2025.[48] Our junk food–filled, overprocessed, industrialized, westernized global diet is responsible for taking the lives of eleven million people every year; an estimated 2.1 billion adults are overweight, and at the same time, 820 million people are globally undernourished. Inflammation associated with obesity has also predicted worsened executive function in both adolescents and adults.[49]

Our children are at a critical phase in neurodevelopment, with lots of hormones (structural and behavioral) and molecular connections; so children, specifically adolescents, are vulnerable to stressors that lead to behavioral changes. When our children's bodies and brains are not getting the nutrients they need to function from real food, how do we expect them to work properly? When we put junk food in our children, we are only going to get out junk behaviors, junk bodies, and junk brains. Bad and fake foods destroy the balance of our children's gut microbiome, lead to inflammation, imbalance their hormones, threaten their prefrontal cortexes, and hamper their ability to function optimally, which creates bad behavior, violence, and impaired intellectual development. Studies show that kids who ate ultra-processed foods had 10 percent smaller brains, and their IQs were seven points lower than those who ate a healthier diet.[50] Remember, food is the single most powerful tool that impacts our children's brains, bodies, and behaviors.

Our Children's Detoxification Pathways Out of Balance

Our children's bodies are little sponges for everything they touch. We are exposed to more and more chemicals, pesticides, pharmaceutical drugs, and radiation than ever before—with more than one hundred thousand new chemicals in the past few years slowly penetrating our everyday lives, most of them invisible. From pesticide exposure to heavy metals, endocrine disruptors, and now even electromagnetic fields, our children's brains and bodies can only handle so much. Their little bodies are not meant to tolerate the eighty-five thousand chemicals our children are exposed to on a daily basis. The blood-to-brain barrier is not fully developed in a growing child, so children are more vulnerable to environmental toxins.[51] Exposures to environmental toxins have been linked to higher rates of behavior issues like ADHD, conduct disorders, and intellectual disabilities.[52]

With one in six children with one or more neurodevelopmental problems, it is even more important to address environmental toxins. The toxins our children are exposed to on a daily basis can slowly accumulate, leading to hormonal imbalances, gut disturbances, a weakened immune system, and brain and body dysfunction.

Our Mental Health/Emotions Out of Balance—The Imbalanced Four *S*'s: Stress, Sleep, Social Health, and Spiritual Health

Increased Stress

With everything going on in the world today and with the accessibility of news at our fingertips, our children are more stressed now than ever before. Now add to that harsh/helicopter/strict parenting, which are externally controlling types of parenting techniques. Our children are living in a world of chronic stress and a flood of negativity. They suffer from a lack of nature, lack of exercise, increased peer pressure, increased screen time, lack of play, over-scheduling, and trying to meet unexpected expectations. The *New York Times* reported that, in 1985, 18 percent of college freshman felt overwhelmed; in 2018, that number has surged to 41 percent! The United States has the highest college dropout rates in the industrial world, with one-third of college students dropping out at the end of their freshman year; leading causes included helicopter parenting, inability to deal with expectations, and chronic stress.[53]

Chronic stress kills brain cells in the prefrontal cortex and makes them grow in the amygdala. From March to October 2020, the proportion of emergency room visits related to mental health increased 24 percent among children between the ages of five and eleven and spiked 31 percent among adolescents between the ages of twelve and seventeen, compared to the previous year. Adolescents between the ages of twelve and seventeen made up the highest proportion of children's mental health–related emergency department visits in 2019 and 2020.[54] A 2021 study published in *Development and Psychopathology* demonstrated that harsh parenting can actually have long-term effects on a child's brain development, leading to smaller brains and even affecting the child's social and emotional development.[55] Harsh, bossy parenting undermines a child's self-confidence and increases self-doubt.

According to the CDC, youth violence is the leading cause of death and nonfatal injuries in the United States.[56] They state that one in five American children between the ages of twelve and eighteen reported being bullied on school property, and one in six high school students reported being bullied electronically in the last year. Forty-nine percent of children in grades 4 through 12 have been bullied by other students at school level at least once, and 70 percent of school staff have reported being a witness to bullying. Bullying is becoming a frequent discipline problem, as nearly 14 percent of public schools report that bullying is a discipline problem occurring daily or at least once a week.[57]

One of the most powerful ways to manage stress is to go outside to play and exercise. Currently, researchers found that kids are spending less time being physically active, with only 18.2 percent of study participants meeting the physical activity guidelines and only 11.3 percent of participants meeting the sedentary screen time guidelines. More than a decade ago, 830 moms across the United States were asked to compare their child's play with their own; 70 percent of mothers said they played outdoors at least three hours or more at a time, but their own children played far less than half of that amount!

When our children are stressed—and have no way to release this stress—it can lead to problems. Our bodies release a hormone called cortisol. During states of stress, the body shuts off the prefrontal cortex access, and the amygdala takes over. We then start to look for a way to lower that stress and pain and increase pleasure. Stress decreases the release of dopamine,[58] which can push us toward bad habits like eating bad food, being stuck on our gadgets, or engaging in other addictions. A study from the Stanford University School of Medicine shows that, in chronically stressed or anxious children, the brain's fear centers in the right amygdala send signals to the decision-making prefrontal cortex, which make it harder to regulate negative emotions.[59] The amygdala activates stress pathways, strengthening its function and impairing prefrontal cortex regulation, which leads to rapid emotional response patterns and impulsive, bad, and irrational decision making. Our children are all falling into this digital world, leading to further chronic stress and inflammation, which in turn influences their internal and external worlds.

Stress weakens the body's immune system; increases insulin resistance, as it leads to blood sugar dysregulation; weakens the gut microbiome; and acts like fuel for the amygdala, promoting new neuronal growth[60] and killing the prefrontal cortex. If your child's amygdala stays in charge, it can make your child more vulnerable to developing bad habits and addictions. Lack of stress management techniques (e.g., meditation, mindfulness, play, and being in nature) and high-stress environments are leading to lower activation of the prefrontal cortex and higher inflammation, which then contribute to the development of a dysfunctional brain and body.

Lack of Sleep

According to the CDC, six in ten middle schoolers and seven in ten high schoolers are not getting enough sleep.[61] Studies show that more than half of children (52 percent) in the United States don't get the recommended nine hours of sleep they need, making American children the most sleep-deprived kids from fifty countries! When we all fail to get enough rest, our bodies cannot complete those important tasks necessary to keep our brains and bodies working effectively. One week of sleep deprivation can alter the function of 711 genes, including the ones that are involved in metabolism, immunity, inflammation, and even stress.[62] This lack of sleep increases the chances of developing problems due to excess toxins, inflammation, and hormone imbalances; influences bad decision making; and contributes to negative emotions and even addictive behaviors.

Lack of Real Social Connections

More kids today are lacking the secure attachments and empathy that they can get from human connection, with studies showing that school-aged children are enjoying only thirty-seven minutes of "quality time" as a family on weekdays.[63] Children with insecure attachment are more vulnerable to mental health problems and have difficulty managing and regulating emotions and interacting with peers.[64] Lack of love and connection leads to increased stress response systems.

One of the reasons for lack of secure attachment is the new age of internet and social media; roughly 70 percent of the world's population has a cell phone.[65] Ninety-five percent of teens are on a digital device; 70 percent say they use social media multiple times a day; and 38 percent use social media multiple times in an hour. More than half feel "addicted" to their devices, admitting that their device distracts them when they should be paying attention to the people they are with. Younger children now spend five and half hours each day in front of screens, and for teens it is more like seven hours. Adolescents are now spending more time using social media and playing video games than they spend sleeping. The statistics are just rising with the pandemic. One study of individuals between the ages of nineteen and thirty-two showed that the more social media they used the lonelier and more depressed they felt.[66] More and more of the younger generation are becoming addicted to the internet,[67] specifically children who grew up with it. Studies have shown that those addicted to the internet may have weaker connections between the anterior cingulate (which is found at the front of the cingulate cortex and wraps around the head of the corpus callosum) and the prefrontal cortex.[68]

Unfortunately, our digital life has disconnected us from those who matter most, leading to lack of secure attachments, lack of self-control, and a lack in family time. We are becoming addicted to the internet and promoting mindless activity, which is disconnecting us from our high-level brains. Studies have shown that excessive screen time can harm a child's health, increasing obesity, lowering self-esteem, creating mood disturbances, and disrupting sleep patterns.

Negative Spiritual Health

Our children are growing up in a world where we all wake up to negativity and fear. In 2019, the kids were scared to go to school because of school shootings, and in 2020–2021, kids are scared to go to school because of the pandemic. Our social media is filled with negativity, our social and work environments are negative, our family lives are negative, and we go to sleep focusing on all the things that are going wrong in our lives. Our children are losing their sense of self, self-confidence, and self-worth, which increases resentment and contributes to a lack of purpose.

Our children's identities are destroyed from the world telling them what they are supposed to have in their lives, what their outward appearance should look like, and what they need to achieve to be truly happy; in the end, they are left feeling inadequate. The lens through which our children view the world is clouded, as negative headlines are 63 percent more prevalent than positive ones. We have access to everything at our fingertips, most people are living in peaceful environments, poverty rates are lower, and crime rates have fallen in the United States from the 1990s to the 2000s,[69] and yet the news, social media, and TV are telling us something different. In one study of college students, as little as fifteen minutes of exposure to negative news was enough to increase symptoms of anxiety.[70] Violence portrayed in films has tripled since 1986. This is the first generation of children to view live acts of bullying, terrorism, global conflicts, school shootings, and daily pandemic death counts.

With negativity or fear constant in our daily lives, our brains—through the science of neuroplasticity (the ability to form and organize synaptic connections)—rewire to respond to this negativity, which threatens our ability to employ the prefrontal cortex and leads to disease and despair. Chronic stress and negativity disconnect the two sections of the brain, leading to decreased empathy, increased impulsivity, and poor decision making. Unfortunately, chronic stress and negativity lead to unhappiness. As a result, we want quick fixes and instant gratification—like checking our messages and e-mails—that give us a dopamine burst. We then rely on these short-term fixes, which leads back to chronic stress, low self-worth, inflammation, and disease. It's a never-ending cycle.

Our children are being raised in a time where the world is hijacking our children's brains and destroying their bodies. Our children's environment, our economy, and our national security—but most important, our children's bodies and minds—are out of balance, leading to impaired brains, bodies, and behaviors. Research shows that our families' decisions and our bodies are being compromised by chronic stress and lack of adequate sleep.[71] When we add a poor diet, increased environmental toxins, unhealthy relationships and negativity, unhealthy digital exposure, and a lack of nature to the mix, it causes further imbalances in our children's brains and bodies, which threatens the prefrontal cortex and leads to selfish behavior and a lack of self-confidence, empathy, sense of purpose, and concern for others and the planet. When our future is imbalanced, and when our future's brains and bodies don't work appropriately, it can destroy the health of our families and our planet.

Holistic parenting can help put a child's body back into balance; alter genes in their favor; optimize the function of his brain, organs, tissues, DNA, and even mitochondria; and allow each cell of the body to function optimally.[72] Holistic parenting can empower and educate our children to be more mindful of their minds, emotions, bodies, and souls; to recognize when they are starting to become out of balance; and to implement strategies to fix the imbalance, which increases resilience. If we don't train kids to take charge of their bodies and brains, someone else will; it's time for parents to help them take the control back.

To understand this situation in more detail, it is important to take a deeper dive into the inner workings of the child's brain. When we are empowered through education on how our children's brains and bodies work, we can then learn to parent our children in a changing world.

• 2 •

The Science of Holistic Parenting

PARENTING HEALTHY, MINDFUL, AND RESILIENT BRAINS AND BODIES

Let's face it: parenting is hard! I am with you! Tiny humans are completely left in your care, when sometimes it's hard enough to just take care of yourself. But guess what?

Healthy, Mindful Children with Better Brains,
Bodies, and Behavior = Easy Parenting

Fourteen years ago, when I found out I was pregnant with my first child, I made it my mission to parent for optimal brain and body health. Since then, the more I learn, the more I implement for the sole purpose of wanting to raise healthy, balanced, self-confident, optimistic, and mindful humans and leaders who will make a difference in this world for the better. I wanted to raise young men or women who would be aware of their emotions and their environment and who would respect every living soul and take care of our planet. Most important, I wanted to raise children with stable and healthy emotions, behavior, brains, and bodies.

I didn't learn it all at once. It was a gradual process. During residency, I was blessed with a healthy child. With blessings come challenges. As a brand-new mom away from family, I was working long hours and not sleeping. I thought I deserved to treat myself to junk food now and then. But "now and then" turned into a daily (even multiple-time-a-day) habit just to survive. I had ice cream every night, as I had free food at the cafeteria. I satisfied all my sugar and junk food cravings. Now add to that all the fake food I was consuming, the increased stress of my husband and I both working eighty-hour work weeks as resident physicians, the lack of sleep, and the bombardment of toxins and sanitizers to my system. And then I became pregnant for the second time.

That pregnancy was my most difficult pregnancy. I was sick all the time and taking acid reducers and nausea medications. I had lots of preterm labor, so I was in and out of the hospital. At his birth, my son's blood sugar levels dropped, and he was taken to the neonatal ICU. As he grew, he continued to become more and more agitated. He had eczema and runny noses, but the most distressing symptoms were his serious anger issues. Oh, my goodness, this child cried nonstop for two hours twice a day for three years! Any little thing would trigger him, from not telling him "good job" after he went to the bathroom to the ritual of washing my hands after cooking. But most of the time, he would cry for no reason whatsoever. He made pools in sinks, stuck forks into toaster ovens and turned them on, and got stuck on the top shelf of the pantry multiple times. Thinking this was his "normal," I continued on my hamster wheel until it came to another screeching halt . . . a mother's worst nightmare unfolded a second time—on my watch this time!

On my day off from work, I would do what all working mothers do—catch up with work and home. One particular day off, I completed my clinic chart notes as I nursed my third child. Ten feet in front of me, my almost four-year-old child played. In a blink of an eye, I heard a screeching gasp and looked up. I saw my four-year-old hanging blue in the face, a curtain cord wrapped around his neck and a chair right next to him! I ran to him and unwrapped him while praying. God saved my child once again! The cords were wrapped above the window sill—how did he get himself into this? What was he thinking?!

After the urgent care visit, I asked him what he was thinking. He said he wanted to be a monkey, like Curious George, so he moved the kitchen chair to the window, unwrapped the cords I had tied up, and wrapped them around his neck and jumped off the chair! He was left with a horrific scar around his neck. This chain of events drove me to see what I can do to optimize his every decision to the best of my ability.

The thought of almost losing my first and second sons haunts me to this day, but I am so thankful that it has motivated me to continue to make it my life's mission to educate and empower other mothers. There is so much more we can do rather than leaving our children's brains, bodies, and behavior up to fate. We can mold our children. We can give them the tools they need to live mindful lives; be in charge of their bodies, their minds, and their decisions; and live life to the fullest with increasing resilience, no matter what life decides to throw at them. As science has evolved, we understand more and more how our everyday decisions impact our children positively or negatively.

Let's dive into first what holistic parenting is and what is going on in our children's brains.

WHAT IS HOLISTIC PARENTING?

We are mind, body, and soul. Our children are mind, body, and soul. Holistic parenting can help nurture our children's minds, bodies, and souls from the inside out and equips them with the skills they need for emotional intelligence, finding enduring deep friendships, making correct decisions, managing stress, and being able to remain resilient all throughout adulthood. Holistic parenting raises mindful children, who are able to pay attention to the present moment, internally and externally, with acceptance and nonjudgment. Holistic parenting is not about control but, instead, autonomy. It's about enabling your mindful child to be fully aware at many different levels of perception and to be able to make her own informed decision. Holistic parenting teaches self-control and builds self-confidence.

If we can help children learn to take care of their bodies, their bodies will take care of them—now and into the future. If we educate children to take care of their minds, they will be able to make good, rational decisions. Holistic parenting can help educate and empower children to be mindful of their bodies, minds, emotions, social lives, and environment; holistic parenting can teach them how to keep their bodies in balance when they start to sway, increasing resilience in any situation and environment.

Holistic parenting can influence our children's DNA, cells, mitochondria, the microbiome, their immune system, and even their brains. Will your child make rational decisions driven by the prefrontal cortex, or irrational decisions driven by the limbic system? To answer this question, let's dive into the science of holistic parenting.

Science of Holistic Parenting

Your child is his brain, and the brain is your child. Anything that changes your child's brain can change who she is for now and years to come. Your new bundle of joy is also a bundle of interconnecting cells, organs, tissues, and muscles that work together in a beautiful and coordinated way. When a child comes into the world, he is made up of millions of cells but limited connections. As the child grows, she develops so many new connections, depending on the circumstances they are living in. Experiences (not just genes) can create, reorganize, and strengthen connections between neurons and eliminate unused neural pathways (called neural malleability or neuroplasticity), which allows the human brain to be shaped and changed during development and throughout a person's lifetime. These experiences are crucial to this early wiring/pruning and enables millions and millions of new connections in the brain to be made.[1]

Experiences alter brain activity, which can change gene expression. When the brain and the body change, your child's behavior changes. When your child's behavior changes, it can change the brain and body. Repeated interactions and communications lead to pathways being laid down that help memories and relationships form and learning/logic to develop. According to a 2006 study by Duke University researchers, more than 40 percent of our daily activities are actually habits.[2] What is known as Hebbian Law tells us that "neurons that fire together wire together."

The first one thousand days of life are important for optimal brain development. The way the brain develops during the pregnancy and the first two years of life can define how your child's brain will work for the rest of her life. Nerves connect, grow, and get covered by myelin (white material that surrounds the brain cells, nerves, and its connections), systems that together decide how a child will think, act, react, and even feel into adulthood, which will affect every system from learning, memory, and impulse control to planning, mood, sensory systems, and everyday decisions. Our children's entire cognitive functions depend on the integrity of the myelin structure in their brains. Their ability to retrieve, store, and process information into thinking, feeling, and behaving depends on how well organized their nerves are and how thick the myelin sheath surrounding the nerves is. When the myelin sheath gets too thin or damaged, nerves will not fire normally. The impulses can slow down and even stop, causing mental health, behavioral, and neurological problems.

The appropriate amount of behavioral control can positively affect child development. In a study of six hundred Flemish families raising a child between the ages of eight and ten, researchers identified different parenting styles. They found that insufficient or excessive behavior control was commonly associated with negative child developmental outcomes such as defiant behavior, misconduct, depression, and anxiety.[3] The adolescents with uninvolved parents fared the worst, while the well-being of kids of authoritarian and indulgent parents scored somewhere in the middle. Holistic parenting is about love, connection, educating, and empowering; it is about using science to nurture kids to be more adaptable, mindful, resilient, connected, and imaginative.

The Human Brain

The human brain is an amazing organ made up of more than one hundred billion brain cells and more than fifty trillion synapses. As we said before, brain development is very rapid in the womb, continues at an accelerated rate in the first two to three years, and then continues to develop for the next twenty years or more. Ninety percent of the growth of the human brain occurs in the first five years of life, when millions of brain connections are being formed, unformed, and then re-formed. At birth, the newborn brain is 33 percent the size of an adult's brain; there are billions of cells and few connections. The brain continues to grow 1 percent per day. At one year, the child has developed

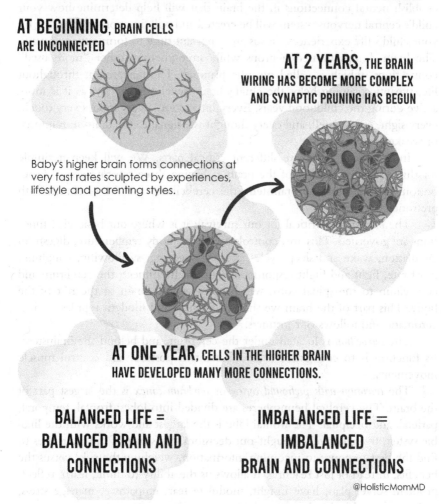

LIFESTYLE AND BRAIN CONNECTIONS

AT BEGINNING, BRAIN CELLS ARE UNCONNECTED

AT 2 YEARS, THE BRAIN WIRING HAS BECOME MORE COMPLEX AND SYNAPTIC PRUNING HAS BEGUN

Baby's higher brain forms connections at very fast rates sculpted by experiences, lifestyle and parenting styles.

AT ONE YEAR, CELLS IN THE HIGHER BRAIN HAVE DEVELOPED MANY MORE CONNECTIONS.

BALANCED LIFE = BALANCED BRAIN AND CONNECTIONS

IMBALANCED LIFE = IMBALANCED BRAIN AND CONNECTIONS

@HolisticMomMD

Figure 2.1.   Our Children's Lifestyle and Brain Connections

more connections in the brain. By the age of two years, the child's brain wiring has become more complex, and synaptic pruning has started. At the end of age one, a baby will develop more than one quadrillion synapses (or neural connections) alone! By the age of three, a child's brain has reached almost 90 percent of its adult size. By the age of seven, this brain sculpting slows down because more and more cells are being myelinated (when a white material starts to surround the brain cells, nerves, and its connections). This rapid brain growth and circuitry has been estimated at an astounding rate of seven hundred to one thousand synapse connections per second in this period.[4]

With twenty-five thousand genes, roughly twelve thousand of them will establish neural connections in the brain that will help determine how your child's central nervous system will be created and will function. Depending on your child's life experiences, this is an important time to form new pathways. The brain dumps unused neurons while strengthening other "more used" connections, which is called synaptic pruning. Though present throughout life, synaptic pruning helps the child's brain develop correctly, as it is more active during the childhood years. Every interaction, every food, every touch, every sight, every smell, and every thought is a signal to the brain to reinforce or weaken a synapse.

In the brain, there are different critical parts. We will keep it simple for this discussion. Think of the brain as having three separate areas.[5] From bottom up these are the brainstem, the cerebellum, and the cerebrum with prefrontal cortex.

The *brainstem* is critical for our survival; it is where our basic vital functions are governed. This area controls breathing, body temperature, digestion, circulation, wake and sleep cycles, arousal, sneezing, swallowing, coughing, heart rate, fight and flight response, and so on. It connects the cerebrum and cerebellum to the spinal cord, which connects our brain to the rest of the body. This part of the brain we share with birds and modern reptiles, so it is automatic and follows our instincts.

The *cerebellum* is located under the cerebrum and behind the brainstem. Its function is to coordinate balance, maintain posture, and control muscle movements.

The *cerebrum with prefrontal cortex* or *cerebrum cortex* is the largest part of the brain. The cerebral hemispheres are divided into lobes: frontal, temporal, parietal, and occipital. The frontal lobe is the largest and works with the limbic system to make well-thought-out decisions. This part of the brain tries to find the best response to incoming information, weighing the risks versus the benefits, instead of just reacting. It allows us the ability to think, learn, reflect, problem solve, plan, have insight, modulate fear, empathize, manage stress, and reason, and it develops as a child grows.

There are two different hemispheres—left and right. The left side controls speech, writing, and comprehension, and it loves order. The right side cares about the big picture and controls musical skills, creativity, emotions, and intuition; manages artistic, nonverbal, and spatial ability; and helps us use our facial expressions for communication. Our "gut feelings" come from the right side. This right side processes the world emotionally and is more dominant in the first three years of life. This part has a strong link to the lower brain and tries to control the impulses of the lower brain. The two hemispheres are connected with a complex band of fibers, called the corpus callosum, that transmits information back and forth. In order to live balanced lives, we need both of these parts of the brain to work in perfect harmony so that we are able to use our memories and emotions in tandem with our logic to understand the whole picture.

The temporal lobe is important for understanding language (Wernicke's area), hearing, sequencing and organization, and especially memory. The occipital lobe is our main vision area. The parietal lobe is for spatial and visual perception; interpretation of signals from vision and hearing; motor, memory, and sensory skills; touch and pain sensation; temperature maintenance; and interpretation of language.

Deeper structures of the cerebrum include the hypothalamus, pituitary gland, pineal gland, thalamus, basal ganglia, and the limbic system. For our discussion, let's dive into the area of the limbic system.

The *limbic system* is the area responsible for our emotions (hunger, fear, anger, pain, pleasure, sleep), memory, and learning (based on sensory input); it sits on top of the brain stem. These responses are mostly reflective and autonomic. The limbic system is associated with the release of the neurotransmitter dopamine and other natural opioids called endorphins. Parts of the limbic system include the amygdala, hippocampus, hypothalamus, and cingulate gyri, which work together to control brain processes.

The hippocampus helps in memory and learning. Working with the prefrontal cortex, it assimilates new memories into preexisting networks of knowledge, leading to memory consolidation and later retrieval. There is an increasing body of evidence showing that a variety of lifestyle factors have a relationship with this brain structure and function in school-aged children, and studies have found that healthy lifestyle factors may improve hippocampal function and academic performance in school-aged children.[6]

The hypothalamus helps control behaviors like hunger, thirst, sleep, body temperature, emotions, blood pressure, secretion of hormones, and sexual response.

The amygdala is involved in emotions like rage and fear, triggering the release of high levels of stress hormones, impulsivity, and rewards. Working with the hippocampus, the amygdala figures out the emotional meaning of everything that has happened in a person's life (real and perceived), modulates the memories of threatening events, and senses whether there is a threat approaching, which is all part of our survival instinct. Brain scans have shown that when we experience feelings of sadness, rage, or fear, there is deactivation of the higher brain areas and activation in the lower and mid parts of the brain. When we feel a sense of danger, the amygdala completely takes over or hijacks the upstairs brain. If this area is damaged, scientists have found that animals lose their aggressive behavior and become fearless.[7] Even in healthy children or adults, this circuit in the amygdala can be altered. When not working in balance with the rest of the brain, damage to the circuit can lead to major problems.

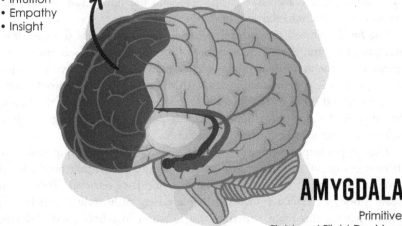

PREFRONTAL CORTEX

- Rational Decision Making
- Examines Pros and Cons
- Ability to Learn
- Plan and Problem Solve
- Fear Modulation
- Intuition
- Empathy
- Insight

- Emotional and Social Intellegence
- Rational Thinking
- Reflection
- Reasoning
- Thinking Before Acting

AMYGDALA

Primitive •
Fight and Flight Decisions •
Rage and Fear •
Triggering Release of •
Stress Hormone
Impulsivity •

IF BOTH WORK TOGETHER→ RATIONAL DECISIONS

IF AMYGDALA TAKES OVER→POOR DECISIONS, DECREASED EMPATHY

@HolisticMomMD

Figure 2.2.   Prefrontal Cortex and Amygdala Connection

The amygdala is very well developed at birth, while the prefrontal cortex (the last to develop) isn't mature yet and slowly starts to develop maturity when the child reaches the middle of his twenties. A normal human being has both parts working in unison, but if your child's prefrontal cortex hasn't even developed yet, it won't be fully functional, so the amygdala frequently reacts, leading to more explosive outbursts where the child is unable to calm himself down. New research is showing that the core of mental illness, the lack of appropriate stress regulatory pathways, and violent behavior are all driven by responses in the limbic system similar to infants and toddlers.[8] Science has shown that this part of the brain can be especially manipulated with lifestyle choices and parenting style, which can interfere with a child's ability to control emotions and make good decisions. The developing cortex is altered by many pre- and postnatal events, including sensory, motor, parent-child relationships, play, stress, hormones, and medications/drugs. Developmental reasons aside, if we can help our child's lifestyle and environment favor a less reactive amygdala, it is a win-win for everyone.

Neurochemicals

Triggered by experiences, neurochemicals can determine a child's behavior. The release of these is governed by the hippocampus, amygdala, hypothalamus, and pituitary gland, which all control our emotional responses. Dopamine, cortisol, endorphins, oxytocin, and serotonin are your child's main brain chemical messengers, which also regulate your child's life and emotions. By understanding these "messengers," we can help our kids learn to fire and wire healthy habits that will leave them feeling satisfied, loved, and empowered.

Dopamine, also known as the "feel-good hormone," has many functions. Dopamine influences our reward systems/circuits, habits, addictions and behaviors, need for instant gratification, and the development of addiction. Pleasure-inducing chemicals like feel-good endorphins are also involved. If there was an experience that triggers this cascade, our body continues to seek out whatever stimuli led to that feel-good moment.

Cortisol is our stress hormone.

Endorphins are released with cardiovascular exercise, laughter, and intimacy, which helps us get some relief from life's hardships, freeing us to try new things. These neurochemicals produce feelings of peace, calm, and bliss.

Oxytocin is released with love, social experiences, and bonding; it makes our children feel loved and safe.

Serotonin is released when you are doing things that you love, as well as during physical activity and sunlight exposure; it produces feelings of contentment and happiness.

Healthy, engaged parents/caregivers are the best brain support a child can have,[9] so your physical and mental health are important.

BALANCED CHILDREN; BALANCED BRAIN, BODY, AND BEHAVIOR

> "The shift away from the prefrontal cortex represents the greatest existential threat for human survival."
>
> —neurologist Dr. David Perlmutter, *Brain Wash*

With imbalanced lives, our children's brains and bodies are suffering, especially when parts of the brain and body start to work out of unison. With this imbal-

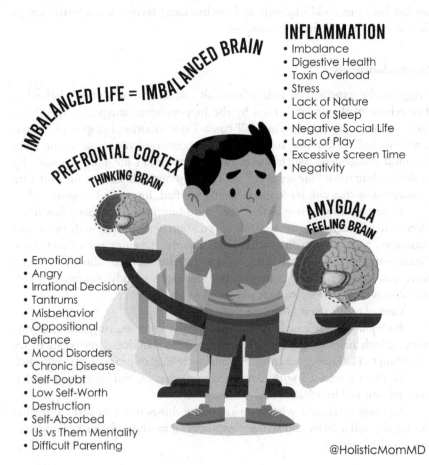

IMBALANCED LIFE = IMBALANCED BRAIN

PREFRONTAL CORTEX
THINKING BRAIN

AMYGDALA
FEELING BRAIN

INFLAMMATION
- Imbalance
- Digestive Health
- Toxin Overload
- Stress
- Lack of Nature
- Lack of Sleep
- Negative Social Life
- Lack of Play
- Excessive Screen Time
- Negativity

- Emotional
- Angry
- Irrational Decisions
- Tantrums
- Misbehavior
- Oppositional Defiance
- Mood Disorders
- Chronic Disease
- Self-Doubt
- Low Self-Worth
- Destruction
- Self-Absorbed
- Us vs Them Mentality
- Difficult Parenting

@HolisticMomMD

Figure 2.4.

ance, the rational parts of the brain (the prefrontal cortex) are hijacked by these lower parts of the brain with alert systems in the driver's seat. But here is the good news: as a caregiver/parent you can help influence the development and interaction of parts of the child's brain, so that all parts of the brain work in unison, which allows the prefrontal cortex to properly manage the lower parts of the brain. Studies in animals and humans have shown that the development of the frontal lobe structure, behavior, and function can be permanently shaped by the experiences.[10] If prefrontal cortex development is precocious during early infancy, this can have important implications for how children's early environments shape the development of frontal circuits important for complex cognitive function.

When our children live balanced lives, all these structures—connected by a network of nerves and brain chemicals, cells, microbes, organs, and tissues—work together like a perfectly playing orchestra, resulting in children who act like real human beings. They are compassionate, loving, empathetic, and caring toward themselves and others; most important, they are physically capable of making better decisions.[11] Now don't get me wrong—they are not going to be perfect all the time. But as a mindful child grows, he will be able to regulate his emotions, think about others, and think before acting as he weighs the risks versus the benefits. By establishing healthy habits and changing negative ones, you can promote healthy neuroplasticity and life habits in your child. With

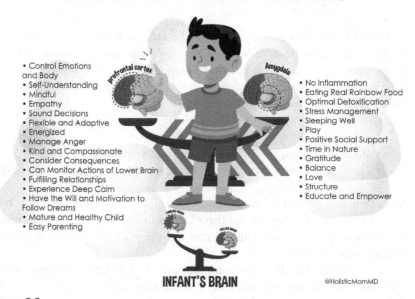

Figure 2.3.

your child's amygdala and her prefrontal cortex in constant communication, depending on her lifestyle and on the parenting style, the connection between the prefrontal cortex and the amygdala will be strengthened.

Brain research is also key in understanding why children misbehave in the first place. The behavior is just the tip of the iceberg; there is so much going on underneath. Research suggests that the prefrontal cortexes of aggressive or oppositional children either haven't developed or develop slower than in typical kids. These children may simply not yet have brains capable of helping them regulate their behavior. In a sense, until a child's prefrontal cortexes are fully mature, we adults must supplement the child's executive function. Executive function doesn't correlate with intelligence; gifted children can also be impulsive or challenging, despite their intellectual strengths and ability to articulate their thoughts.

Children can learn and practice skills that support the desired behavior. When you love, let go of control and bond with, nurture, and care for your child, and when you offer healthy foods and focus on gratitude, meditation, prayer, and sleep, your child's brain will be more stimulated. This balanced lifestyle also multiplies the neuroglial cells, increasing the pathways between areas of the brain; optimizes digestive function; strengthens the mitochondria; optimizes gut bacteria; and lowers stress and overall inflammation, which heals and prevents chronic disease in a child. When children feel better, they do better.

FOUNDATIONS OF HOLISTIC PARENTING

A child's brain and neural connections take time to form, so as a child's prefrontal cortex is unfinished, his limbic system will take over most of his or her emotions. It is our job as parents to help guide the child to help her form these connections. Among the factors that have the most profound effects on brain development are[12]

- inflammation;
- digestive health, nutrition, and detoxification; and
- the four S's: stress management, sleep, social health, and spiritual health.

According to the Centers for Disease Control and Prevention (CDC), how well a brain develops depends on these factors in addition to genes; nurturing and responsive care for the child's brain and body are also key to supporting healthy brain development.[13]

Let's briefly dive into the important pieces of holistic parenting, which will lower overall inflammation and optimize hormones and gut bacteria, the ability to detoxify, brain health, and cognitive and executive function.[14]

Digestive Health and Detoxification

Your child's brain actually starts in in the gut. The gut is the house of the immune system and is home to trillions of microbes that dictate you child's health and her brain. The gut houses the enteric nervous system that lines the gut and stretches a web of about 500 million neurons that send messages back and forth across the vagus nerve, which runs from the abdomen to the brainstem. Changes in the gut microbiome have been linked to changes in behavior and brain function. A 2021 study that followed more than four hundred infant boys found that boys with a gut bacterial composition that was high in the bacteria Bacteroidetes at one year of age had more advanced neurodevelopment, cognition, and language skills one year later.[15]

Nutrients regulate every single chemical reaction in your child's body. Studies have shown that children who eat a rainbow of whole foods packed with color, fiber, nutrients, minerals, and good fats actually have healthier brains, are less violent, and show improvement in cognition, behavior, academic performance, attention, and focus. Real food lowers inflammation, balances hormones and blood glucose control, optimizes mitochondria, and improves the immune system. Real food also restores our dying ecosystem and protects our planet.

When most chronic conditions are due to an imbalanced immune system, it is important to optimize the house of the immune system—the gut! Your little one's gut has a trillion bugs that keep your child healthy. Educating the child about taking care of the "friends" in his gut is important to optimize his immune system and lower inflammation, which in turn optimizes his brain and body function to heal and prevent chronic conditions now and years to come! Role model a healthy, nutrient-dense lifestyle for your children by focusing on real rainbow nutrient-dense foods and optimal hydration. Real food gives a child control over their minds and bodies to make mindful decisions, as they are no longer "slaves" to the junk food industry. A mindful, resilient child has full autonomy to make educated food choices, read labels, reflect on how the food affected her body, and adjust intake according to how her mind, body, and soul feel.

Detoxification

Pesticides and other environmental toxins can lead to neurodevelopmental damage while disrupting the endocrine system. Lowering the toxic load can help optimize your child's brain and body function. Incorporating foods that will help the body detoxify—keeping bodily fluids moving and swapping out toxic for clean—can help lower overall inflammation, so that the child can optimize his brain and body function. A mindful, resilient child can make environmentally conscious decisions, lower the toxins that she is exposed to, and optimize her body's detoxification systems.

Optimize the Four *S*'s: Stress Management, Sleep, Social Health, and Spiritual Health

Stress Management

Managing stress is essential in any healing and disease-prevention program, as our thoughts, feelings, and emotions directly affect our children's physical health; research has shown that 90 percent of illnesses and disease are stress related. Educating our children about the importance of stress management is essential. Parental burnout hits Western countries the hardest, and, as parents, it is important to be aware and honest about our own stressors and emotions, as children are like sponges and can sense and absorb even subtle changes in mood or behavior. Decrease control over your child, let go of unrealistic expectations, and stop overscheduling yourself and your child. A child mirrors our emotions and takes in our stresses and worldview.

It is easy for our children to get stuck in the "dopamine traps" of internet surfing. Creating family rules for social media and cell phones is important to prevent addictions. Replace these traps with regular routines of prayer, mindfulness, and other stress management techniques to lower overall inflammation, optimize the gut microbiome, balance hormones, and enhance brain health, so that our children can make better decisions.

For optimal stress management, it is important for your child to feel loved, respected, safe, and secure in his environment; have clear structure and rules; perform chores and work together as a team; spend time in nature with the family; and engage in unstructured play and exercise, with less child-centered activities. Older children can learn to manage stress and reduce the effects of stress by practicing abdominal breathing, meditation, mindfulness, and prayer. Studies have shown that mindfulness can literally change the brain; as little as eleven hours of mindfulness over one month can create measurable changes on brain scans.[16] A mindful child is able to incorporate these stress management techniques into her daily routine and increase these practices in times of stress.

Sleep

When a child sleeps, the body restores itself, and essential processes take place. Establish proper bedtimes so that the adrenal glands don't go into overtime and cause undue stress. During sleep, the child's body can work to lower overall inflammation, build and release hormones to help growth, repair itself, produce white blood cells, rebalance ghrelin and leptin, control appetite, optimize detoxification, support memory and learning, direct blood to developing muscles, and improve the immune system. It is important to help your child live a life that will support sleep, develop a sleep routine, and create an environment that is conducive to sleep. A mindful child prioritizes his body's needs, including sleep. If struggles occur during sleep, a mindful child will try to identify the reason for sleep disturbances and find ways to correct it because he is aware of the importance of sleep for the brain and body.

Social Support: Love Heals

Developing bonds of love, respect, and honor and being involved in a child's life can help activate a sensory nerve in the child's brain that releases oxytocin and natural opioids, which decrease stress response systems and provide the child with feelings of well-being and help the brain develop. Feelings of love can help grow more connective neural fibers in a child's brain, which play a role in increasing cognitive function.

Forming secure attachments with your children through unconditional love and eye-to-eye communication, educating them on empathy, and having family (and extended family) time will empower them to connect their feelings with what is going on in their lives and help them label their emotions. In part II, we will discuss discipline, bullying, social curve balls, and tips on parenting teens about addictions and sex. A mindful child will be able to engage in self-reflection, acknowledge his feelings and emotional needs, and create and nurture loving friendships that will serve him, instead of filling empty voids with destruction.

Spirituality: Power of Positivity

Science has proven the importance of spiritual health and our children's overall health. Gratitude and optimism strengthen the connections between the amygdala and prefrontal cortex, improving overall health and well-being. In a world of negativity, it is even more critical to "train" our subconscious to be more positive. Incorporating gratitude, using targeted and thought-out words of appreciation/encouragement, teaching forgiveness, and helping a child find purpose can optimize his brain/body connections and increase self-confidence. A positive sense of identity will build self-confidence and will lead to better academic performance, happiness, sense of well-being, and increased resilience. A mindful child is a more grateful, confident, less resentful child who is constantly aware. When this child notices that his mind is becoming negative, or has increasing resentment in his heart, the child is able to reflect and adjust by incorporating techniques to build positivity, confidence, and love for a higher purpose than himself.

When a child's life is balanced, the child benefits humanity. When a child's life is imbalanced, humanity is at a loss.

A CHILD'S BALANCED LIFE VS IMBALANCED LIFE

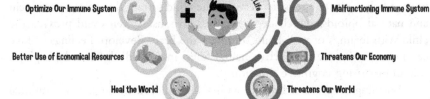

Positive Impact on Decision Making   Negative Impact on Decision Making

Decrease Chronic Disease   Increase Chronic Disease

Optimize Our Immune System   Malfunctioning Immune System

Better Use of Economical Resources   Threatens Our Economy

Heal the World   Threatens Our World

@HolisticMomMD

Figure 2.5.

THE POWER OF HOLISTIC PARENTING: A GLIMPSE INTO MY LIFE

After twelve years of research (which included thousands of parenting and functional medicine books, podcasts, lectures, and seminars), I took what I learned and changed my family's entire lifestyle. Educating and empowering my children to be autonomous and in charge of their own health, brains, bodies, behavior, and decisions has made them the easiest children to parent!

Don't get me wrong—parenting is still hard. My children still make "crazy" decisions because their prefrontal cortex isn't fully developed yet, and they still need guidance. I'm not perfect, and they are not perfect. I am still growing, and my children are still growing. We are still learning daily. In the rest of this book, I am going to teach you that when you educate and empower your children to be mindful and help them develop their individual "healing" routines, we can lower overall inflammation and put their brains and bodies back into balance to make better decisions on their own. They will be more resilient, in charge of their own lives, and able to grow in adversity.

This didn't happen overnight. It took time—one day at a time and one task at a time—but now we work together as a family and as a team. Starting from a very young age, my kids have taken charge of the cleaning before they leave for school; they unload and load the dishwasher, mop the floors, fold laundry, and do anything else that needs to be done—all by themselves with minimal guidance and no complaining. They play all day long together with limited arguments. I stock up the pantry and the fridge with everything they can eat, so they eat what they want, making mindful, healthy choices. They are educated on what ingredients are in products they use and are able to make well-informed decisions on how to limit the toxins in the world around them. By limiting my own stress, role modeling stress management techniques, showing love and positivity, and decreasing child-centered activities, I am able to involve them in my life. They help me write my books, help me make my videos, and help me speak to audiences. They also started their own podcast called *The Holistic Kids Show*! All of this maximizes their exposure to real life and real-life consequences. With limited electronic devices, they love to play all together (they are currently obsessed with Pokémon) indoors and outdoors; they are able to entertain themselves and resolve their own conflicts. The older children look after the younger ones. They are able to help us come up with family rules. We are blessed to live in an extended family home, surrounded by unconditional love from aunts, uncles, and grandparents. They help me raise my children and follow the rules our family has set (I know, I am spoiled), though that can come with its own challenges. But when we focus on all the positives it brings into our lives, living with grandparents is one of the biggest blessings. They model positivity, balance, and connection. When there is less control, there is less resentment and stress.

When children don't argue, don't complain, and are happy overall with no tantrums, doesn't that make life so much easier? Wouldn't that make parenting so much easier? But that's not all. I am now trying to raise children who are informed, autonomous, mindful, grateful, confident, and resilient; have self-control; and are able to make good decisions. They are able to recognize that something is "off balance" and look into their lives to see where they can help put their bodies back into balance.

If my five-year-old feels a little "off"—he's a little bit more agitated or a little bit tired, or he has some diarrhea, for example—he will immediately think back in his day to determine when he went "off balance." One day, I found my seven-year-old, on his own, eating sauerkraut. When I asked why, he said, "I was feeling a little agitated, and I think the ketchup I had yesterday at Grandma's had organic sugar, so I think that is making me feel a little agitated; I want to feed my gut bugs good foods so I can feel less agitated!" What?! It's the same with my thirteen-year-old and ten-year-old; they are now able to adjust their lives to make sure their emotions, bodies, and brains are working as best as they can get them to work. When you empower children with education, we empower them to take care of their own health. When we raise children, or tiny adults, with the power of mindfulness, they are able to constantly look within themselves and fix their imbalance on their own before it even becomes a problem! They are mindful of their own behaviors, and they look deep within to adjust as needed. It is a learning processes, and they get better with time

Holistic parenting is all about loving, connecting with, educating, and empowering your children and guiding them along the way; it's about giving them the positive mind-set and life skills to navigate our rapidly changing world. Every conversation you have with your children, every hug, and everything you do—from the food you put in their bodies to how they manage their stresses to their sleep, social health, and spiritual health—has the power to mold our children's brains and bodies for the better. By focusing on the key foundations of holistic parenting, which can easily be incorporated into your family's daily routine, we will be able to help our children thrive and make better, everyday decisions for their bodies and the planet. You will have ups and downs. No one is perfect, and no child is the same. But the tools in this book will help you maximize success in whatever you and your family are dealing with.

Let's dive into these principles in a little bit more detail, then address common parenting dilemmas and what to do if your child does get sick.

Holistic parenting puts children back in the driver's seat of their lives while they navigate through all of life's ups and downs. Isn't this exciting? Remember, if I can do it, you can do it, too!

Part II

FOUNDATIONS OF HOLISTIC PARENTING: REAL-LIFE PARENTING SOLUTIONS FOR THE WHOLE MINDFUL, RESILIENT CHILD

• 3 •

Digestive Health and Detoxification

DIGESTIVE HEALTH AND NUTRITION

As parents, feeding ourselves is hard enough, let alone trying to feed a whole household! With our busy schedules, it is easier to give our family something quick and easy, something that will satiate and delight, so we can quickly get back to our busy schedules. By trying to make our lives easier, did you know that this "quick" meal is actually making your life more difficult, not easier?!

I know it sounds crazy, but food is information; food talks to our genes, but food also transforms our children's brains, bodies, and behavior—for better or for worse! More than 90 percent of the genetic switches in our DNA associated with longevity are significantly influenced by our lifestyle choices, including the foods we eat.[1] Food is the most powerful tool we have to impact our children's health and minds.

Imbalanced Nutrition Leads to Imbalanced Children

Have you ever wondered why there is a separate "kids' menu" at restaurants? Most of the time, the kids' menu is packed with very highly processed foods like chicken nuggets and grilled cheese sandwiches. Our children are eating more and more "fake food" than ever before, and it is coming with a consequence. With every bite, these foods are changing our biochemistry, constantly influencing how our children feel and behave. These energy-dense, nutrient-poor foods are destroying their health and brains and affecting every cell in the body.

The food our families are eating is not the same food our ancestors used to eat. In the first part of the twentieth century, chemically altered food substances replaced real food with bioengineered food that lacked nutrition. Food science

51

has never been more complicated, as large companies modify foods in their chemistry labs with engineered substances that have unpronounceable names. Food companies are adding in addictive and toxic substances, calling them food and getting us all hooked and enslaved.

The government supports the production/sales of foods that are biologically addictive, providing way too much of the food that hurts us and not enough of the food that benefits us. The food monopoly is made up of "Big Food" companies, fertilizer companies, "Big Seed" companies, and "Big Ag" companies that control everything from how our food is grown to how it ends up on our plates.

Our food system and the education we receive about food is being manipulated. Using the latest research on how our brains work, our food system is spending billions of dollars on colorful advertising of "fake foods" to appeal to our children, especially to minority groups. Junk food advertisements are on TV and social media, and it is given out as a reward or gift in schools and in lunch rooms; this gets our children hooked on junk food and, ultimately, creates customers for life. Studies show that if a child sees a commercial for a particular food, the child will consume 45 percent more food.[2] In 2019, a study at Dartmouth College found that children who watched more ads for high-sugar cereals consumed more of the product.[3] The food system gets us addicted young and promotes sickness into our old age.

The food we all eat (fake, processed foods) or don't eat is the single biggest cause of death and suffering worldwide. Globally, one in five deaths in 2017 was associated with a poor diet.[4] For every 10 percent of a person's diet that comes from processed, artificial, and impure foods, the risk of death goes up by 14 percent of "all-cause mortality."[5] For the first time in history, there are more overweight people than there are underfed adults and children on this planet,[6] mostly in low- and middle-income countries. The World Health Organization (WHO) has formally recognized obesity as a global epidemic.[7]

In 2019, *Lancet* published the findings of the most comprehensive study of people's diets. The study followed people in 195 countries over a twenty-seven-year period and determined dietary risk factors based on the effect of diet on health.[8] Despite limitations, the researchers concluded that a diet without enough healthy foods and with too many bad foods accounted for eleven million deaths and 255 million years of disability and life years lost. Most striking was the finding that the lack of protective foods (whole, real unprocessed foods) was as (or more) important in determining risk of death as the overconsumption of processed foods.[9]

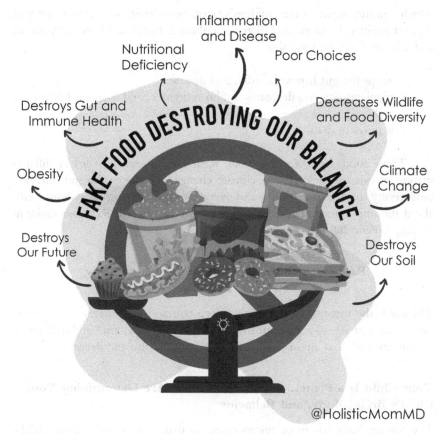

Inflammation and Disease

Nutritional Deficiency

Poor Choices

Destroys Gut and Immune Health

Decreases Wildlife and Food Diversity

FAKE FOOD DESTROYING OUR BALANCE

Obesity

Climate Change

Destroys Our Future

Destroys Our Soil

@HolisticMomMD

Figure 3.1.

Balanced Nutrition, Balanced Digestive Health, Balanced Brains, and Balanced Bodies

The food world is confusing. Most nutrition research is obtained through surveys and questionnaires, and most aren't even that accurate. Other studies are funded by those who have a conflict of interest. It is difficult to make real sense of the studies and what they say about our consumption and our eating habits. As a mom of four boys who feeds a family of eight daily (with up to even twenty on most weekends), I get it . . . my secret to clear the muddy water is this: simplicity is key to success.

As parents, we need a way of life, not a diet. We talked a lot about inflammation, so with that in mind, we need to limit the foods that will cause inflammation and increase foods that lower the overall inflammation, give our children energy, and optimize the immune system and the mitochondria, which will turn genes in our children's favor, build brain connections that will support healthy decisions, and increase resilience. For that, I have my patients and families focus on food that

- keeps the gut happy, healthy, and diverse;
- regulates glucose, decreases insulin resistance, and balances hormones; and
- is nutrient dense.

Those foods are *real, whole foods.* Real food doesn't just lower inflammation, it can also help reverse climate change, regenerate the soil, increase biodiversity, protect our waters, and even restore our dying ecosystem! I talk about the importance of real food in depth in *The Holistic Rx: Your Guide to Healing Chronic Inflammation and Disease.*

Real Food Keeps Our Children's Guts Happy, Healthy, and Diverse

The gut is the first line of defense between you and the universe. The gut is home to about 70–80 percent or more of the immune system[10] and trillions of microorganisms that are in charge of your child's health and decisions!

Your Child Is a Planet, and Its Inhabitants Are Determining Your Child's Brain, Body, and Behavior

The human body has more microorganisms than human cells! Your child's gastrointestinal tract, mouth, skin, and reproductive systems are packed with bacteria, viruses, parasites, fungi, protozoa, amoebae, archaea, and even bacteriophages; all of these combined are known as the microbiome, a collection of trillions of microbes that live inside and on the human body. Each one of these microbial categories has its own community, all mingling together. Starting from conception, we are exposed to trillions of bacteria daily, and our microbiome continues to grow with us, constantly changing.[11] Our inner garden contains a unique composition of good bugs (mutualists), bad bugs (pathogens), and neutral bugs (commensals) that are involved in most, if not all, biological processes that constitute human health and disease by directly affecting our family's epigenetics, minds, and immune system. Our human cells are outnumbered ten to one, and there are roughly 360 million microbial genes for every human gene.[12]

Newborns are born with low microbial diversity, which gradually increases as they get older. A 2020 study shows that the infant gut microbiome undergoes dynamic changes in the first thirty-six months of life. During the first three years of life, the development of the microbiome is influenced by neonatal and maternal exposures[13] and the child's diet, lifestyle, and environment, which play a major role in the shifting of the gut microbiota in early life. The diversity of the microbiome is key to determining the health of a child's brain, body, and behavior.

What Influences Our Children's Microbiome?

Any environmental insult—including stress, infections, inflammation, and dietary deficiencies—can affect the gut microbiome, which can lead to brain disorders later in life.[14] Factors that put your child's microbiome out of balance include the following:[15]

- *Mode of delivery:* The initial colonization of the human gut microbiome is influenced by a wide range of factors that may have long physiological consequences.[16] A relatively lower gut microbial diversity was reported in C-section-delivered infants at the age of two years.[17] Babies delivered by C-section had decreased gut microbiota diversity, delayed Bacteroidetes colonization, and reduced Th1 responses.[18]

- *Fake food:* What our children eat can directly affect the composition of their microbiomes; diet can either hurt them or help them. Diet composition and patterns during the first three years of life can impact diversity of the gut microbiome with potential effects on infant development and risk of disease,[19] starting with breast milk. Breast milk contains indigestible fibers, called oligosaccharides, that have no nutritional value but are designed to feed the microbiome. Breastfed babies actually have lower risks for colds, RSV infections, digestive issues, metabolic issues, autoimmune diseases (e.g., type 1 diabetes and celiac disease), cancer, and obesity.[20] Breast milk protects against harmful bacteria[21] and makes the gut wall impermeable[22] because it contains a prebiotic that promotes the *Bifidobacterium longum* and enhances immune function.[23] A 2021 study examined more than nine thousand children and found that breastfed babies also scored higher on neurocognitive tests at the age of nine and ten.[24] As a child grows, a high-fiber, nutrient-rich, and anti-inflammatory diet filled with colorful, unprocessed foods promotes beneficial bacteria, which enriches the microbiome. Processed foods that contain artificial sweeteners, additives, colors, flavors, and other chemicals serve to throw off bacterial balance.

- *Toxic environment:* Daily toxic environmental contaminants can kill off many beneficial microbial strains. A 2020 study published in

Environmental Science and Technology Letters found a correlation between the levels of beneficial bacteria and fungi in the gastrointestinal tract of children and the amount of common chemicals in their homes. Researchers found that children who had higher levels of chemicals (semivolatile organic compounds like phthalates and PFAS [polyfluoroalkyl substances, a group of man-made chemicals]) in their blood had a reduction in the amount of bacteria, and children with increased phthalates had a reduction in fungi populations.[25]

- *Chronic stress:* In healthy children's populations, chronic stress can negatively affect the microbiome. A study linked behavior issues and socioeconomic stress to a distinct microbiome pattern.[26] The researchers recruited forty families with children between the ages of five and seven from a variety of socioeconomic groups. They found that children at higher socioeconomic risk had different microbiome profiles compared to their peers at lower socioeconomic risk.[27] When researchers looked at their behaviors, they saw that the children with certain types of behavior dysregulation, such as the ability to inhibit impulses and depression, had distinct microbial profiles. *Akkermansia muciniphilia* is a type of beneficial bacteria found in the intestine, and its deficiency can increase the likelihood of developing obesity and type 1 diabetes. Stress hormones like cortisol and catecholamines like epinephrine and norepinephrine will reduce the levels of *Akkermansia muciniphilia*. Stress can negatively affect the microbiome and has lasting effects in children.[28]

- *Medications:* Though some medications can save your child's life, they do come with a side disadvantage, so you need to weigh the risks versus the benefits when it comes to medications, specifically antibiotics. Antibiotics given during labor and pregnancy, and antibiotics given directly to the child, have a negative impact on the newborn intestinal flora, which has been linked to physical, behavioral, and memory function.[29] Some other medications—especially NSAIDs, other pain killers, birth control pills, steroids, chemotherapy drugs, acid-blocking medications, opiates, antibiotics, and sleep medications—can negatively affect the microbiome.

- *Other factors:* Infections or exposures that were never resolved (e.g., bacteria, viruses, fungi, or parasites) and overly strenuous exercise may increase pro-inflammatory cytokines in the bloodstream and harm the lining of the intestinal wall, which will affect the microbiome.

People with a higher-than-average number of different microbial species tend to be the healthiest. The presence of fewer species and the absence of healthy gut bacteria alter genes (leading to inflammation) and alter signaling pathways involved in learning, motor control, and memory. Additionally, you crave the wrong types of foods.

The Microbiome and Its Function

The gut microbiome influences the endocrine system, the immunological and neural pathway that plays an important role in infant development.[30] Our child's microbiome is a critical player in multiple physiological functions: it promotes normal gastrointestinal function by digesting multiple nutrients, synthesizes hormones and vitamins, balances pH, helps extract energy and harvest calories from undigested food particles as they pass through the digestive tract, absorbs food, manufactures neurotransmitters, controls blood sugar balance, and helps maintain a healthy weight and metabolism. The bacteria interact with the immune system, influence the T cells (a critical part of the immune system), help fight off colds and infections, help organize the right level of response to an invader, have antitumor and anticancer effects, and break down bacterial toxins.

The microbiome helps shape your child's brain, mood, behaviors, and decisions. The gut contains the same neurotransmitters found in the brain. Three-fourths of the body's neurotransmitters are found and made in the gut, including 50 percent of the body's dopamine and 90 percent of the body's serotonin. Negative changes to the microbiome can lead to cytokine release; it can also increase stress and inflammation, leading to mood disturbances, bad decisions, and even bad food cravings, partly via the vagus nerve. Positive changes in the microbiome create a calming response.

Our gut is naturally permeable to allow vital nutrients, like proteins, starches, and digested fats, to pass through the tight junctions and enter the bloodstream. The intestines are covered by intestinal epithelium, a single layer of cells that separates our body from the stuff in the intestines. Normally, the cells that line the intestine stick together very tightly to form a protective barrier that is very hard to penetrate, keeping the bigger particles that could damage the system out of the body. It also acts as a relay switch for the messages coming from the rest of the body to the good bacteria in the gut.

When our children's internal and external worlds are balanced, everything works better. But this balance of gut bacteria can be disrupted when we constantly add in fake foods and other negative environmental factors (discussed earlier in the chapter). If an imbalanced gut microbiome (or dysbiosis) goes on for a while, pathogenic microbes or improperly digested proteins may activate the immune system, creating a fire or war in the gut as they trigger the immune cells. This situation leads to inflammation and damage to the gut wall epithelial cells, and the junctions become leaky and increasingly permeable.[31] Eventually, this leads to increased intestinal permeability, or leaky gut syndrome.[32] When your child's gut becomes permeable, weak, and compromised, it allows things to pass through the membrane into the bloodstream that normally would not, such as undigested food particles, gluten, viruses, bad bacteria, and toxins that trigger the immune system,[33] which imbalances the gut microbes further.

For short periods of time, acute inflammation isn't bad, but when the immune system is constantly in the "on" position for months, it can turn into chronic inflammation. Over time, the immune system becomes highly reactive, responding to stimuli that it previously would have ignored, such as foreign substances like zonulin (a protein that modulates the permeability of tight junctions between cells of the wall of the digestive system), and keeps the gates open. When this continues for months and becomes chronic, it can lead to translocation of bacteria, and bacterial products like lipopolysaccharides (also known as an endotoxin), penetrating the bloodstream, activating the immune system and releasing cytokines that instigate inflammation through the body and central nervous system. An imbalanced microbiome creates an inflammatory environment that will create intestinal permeability.

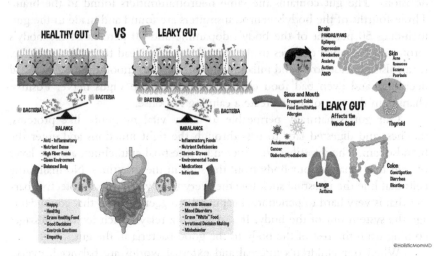

Figure 3.2.   Leaky Gut, Leaky Brain, and Childhood Illness

Leaky Gut and Leaky Brain: The Gut and Brain Connection

Your child's gut and brain are constantly talking to each other. A leaky gut can cause brain inflammation and can affect brain hormone production.

For every message from the brain that goes down to the gut microbiome, there are nine messages from the gut going up to the brain. These messages can influence the brain's response to a stressful situation, activation of the brain's immune system, the adaptability of these new cells to learn (neuroplasticity), brain hormone production (which controls how the brain works), and the growth of new brain cells (neurogenesis).

An imbalanced microbiome leads to increased immune cells that release cytokines to talk to other immune cells, messages that cross the blood-to-brain barrier to activate the brain's immune system. The specialized immune system in the brain (glia cells) is activated to fight the invaders, leading to more inflammation. These cytokines can even act as neurotransmitters, and when they travel to the brain, they can trigger the body's own protectors, the microglia (that outnumber neurons three to one), which normally help the brain restore, prune unused connections, and stimulate new connections to form. But when the cytokines activate the microglia, they shift into "alert inflammatory mode,"[34] leading to dysregulation, which is fine for a short time; however, if it gets stuck in this mode (microglial activation) in the long term, it can lead to further inflammation. The microbiome controls the development and maturation of the microglia.

This process can actually begin in utero, especially if the mom was in a state of chronic inflammation or had an infection.[35] Breaches in the blood-to-brain barrier can also come from head trauma and the internal and external environment. Diet alterations and infections in children have all been associated with brain function and behavior abnormalities.[36] Dysbiosis of the maternal gut microbiome in response to changes in stress can affect the child's brain and behavior.[37] The system is so sensitive that even one abnormal bacterium entering the gut has the potential to change the way the brain fires within a couple of hours.[38] This inflammation leads to a dysregulated connection between the amygdala and prefrontal cortex, leading to irrational decision making and symptoms leading to brain fog, mood swings, mood disorders, tics, anxiety, sleep issues, mood disorders, and even autism in those with gut dysfunction. A thriving microbiome promotes learning, memory, good behavior, and a good mood.

Your Child's Chronic Symptoms Start in the Gut

The gut microbiome is a large contributor to the health of the child;[39] an unhealthy microbiome makes kids more vulnerable to allergies, autoimmune diseases, and even type 1 diabetes.[40] Even symptoms beginning in the first few weeks of life, like colic, can be improved with a probiotic (*Lactobacillus reuteri*).[41]

Progressive changes in microbial diversity of the infant gut microbiome are likely to reshape metabolic functions over time. These children tend to have more health issues, such as obesity, high cholesterol, insulin resistance, increased inflammatory markers, chronic diseases, allergies, diabetes, psychiatric issues, inflammatory bowel disease, and inflammation, and they even show signs of bad decision making. Gut microbial alterations in early infancy have been shown to affect the risk of childhood obesity, nonalcoholic fatty liver disease, allergies, hives, urticaria, food sensitivities, asthma, and even type 1 diabetes.[42] Leaky gut has been implicated in most chronic health conditions, food sensitivities,[43] autoimmune diseases,[44] digestive issues, skin problems, estrogen dominance (which can lead to painful breasts and heavy periods), insulin resistance, autism,[45] attention-deficit/hyperactivity disorder (ADHD),[46] and so many more.

We have so much power as parents. Through diet and lifestyle, you can manipulate the environment in which these microbes exist; you can make them work for you, instead of against you, and your child will be healthier. If you take care of these microbes, these microbes can take care of your child. We depend on them, and they depend on us. When parenting your child for better brain and body health, real food balances your child's microbes, thereby balancing the brain, body, and hormones.

Balanced Insulin and Leptin = Balanced Brains and Bodies

More and more children today are becoming hormone imbalanced—and even prediabetic. Our children are eating more of the wrong food, which contributes to insulin and leptin resistance. This state of hormonal imbalance leads to overeating and inflammation. Insulin manages glucose levels, and leptin helps with satiation.

Fake Foods → Insulin and Leptin Resistance →
Overeating, Dysfunctional Brain, Body, and Behavior

What Is Insulin Resistance?

When our children take a bite of food, it is absorbed and enters into the bloodstream. The glucose in the body is needed for the cells for energy and fuel. But glucose can only enter the cell if it has a key—insulin. Insulin is a storage hormone produced by the pancreas; it controls blood sugar levels and determines our metabolism. Over time, the flood of inflammatory signals starts to wear down this key because it keeps on using the key over and over again as the body stops listening to the insulin. Eventually, the key stops working,

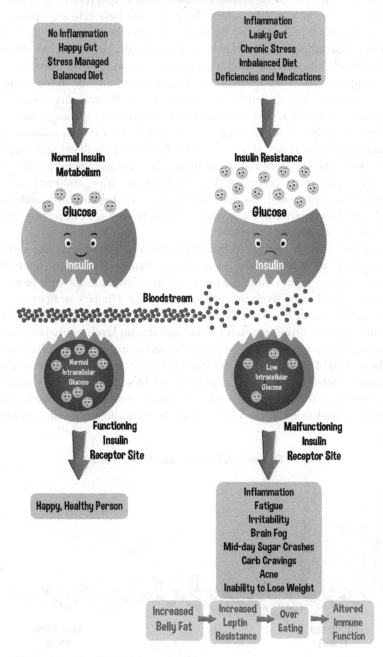

Figure 3.3.   Insulin Resistance in Kids

and the cells don't open their doors to insulin and are unable to absorb glucose adequately, which leads to insulin resistance. To keep everything in balance and the glucose in a healthy range, the pancreatic beta cells start producing even more insulin. Over time, the beta cells can't keep up with the body's increased demand for insulin; this leads to excess glucose in the bloodstream, which disturbs this delicate balance and makes the body uncomfortable.

Symptoms of insulin resistance are fatigue, irritability, brain fog, memory or concentration issues, weight gain around the midsection, sugar crashes in the middle of the day, and an inability to lose weight. Missing a meal can lead to irritability and fatigue. After meals, people with insulin resistance feel sluggish and sleepy. They also can be addicted to carbohydrates and have hypoglycemic attacks. They can suffer from acne, irregular periods, infertility, cysts, polycystic ovary syndrome (PCOS), poor sex drive, and increased hair growth. The skin around the folds and creases can become dark and thick, called acanthosis nigricans. Sadly, this problem is now present in very young children and is constantly overlooked.

An imbalanced lifestyle can lead to prediabetes/insulin resistance and diabetes, which can in turn lead to more chronic illnesses. Diets now full of fake foods are raising insulin more than ever before. Cereals made with processed corn raise blood sugar levels more than sugar does! The lack of fiber can lead to increased visceral fat, and artificial sweeteners have been linked to weight gain and diabetes. Stress increases cortisol and insulin levels, worsening insulin resistance. Leaky gut, or dysbiosis, increases inflammation, worsening obesity and belly weight. Toxins in our environment are now making our cells numb to insulin. Deficiencies due to our food and lifestyle (especially vitamin D and magnesium deficiency) are leading to insulin resistance. Medications like steroids can lead to an elevated blood sugar level, leading to insulin resistance.

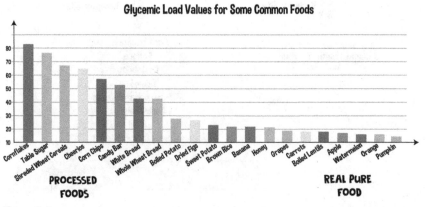

Figure 3.4.

Let's Talk Leptin

Leptin is a metabolic hormone, also known as the hunger hormone produced by our fat cells that tells us when we are satiated and to stop eating. It is the gatekeeper of fat metabolism, monitoring how much energy an organism takes in. When the stomach starts to fill up, fat cells release leptin to tell the brain to stop eating. The more fat a child has, the more circulating leptin a child has. Leptin also tells the brain there's sufficient body fat to sexually develop, so leptin increases the production of gonadotrophin-releasing hormones from the brain, initiating puberty.

Eating more artificial and processed foods can lead to quicker leptin resistance, so we continue to overeat, as our bodies don't know when we are full. This is why restaurants give you bread at the beginning of a meal. The processed bread inhibits leptin (which then leads to overeating); the body then becomes numb to insulin and leptin, further increasing leptin and insulin resistance. Lack of sleep, high stress levels, high fructose corn syrup, high insulin levels, and overeating can all lead to leptin resistance. Studies show that the majority of overweight individuals who are having difficulty losing weight have leptin resistance;[47] the constant surges of leptin can overwhelm the system. Like insulin, over time the body's receptors start to turn off and become leptin resistant, and we stop listening to the leptin signal. As with all hormone issues, leptin resistance is a complex issue.

Consequences of Insulin and Leptin Resistance

More and more children today are insulin and leptin resistant. This is a growing problem that leads to inflammation and is an integral part that needs to be addressed when looking to optimize our children's brains and bodies. Studies have shown that the amygdala was more active when inflammation was high,[48] and the most active amygdalas were by far the most likely to develop type 2 diabetes (with or without obesity). Our children's brains are complex organs that are constantly growing and changing throughout their lifetime.[49] The brain has high metabolic activity; although it only contributes to roughly 2 percent of total body weight, it uses 20 percent of the total energy generated from food consumed.[50] The preferred source of energy in the brain is glucose, but the brain can't store glucose;[51] the impact of glucose on brain functioning generalizes to the cognitive processes involved in learning.[52]

A study of 2,519 children aged eight to sixteen years found that childhood obesity has negative psychosocial and cognitive impacts on children's academic performance.[53] Inflammation associated with obesity has also predicted worsened executive function in both adolescents and adults.[54] These fat cells are blocking us from connecting to our prefrontal cortex and making good decisions.

Insulin resistance and leptin resistance can also negatively influence puberty. The transition from childhood to adulthood is a period of intense hormonal, metabolic, and physical changes. In the 1800s, puberty occurred around age sixteen for girls; in the late 1900s, the average age dropped to twelve; now the average age of puberty is under ten years old! As insulin rises, it also stimulates the production of leptin from fat cells, which then activates the production of a precursor sex hormone in the brain and gonads. Our children's nutrition and metabolic health have a strong influence on when puberty begins. According to a 2007 study of girls between ages two and eight, for every one unit increase in body mass index, the onset of puberty is one month earlier![55]

Eat Nutrient-Dense Food

We talked about healing foods that optimize the gut bacteria and hormone levels; these are the most nutrient-dense foods you can give a child. When children consume less nutrients and more high-calorie foods, their bodies are malnourished but overfed. With this giant shift in nutrition to a diet lacking in diversity, more than 90 percent of Americans, including our children, are lacking in one or more nutrients at levels that are creating alarming vitamin and nutrient deficiencies. B vitamins, magnesium, vitamin D, selenium, vitamin K2, vitamin E, and potassium are lost from the modern diet. In fact, the number one cause of disease is the lack of vegetables and fruits in our diet, which leads to nutritional deficiencies and creates imbalances in the body.

Nutrition affects a child's cognitive development and performance, and a bad diet is now a more accurate predictor of future violence than past violent behavior.[56] Supplementing nutrient deficiencies has been shown to reduce violent acts by as much as 91 percent.[57]

Research on individual nutrients indicates they have roles in cognitive function and the potential for learning. For example, research has shown that childhood iron has a large role in mental, motor, and general behavior; deficiencies can lead to impairments in both motor and cognitive functioning in children, negatively impacting academic performance.[58] Other important micronutrients for brain development and function are iodine, folate, vitamin B12, and zinc.[59] Great levels of carotenoids have been associated with higher scores on cognitive tests.[60] Lutein, one of the three major dietary carotenoids, is present in the brain and has a functional importance on cognition and infant brain development.[61] Vitamin and mineral supplementation has been shown to reduce antisocial behavior and aggression.[62] In a sample of more than thirteen thousand children and adolescents, the frequency of junk food consumption was significantly associated with violent behaviors and psychiatric distress.[63]

Parents and our parenting habits can help build our child's brains/bodies or break it down. If we feed our children real food, we can help them heal their guts and balance insulin and leptin levels. These real foods optimize the immune system and the mitochondria, and they lower overall inflammation. These real foods are the most powerful factors in brain and body health.

The Healing Plate: Eat the Rainbow!

As we discussed, our children need food that will enhance gut health, balance hormones, and provide their bodies with the best nutrition possible to optimize brain, body, and behavior. There are a lot of "diets" out there, but I believe in a whole lifestyle. Every child is different, so whether your family is vegan or vegetarian, or whether your family eats animal protein, at every meal your child needs to be "eating the rainbow." This means you need to provide your child with the following:

Rainbow vegetables
Clean protein
Healthy fats
Adequate hydration and fruit

Child's Healing Plate

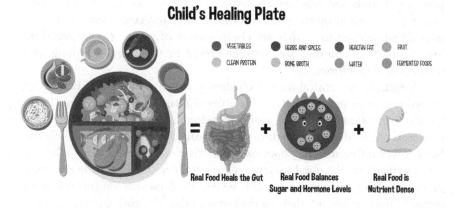

| VEGETABLES | HERBS AND SPICES | HEALTHY FAT | FRUIT |
| CLEAN PROTEIN | BONE BROTH | WATER | FERMENTED FOODS |

Real Food Heals the Gut = Real Food Balances Sugar and Hormone Levels + Real Food is Nutrient Dense

@HolisticMomMD

Figure 3.5.

I find that lists help my children focus on what they can have instead of what they can't have. I know they might want all the carbs and sweets first, but remember, your children's taste buds are being manipulated! Their cravings for the food they are always asking for are being dictated by their gut bugs that manipulate their minds. How? Because the gut and the brain are so intricately connected, they work by changing the neural signals along the vagus nerve, to the point that they alter the taste receptors to make them crave foods that will allow those bugs to thrive. Isn't that crazy?!

If our children eat processed carbs first, they deprive their bodies of the nutrient-dense foods they really need to function optimally. To make it fun, focus on lots of real *color*! Kids love color, and each color has a specific benefit for their little bodies. An added bonus is that all these meals quickly satiate, enhance gut health, and decrease insulin resistance by improving the immune system and metabolism, which in turn optimizes the connections between the amygdala and prefrontal cortex and, most important, heals and prevents chronic disease.

Rainbow Vegetables

Unfortunately, vegetables don't factor in our diets as much as they should. About three-quarters of the world generally only eat twelve plants and five animal species. And with about 250,000 to 300,00 known edible plant species, humans only consume between 150 and 200 of them. Seventy-eight percent of the world's population doesn't eat the minimum of five servings of fruits and vegetables a day, and children are actually no different. Only 12.2 percent of girls and 9.4 percent of boys consume the recommended five portions of fruits and vegetables a day.[64] Sixty percent of the world's calorie intake is dominated by three crops—wheat, rice, and corn—that are turned into ultra-processed food; they are cheap sources of energy but are relatively low in nutrition, and they are consumed more by the poor, the young, and less educated minorities.

Vegetables are critical for our children's bodies and health, as they affect everything, even genetic code. Vegetables regulate our genetics, and long-term consumption can protect against development of cancers, diabetes, osteoporosis, neurodegenerative diseases, and heart disease.[65] Vegetables help the body lower inflammation,[66] optimize detoxification, keep the body alkaline, act as fertilizer for the good bacteria in the gut, keep things moving smoothly in the gut, help maintain a healthy weight, and prevent cancer and heart disease;[67] most important, they are packed with disease-fighting phytonutrients (*phyto* means plants),[68] minerals, and vitamins.

Eat the rainbow: Focus on eating lots of color and lots of different variet-ies of veggies. Some will actually have a more powerful effect when eaten together (check out my book *Adam's Healing Adventures: The Power of Rainbow Foods* for a fun way to get your kids to eat the rainbow).

Red veggies (like tomatoes, bell peppers, beets, and carrots) contain lycopene, which protects against genetic damage (antioxidant) that can cause cancer and even protects against heart disease. Beets contain phytonutrients called betalains, which are antioxidants, anti-inflammatory, and important for detoxification support.

Orange veggies (carrots, pumpkins, sweet potatoes, orange bell peppers and squash varieties) have alpha carotene and beta carotene (antioxidants). Alpha carotene protects the skin and vision and protects against cancer; beta carotene is converted to vitamin A, which may also slow cognitive decline.

Yellow-green veggies may not look yellow to the eye but include greens (e.g., spinach, mustard, turnip greens, yellow corn, and avocado); they signal the carotenoids lutein and zeaxanthin, which are beneficial for our eyes and protect against atherosclerosis (hardening of the arteries). Yellow summer squash is a good source of dietary fiber that aids digestion.

Green veggies (e.g., greens, collards, broccoli, bok choy, cabbage, kale, arugula, watercress, mustard, fennel, broccoli rabe, and sprouts) have phy-tochemicals, isocyanates, indoles, and sulforaphane, which raise glutathione, boost detoxification, and inhibit carcinogens. Sea vegetables like seaweed or edible algae are rich sources of iodine and strengthen the immune system; they contain important antioxidants and nutrients to fight inflammation and even cancer. Cruciferous vegetables have so many nutrients (like A, C, and K) and are packed with fiber; they also have glucosinolate, which can reduce inflam-mation and fight cancer.

Pale green-white veggies (e.g., garlic, leeks, onions, and cauliflower) contain allicins, which have powerful antimicrobial and immune-boosting properties. They are anticancer and antitumor, and they also contain antioxi-dant flavonoids. Sulforaphane is a phytochemical found in cruciferous veggies and may help prevent cancer by improving antioxidant activity in the body and contribute to detoxification. Cauliflower is rich in glucosinolates, sulfur-containing phytonutrients that have antioxidant, anticancer, and detoxifying properties.

Blue-purple veggies, such as purple potatoes, red cabbage, and eggplants, prevent cell aging, improve vascular and cognitive function, increase blood flow, reduce inflammation, and inhibit DNA damage in the brain.

Brown foods like mushrooms can enhance the microbiome and are a great source of vitamin D; they protect the nervous system and are even anticancer. Different types of mushrooms have other benefits; reishi mushrooms, for example, promote self-repair and cellular resistance.

Vegetables have lots of fiber, specifically broccoli, kale, green beans, artichokes, sweet potatoes, carrots, and butternut squash. Fiber is important because it helps suppress appetite, control cravings, stabilize blood sugar and insulin levels after a meal, lower blood pressure, fight chronic disease like cancer, remove toxins, feed healthy bacteria, and decrease overall inflammation. Some vegetables also have resistant starches (that are not digested in the small intestine), which regulate blood sugar and metabolism as well as optimize gut flora—for example, psyllium husk, inulin from chicory or Jerusalem artichokes, or high amylose plants like potatoes, plantains, and green bananas.

Do not remove the skins from fruits and vegetables, as they are highly nutritious, regulate appetite, affect fat storage,[69] control blood sugar,[70] regulate insulin release,[71] and optimize detoxification. When possible, focus on eating local, whole organic vegetables (heirloom varieties are best) as the whole plant is full of vital nutrients. They can be eaten raw, juiced, cooked (some are great cooked and cooled, as that process creates resistant starch), and cultured. Wash vegetables and fruits with skins, but don't go overboard: a tiny bit of organic soil adds diversity to the microbiome.

Clean Protein: Quality over Quantity

Our children's bodies need protein to help them grow, thrive, heal, optimize the immune system, control appetite, synthesize muscles, and construct the gut lining. Protein is the building material for enzymes; it increases metabolic fire and the ability to burn calories, and helps you feel full. Lack of protein results in a cascade of negative consequences at the brain level, like decreased brain volume and altered hippocampal formation.[72] Preclinical trials have shown that early life malnutrition indicates that protein or protein energy restriction results in smaller brains with reduced RNA and DNA contents, fewer neurons, and reduced concentrations of neurotransmitters and growth factors.[73] Supplementing undernourished children with protein has been shown to improve children's cognitive performance and is most effective in the first two years of life.[74]

Seafood lowers the risk of type 2 diabetes, autoimmune diseases, and even cancer,[75] depression, aggression and other mood disorders,[76] and ADHD;[77] symptoms of inflammatory disorders improve with omega-3 consumption, including asthma,[78] cardiac disease, and diabetes. Seafood is also a great source of dietary protein, vitamin D, vitamin B12, iodine, and selenium. Poultry is a good source of some critical nutrients like protein, B vitamins, and minerals, and the dark meat contains vitamin K2. Pasture-raised protein has more EFAs (essential fatty acids). Eggs are a great source of choline, which is needed for brain health and detoxification.

When it comes to protein, quality is more important than quantity. Choose grass-fed, pastured, organic, wild-caught protein that have not had any antibiotics and/or genetically modified (GMO) feed. Meat from grass-fed animals is full of micronutrients.[79] If you are going to consume canned fish, sardines, clams, oysters, and salmon are great options as long as they are in non-BPA cans and packed in olive oil. Wild-caught seafood contains healthy sources of EPA and DHA, and children need fatty acids, as they are critical for all cells of the body and for brain health. Wild-caught fish is best, as farmed fish contains higher levels of toxins like polycholorinated piphenyls (PCBs) and persistent organic pollutants (POPs).[80] Small wild-caught fish are highly nutrient dense. Consume smallish fish, wild or sustainably raised cold-water fish, including wild salmon, mackerel, sardines, herring, small halibut, anchovies, and sable (black cod). Pregnant women should consume eight ounces of fish per week that is low in mercury (e.g., sardines, herring, anchovies, wild salmon, and mackerel), but fish oil supplementation may be better. Plant protein contains low levels of leucine compared to animal protein,[81] so your child might not be able to get the protein the body needs just from plants. Sources of protein like hemp seed protein, chia protein powder, pea protein powder, lentils, and beans are also great sources of fiber. Beans contain resistant starches that feed our good bacteria, which keep the colon healthy.[82] Soak them overnight, sprout, ferment, pressure cook, and obtain organic when possible; use non-BPA cans, and remember that some people may also not be able to tolerate them, as they do contain lectins and phytates.

Vegetarians and vegans end up with deficiencies of vitamin K, omega-3 fats, vitamin B12, vitamin A, iron, and even calcium,[83] so they can be at a significant disadvantage nutritionally, specifically if they are consuming large amounts of antinutrients that bind the minerals they actually need.[84]

Healthy Fats

Our children's brains and bodies need fat; every cell of the body needs fat, and the nervous system is more than 60 percent fat. Healthy fats are necessary for brain function (specifically for infant brain development) and cellular function, as they are essential for absorbing fat-soluble nutrients required to make HDL (or "good") cholesterol, which is important for properly functioning neurons. Fat aids in the body's important metabolic and immune system functioning and is required for cell structure; it also balances mood, aids in dementia prevention, and optimizes bone and digestive health. Fat is likewise required to make hormones like testosterone and estrogen and for metabolizing vitamin D. Fat satiates us by turning on leptin, the hormone that regulates feelings of fullness, which is often disrupted by eating too many processed and refined carbohydrates and bad fat. Omega-3 fatty acids actually reduce inflammation, protect the brain, help with memory, and improve the brain's processing speeds;[85] they are also important in preventing and healing chronic conditions.[86] Children's long-chain omega-3 fatty acid intake has been positively associated with relational memory, and adolescents' fatty fish consumption has been associated with faster processing speeds compared to those consuming meats or supplements. Omega-3 should be eaten in the correct ratio to omega-6; ideally, the omega-6 to omega-3 ratio should be somewhere between a four to one ratio and a one to one ratio to optimize health, fight disease, and stop premature aging. The imbalance between omega-6 and omega-3 has been shown to depress the immune system function, contribute to weight gain, and lead to inflammation. Healthy fats, including omega-3s, are actually protective and important in reversing every single indicator of heart disease risk, including LDL (or "bad") cholesterol, hypertension, diabetes, and inflammation, and they protect against autoimmune disease and depression.

About 90 percent of Americans are deficient in omega-3 fatty acids, and a deficiency has been linked in mood disorders like violent behaviors, bipolar disorder, depression, autism, ADHD, seizures, and schizophrenia. Deficiencies in HDL (or "good") cholesterol have been linked to brain disorders like autism,[87] violent behaviors, and even suicide. Those with lower HDL cholesterol actually have more allergy disorders like asthma.[88]

There are different types of fats: saturated (butter and coconut oil), monounsaturated (olive, avocado, and many nuts), polyunsaturated (omega-3 and omega-6), and trans-fats. You want a healthy ratio of omega-3 to omega-6. Elevated omega-6 fatty acids have been linked to violent behavior, allergies, asthma, autism, cancer, and other neurological conditions.[89]

Examples of good fats include the following:

- Olive oil is packed with antioxidants. Look for extra virgin organic olive oil.
- Fats found in butter from grass-fed animals with their fat-soluble vitamins have anticancer properties, lower obesity, reduce inflammatory markers and autoimmune diseases,[90] and help heal the damaged gut and celiac disease. Look for organic raw butter from pastured animals.
- Grass-fed ghee is full of vitamins D, A, E, and K; omega-3s; CLA; and butyrate, which promotes intestinal health, healthy skin, and vision. In ghee, the milk solids have been removed, so it is casein and lactose free; it can easily be tolerated by those with lactose intolerance or those with dairy allergies.[91]

- Nuts are a great source of proteins, minerals, fiber, and essential fatty acids. They also contain potent antiangiogenic omega-3 PUFAs (poly-unsaturated fatty acids). Studies[92] have proven that nuts lower the incidence of cardiovascular disease and cancer, improve brain function, promote weight loss, improve cholesterol, prevent blood glucose from spiking, decrease the risk of type 2 diabetes, and even lower the risk of death.[93]
- Seeds contain protein, fats, fiber, minerals, antioxidants, and omega-3s (flaxseeds) that can reduce inflammation, improve gut function, and prevent autoimmunity and heart disease.
- Avocados are full of good fat. They help build lean muscle mass; detoxify; build healthy skin, hair, and eyes; aid in digestion; protect against insulin resistance; and help burn fat. Avocados are healthy fats that are good for the brain, as the brain is mostly made of fat.
- Coconut oil can be a healthy addition to your child's diet. It has anti-inflammatory, antifungal, and antimicrobial properties; improves digestion, brain health, and metabolism;[94] lowers insulin[95] and sugar levels; and acts as an antioxidant.
- Animal sources of fats from tallow help lower overall inflammation in fat tissues.[96]

Focus on eating the pure oils that our ancestors have eaten, and avoid processed toxic oils and fats. Healthy fats are a great snack; they satiate, keep blood sugar balanced, and increase metabolism. A typical serving of fat is about a tablespoon of oil, handful of nuts, or four ounces of fish or other animal protein. Don't eat fats with carbohydrates, sugar, or starches, as that can just lead to weight gain. Do your best to look for organic, non-GMO oils in glass jars whenever possible.

Respect the oil: Oils begin to get damaged at certain temperatures, destroying valuable nutrients (smoke point), and even good oils can start to go bad if not treated properly. Oils that contain saturated fats have strong double bonds, so they are more stable during cooking and have less chance of releasing toxins. Oils can be divided into two categories according to their optimal temperature (i.e., high-heat/medium-heat oils versus low-heat/no-heat oils). The following lists will help you differentiate the oils; the smoke point in Fahrenheit (F) and Celsius (C) is listed for each oil.

High-heat/medium-heat oils include the following:

Coconut oil (350F/176C)
Butter (350F/176C)
Ghee (450F/204C)

Avocado oil (520F/271C)
Beef tallow (400F/204C)
Duck/chicken fat (375F/190C)

Low-heat/no-heat oils include the following:

Extra virgin olive oil (320F/160C)
Flaxseed oil (225F/107C)
Walnut oil, macadamia oil, sesame oil, almond oil, tahini, and hemp oil
(all of these can be used raw)

Water/Drinks

Optimal hydration is key in decreasing inflammation and optimizing cell function; proper hydration flushes out toxins through the kidneys, promotes weight loss, increases energy, and promotes healthy bowel movements. Drink water that is filtered. Try adding slices or wedges of orange, lemon, or lime to water or teas. Throw in a mint leaf for an extra refreshing flavor along with stevia. Also try carbonated water.

Bone broth contains calcium, magnesium, phosphorus, collagen, and other nutrients that can be easily absorbed; it can help heal and seal the gut lining, promote growth of good bacteria, and reduce inflammation and food sensitivities. Fresh, raw vegetable juice and smoothies are also a great option for a fast meal. For a smoothie, add all the key nutrients: fruit; veggies; non-dairy milk or water; smart fat like chia, flax, or coconut oil or MCT oil; and a protein powder. Organic teas (black, white, green, herbal, or yerba mate) are a great drink to enjoy with lots of benefits; green tea, for example, is anti-inflammatory and has antioxidants, phytonutrients, and detoxifying properties.

Vinegar/Fermented Foods

Adding fermented foods to your child's diet will optimize health and healing by supporting digestion and liver detoxification and by strengthening the immune system. Apple cider vinegar promotes heart health by decreasing LDL cholesterol; it is rich in glutamine, improves inflammation, and helps regulate the glucose level. It has been shown to enhance vitamin K2, boost the immune system, and support cardiovascular health. Apple cider vinegar also contains *Bacillus subtilis*, a soil-based organism that provides beneficial bacteria, supports healthy immune system functioning, and helps reduce occasional diarrhea. Other fermented foods your children can try are miso, kombucha, kvass, pickles, pickled ginger, and homemade ketchup.

Fruit!

Most kids love fruit, and it provides endless health benefits. Eating the rainbow of fruit can be fun and beneficial, as every fruit and veggie color represents a different family of healing compounds (see the benefits of vegetables earlier in this chapter). Eating fruit prevents cancer and diabetes; improves blood pressure, insulin levels, cholesterol, and triglycerides; and lowers overall mortality risk.[97] They are packed with antioxidants, minerals, and vitamins that lower inflammation and improve detoxification. Fructose can increase triglycerides. Fructose with fiber, like in fruit, can slow absorption of fructose and feed the good bugs in the gut, which cleans the intestine.

Red fruits like pomegranates are powerful fruits that lower oxidative stress and even the risk of cancer by lowering overall inflammation. Pomegranates heal from the inside out, as they are anticarcinogenic; by altering our microbiome, they reduce arthritis and joint pain, lower blood pressure, and protect the heart. A bacteria in the gut called *Akkermansia muciniphila* makes up 1–3 percent of all gut bacteria, but it has a huge impact, as it can help improve glucose metabolism, decrease inflammation, and combat obesity.[98] Other red fruits like berries, watermelon, red grapes, apples, cranberries, goji berries, lingonberries, red pears, red plums, and cherries are all great for immune health. Orange foods are packed with vitamin C and beta carotene; examples are stone fruits like peaches, apricots, cantaloupe, and mangos, which are all DNA protective, packed with antioxidants, and great for reproductive health. Yellow fruits like bananas, apples, golden raisins, starfruit, and pineapple are great for digestive health. Green fruits like kiwi, green grapes, and green apples are great for heart health, and blue-purple foods like berries, grapes, acai berries, plums, and figs are great for brain health. Brown fruits like dates can inhibit cancer and boost energy.

Remember to enjoy local, organic, and seasonal fruits in moderation. You can also combine fruit with protein and a fat source to keep inflammation at bay and avoid glucose spikes.

Sweeteners/Sweets

Honey is a natural, less processed sweetener and is full of antioxidants, vitamins, and minerals; it contains a high concentration of enzymes (more than five thousand), which lowers inflammation, promotes detoxification, and supports wound healing.[99] Honey has powerful antimicrobial properties, and it also helps improve conditions like allergies, coughs, and asthma; decreases complications of type 2 diabetes;[100] and protects the liver and kidneys from the effects of numerous toxins, including Tylenol.[101] It is best to choose cold expressed raw organic honey, or manuka honey, but use it sparingly to keep glucose levels under control. One should not give honey to children less than one year old because it can cause botulism.

Maple syrup also contains lots of beneficial antioxidants;[102] it decreases the plasma glucose, protects the microbiome, and protects against cancer.[103] Date sugar is packed with antioxidants. Organic stevia whole plant extract can also be used, as it doesn't raise glucose levels. Dark chocolate (higher than 70 percent cocoa is best) has numerous health benefits. It contains bioflavoids that promote relaxation, lower blood pressure, protect the heart, improve lipid profiles, enhance cognition, and protect against inflammation and cancer.[104]

Herbs and Spices

Herbs and spices are powerful antioxidants and detoxifiers; they are anti-inflammatory and protect DNA. Garlic decreases blood pressure, prevents clots, and improves cholesterol (crush and chop to release its secret power: allicin). Turmeric is anti-inflammatory. Green herbs like oregano have antifungal, antibacterial, antiparasitic, and antioxidant properties; others like mint, basil, dill, chives, paprika, rosemary, and parsley are also beneficial. Thyme has powerful antiseptic, antioxidant, and anti-inflammatory properties; it aids in digestion and is good for lung function. Sage, an antioxidant, lowers blood sugar and improves blood pressure; it is good for the brain and is anti-inflammatory. Cumin is anticancer and helps the immune system. Focus on organic spices in glass bottles.

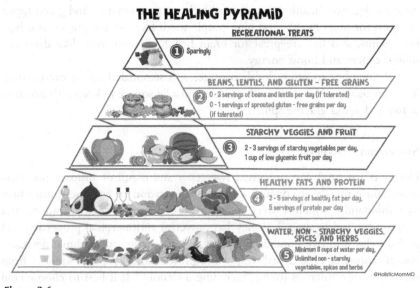

THE HEALING PYRAMID

RECREATIONAL TREATS
1. Sparingly

BEANS, LENTILS, AND GLUTEN – FREE GRAINS
2. 0 - 3 servings of beans and lentils per day (if tolerated)
0 - 1 servings of sprouted gluten - free grains per day (if tolerated)

STARCHY VEGGIES AND FRUIT
3. 2 - 3 servings of starchy vegetables per day,
1 cup of low glycemic fruit per day

HEALTHY FATS AND PROTEIN
4. 2 - 5 servings of healthy fat per day,
5 servings of protein per day

WATER, NON – STARCHY VEGGIES, SPICES AND HERBS
5. Minimum 8 cups of water per day,
Unlimited non - starchy vegetables, spices and herbs

@HolisticMomMD

Figure 3.6.

Salt

Table salt is different from sea salt. Table salt is toxic, as it has been overly processed, altered, and stripped of its nutritional benefits, which causing fluid retention. But sea salt, Celtic salt, and Himalayan salt are the real deal. These are full of trace minerals (including, among others, magnesium and calcium), which are all needed for the body to function optimally.

To Go Organic or Not to Go Organic?

Is the price increase worth the benefits? Unfortunately, the way the agricultural industry has evolved, most farmland was pesticide free, but after World War II that changed. Today we use more than 5 billion pounds of pesticides in farming every year!

The difference between the two is how the crops are grown. For organic foods to carry the USDA label, the guidelines prohibit the use of pesticides, herbicides, hormones, genetic engineering, and antibiotics, and there are certain standards in the humane raising of animals; conventional produce, however, doesn't have to follow any of these restrictions. In a study published in the *Journal of Applied Nutrition*, organically and conventionally grown apples, pears, potatoes, wheat, and sweet corn were compared and analyzed for their mineral content over a two-year period; organic produce was found to be more nutrient dense.[105]

Studies have shown that pesticides are carcinogenic[106] and neurotoxic;[107] they also are linked with depression and respiratory issues.[108] Pesticide exposure cripples the mitochondria and reduces liver enzyme activity needed for detoxification.[109] A study of more than one thousand American children showed that children with higher organophosphate pesticide traces in their urine were twice as likely to have an ADHD diagnosis compared to those with lower levels.[110] Exposure to pesticides around the time of birth disrupts neurotransmitter function, disrupts the baby's thyroid, and is associated with autism spectrum disorder and ADHD. Pesticide exposure during childhood affects children's health and has been linked to obesity, food allergies, abnormal or delayed development, asthma,[111] ADHD, and even cancer.[112] Pesticide exposure during pregnancy may lead to an increased risk of birth defects, low birth weight, and fetal death.[113]

Choosing from organics is best, but if you can't, the Environmental Working Group (EWG) has a list of the "dirty dozen" and the "clean fifteen" (foods with and without pesticides). Stick to purchasing organic with the foods on the dirty dozen list. Studies have also shown that organic vegetables have higher levels of vitamin C, antioxidants, polyphenols, and carotenoids, and they even taste better! To try to eliminate the pesticide residue, rub the fruit or wash and soak in a diluted solution with 3 percent hydrogen peroxide for about twenty minutes.

Foods to Limit . . . Who and Why?

If you are dealing with a chronic issue, tantrums, agitation, oppositional defiant disorder, or anything else that is off balance with your child, watch your child closely after each meal. Do certain foods seem to trigger unwanted behaviors? Could your child have a food sensitivity?

There is a difference between food allergy and sensitivity. If your child eats or is exposed to a food and the body then develops IgE antibodies to the food, she can experience an immediate response like hives, swelling, or difficulty breathing, and she is allergic to the exposure. Some foods create IgG antibodies to that food, which lead to leaky gut, irritable bowel syndrome (IBS), depression, headaches, heart palpitations, fatigue, brain fog, post-nasal drip, sinus issues, change in mood and behavior, and other symptoms of inflammation; this is also known as developing a food sensitivity or intolerance to that specific food. Because these reactions can be outside the realm of the digestive tract, and often are delayed, it can be hard to connect a particular food to your child's condition. The following foods are the major common culprits in allergies or sensitivities, inflammation, mood/behavior changes, and chronic conditions.

I would highly recommend removing these foods from your child's diet, as it can greatly improve health. When dealing with an illness, I have seen most children do really well and their symptoms improve immediately once they remove all processed foods (sugar, processed/artificial foods, soy), and some of the foods like dairy and grains, specifically wheat/gluten, from their diet. An elimination diet or even a blood test can help determine which foods your child could be sensitive to. The following are some that are frequent culprits.

Gluten and Grains

Unfortunately, we are all eating more starches and carbs than ever before. When our children are eating legumes and grains as the foundation of every meal they eat, they start to limit the variety of the foods they eat.[114] Whole grains can be a great source of fiber, minerals, and vitamins, but once they have been turned into processed flour, they lose their nutritional value. When 88 percent of Americans are metabolically unstable, one in every two people has diabetes/prediabetes, and one in every four teenagers is prediabetic/diabetic, I recommend limiting/eliminating processed grains, specifically gluten, to lower inflammation, stabilize blood sugar levels, and optimize/expedite healing.

Gluten and Your Kid

We have all heard of gluten. But why are adults and children trying to avoid it if they don't have celiac disease? Gluten is a protein found in grains such as wheat, barley, rye, kamut, and spelt. Unfortunately, the wheat today is much different from the wheat of our ancestors and can trigger troubling symptoms in children and adults.[115] The average human body reacts to today's gluten, prompting an immune response and leading to inflammation and other health issues.

In the last fifty years, modern wheat has been hybridized and manipulated to contain a "super starch" called amylopectin A, which raises our blood sugar, leading to insulin resistance;[116] wheat is also sprayed with massive amounts of chemical fertilizer and pesticides.[117] This high-yielding dwarf wheat has a much higher amount of gluten, more phytic acid, and amylopectin, but it has fewer nutrients. This new gluten protein molecule is large, and we lack the specific enzymes to fully break it down. When the partially digested molecules come into contact with the small intestine, they spark the immune system and create inflammation. Zonulin controls the tight junction in the gut wall. Gluten can cause the gut cells to release zonulin (the protein that can loosen tight junctions in the intestinal lining), creating a permeable barrier and leading to leaky gut syndrome or increased intestinal permeability. Gluten can not only lead to leaky gut syndrome and food sensitivities but also cause large spikes in blood sugar, contributing to blood sugar dysregulation, insulin resistance, obesity, and further inflammation. Gluten binds to opioid receptors in the gut, the same receptors to which morphine and heroin bind, making our kids' bodies crave it; there is even a withdrawal effect when one stops eating it.

Studies have shown that young children who eat gluten have a 46 percent increased risk for developing type 1 diabetes for each ten grams of gluten consumed;[118] eating gluten also has been found to increase the risk of other autoimmune conditions like celiac for those predisposed children.[119]

Examples of foods with gluten are barley, rye, wheat, durum, graham, kamut, semolina, spelt, oats, and soy sauce, and it can be hiding in other products like ketchup. Avoid foods that are packaged, processed, and canned with "natural flavors." Gluten can be hiding in anything, including body products, so if you are sensitive, make sure it is marked "gluten free."

Other Grains

Whole grains can provide minerals, nutrients, fiber, and vitamins, but not as much as compared to other categories discussed earlier; they are not needed to sustain a healthy existence free of disease. The truth is that grains are anti-nutrients (as they contain phytates). They prevent the body from absorbing their nutrients and minerals (like calcium, magnesium, iron, zinc, and potassium); decrease the digestion of fats, protein, and starches; lead to nutrient deficiencies; promote leaky gut; and feed unfriendly bacteria. Grains also damage the intestinal cells, as they contain amylopectin, which causes blood sugar spikes that lead to insulin resistance; this increases belly fat and inflammation,[120] interferes with cell function, and makes it hard to digest. Corn is also one of the most commonly genetically engineered foods, with about 90 percent of corn being genetically modified.[121] Brown rice contains the hull of the grain, which has more phytonutrients than white rice; white rice is typically fortified with other vitamins because the hull has been stripped away, which actually is associated with increased risk for type 2 diabetes. If you are going to have rice, make sure to eat traditional colored varieties of rice, as they have more antioxidants and antiallergic protection.[122] Rice also contains arsenic, which may cause cancer.[123] Oatmeal has been shown to spike blood sugar; elevate insulin levels; increase sugar, adrenaline, and cortisol levels;[124] and make you hungrier.

If your child is dealing with a chronic health condition, prediabetes, seizures, neuropsychiatric symptoms, or mood or behavior issues, he may see dramatic results when he removes all grains from his diet. Once your child is able to tolerate them, less processed, sprouted grains can be added back to his diet. Examples of grains that can be added back into the diet include organic sprouted grain flours like buckwheat, sorghum, quinoa, millet, amaranth, corn, oats, red or black rice, and even sourdough. Personally, I have noticed that if I feed my kids grains regularly, they don't eat their veggies. If I want to fill their bellies up with the most nutrient-dense foods that heal, I make sure they have veggies, protein, healthy fats, and fruit, and usually by that time they are almost full, so they don't need any more food. In my house, grains are consumed as a treat.

Dairy

Dairy products are packed with magnesium, calcium, vitamin A, vitamin B6, vitamin B12, added vitamin D, zinc, and selenium, and A2 milk boosts glutathione and so much more. Milk from cows that graze outside is packed with healthy fats, including CLAs.[125] But, unfortunately, about 70 percent of the world's population has milk-related digestive issues.[126] Studies show that increased premature dairy intake can lead to weakened immunity, allergies, and respiratory infections.

Why? For too long, we have been drinking the processed, more toxic form of dairy that comes from these genetically improved cows. Their milk has a high level of A1 casein, which tends to be digested in our bodies into opiate fragments called BCM7 that can trigger significant inflammation in vulnerable individuals and is associated with an increased risk of developing diseases. Dairy (in any form) triggers an inflammatory response capable of attacking the body's own tissues. Normally, milk should separate easily for easy digestion, but now it's been modified (by pasteurization and homogenization) to kill the bad bacteria. Pasteurization destroys[127] healthy probiotics, vitamins, minerals, enzymes, and nutritious proteins; makes lactose difficult to digest; creates free radicals; and alters the casein protein, creating a molecule that resembles gluten. After the age of five, the body stops producing the enzymes that break down the macromolecules in milk (lactose and milk proteins). Commercial milk is also fortified with vitamin D, but studies have shown that it may actually inhibit activation of vitamin D receptors and limit potential health benefits. Industrial cows are separated from their calves and given ongoing doses of hormones like Monsanto's rBGH (recombinant bovine growth hormone) to maintain milk production; this hormone may alter puberty in children.[128] Other causes of altered puberty include increased processed foods (specifically soy), obesity, and even endocrine disruptors in our environment.[129]

Commercial cow's milk contains cancer-causing growth factors, insulin-like growth factors (IGF-1),[130] reproductive hormones, antibiotics, and milk allergens.[131] In children, cow's milk is a common food sensitivity/allergy[132] and can be associated with recurrent ear infections, congestion, and sinus problems during childhood.[133] Cow's milk produces an opioid that can create a shortage of antioxidants in the brain; additionally, cow's milk has been linked to schizophrenia,[134] ADHD, and autism,[135] and it can also trigger autoimmunity and diabetes.[136] Children with eczema, asthma, and epilepsy are more sensitive to dairy,[137] which can lead to leaky gut syndrome and cause an inflammatory response, and dairy creates more problems for those with IBS. A high intake of cow's milk (thereby protein intake early in life) can increase the risk of being overweight and obese later in life, limit diversity in the diet, and result in iron deficiency.[138] Don't even get me started on how cows are treated on these factory farms. Can you imagine the impact of stress on their milk production?

Once your child improves gut function, you can gradually start adding raw A2 dairy back in, and see how your child responds. Start with raw, organic, pastured goat and sheep milk. One can also make goat's milk kefir to boost healthy fats and improve gut flora. Raw milk is different and can actually transform a child's epigenetics,[139] which can increase microbial diversity; reduce allergies; lower the risk of cancer, inflammatory bowel disease, obesity, and diabetes; and optimize the brain, gut health, and the immune system.[140] Low-heat boiling preserves the milk benefits better than high-heat boiling. If your child has been drinking commercial milk all his life and is sensitive to it, he might still have symptoms with raw milk and cultured dairy products.

Alternatives to cow's milk include coconut milk kefir, with its wonderful antifungal and antiviral properties to help heal leaky gut, and almond milk (the milk should have no additives; it should be simple ingredients like almonds and water). Most people can tolerate butter and ghee from grass-fed cows. Remember, milk can actually weaken the bones, and there are far better calcium sources that are necessary for optimal bone health. For good general health, focus on these foods: flaxseeds, spinach, sardines, walnuts, Brazil nuts, greens (e.g., mustard and collard), sesame seeds, wild salmon, broccoli, and kale.

Foods That are Destroying Our Future and Our Health

Genetically Modified Organisms (GMOs)

Genetically modified organisms (GMOs) are created through biotechnology, also called genetic engineering. GMOs are organisms (for example, plants, animals, viruses, or bacteria) in which the DNA has been artificially manipulated in a lab to produce foreign compounds that cannot occur in nature. GMOs were engineered to withstand exposure to herbicide and/or to produce an insecticide, but now new technologies are being developed to create new organisms via synthetic biology and to artificially develop other plant traits. In addition to engineering crops to withstand Roundup, scientists engineered crops like cotton and corn plants to produce their own toxic insecticide/ pesticide called Bt toxin; this toxin breaks up tiny holes in the gut walls of the insects, which destroys their digestive lining and kills them. Foods are altered to become herbicide-tolerant crops, which means that farmers can spray the plant directly with more weed killers without actually killing the plant. Unfortunately, 80 percent of all products on the supermarket shelves contain GMO ingredients, such as soy, canola, corn, and sugar beets, and more than 750 different products sold in the United States contain high levels of glyphosate, an active pesticide in the weed killer Roundup (made by Monsanto), which is the most heavily used weedkiller in global agriculture and second-most popular pesticide for home use.

Since glyphosate's introduction in 1996, its use has increased fivefold. These plants become less nutritious and more vulnerable to pests. Glyphosate accumulates in the growth points and accumulates in our tissues.[141] Glyphosate works by the shikimate pathway in plants and our gut microbes. This chemical is very active in disrupting beneficial bacteria, leading to leaky gut and imbalanced gut bacteria; it doesn't kill the bad bacteria, which instead multiply and cause damage to the intestinal wall. As a chelator, glyphosate can take out metals and minerals from the body, specifically amino acids like tryptophan and tyrosine that the gut bugs need to make dopamine and serotonin. Glyphosate may negatively affect vitamin D3 activation in the liver, potentially explaining the epidemic levels of vitamin D deficiency. Glyphosate exposure has been linked to increased cancers,[142] allergies, various digestive issues, and an altered immune system. Even at very low exposure, glyphosate kills umbilical, placental, and embryonic cells,[143] and it is associated with genetic damage.[144] The herbicide acts as an endocrine disruptor that can affect children's future reproductive health.[145] Glyphosate has been implicated in the development of autism and neurobehavioral problems in children, as well as other diseases like Parkinson's and Alzheimer's, and it impairs detoxification.[146] Glyphosate may help kill some weeds, but the crops have fewer earthworms and nutrients,[147] which ultimately affects the soil and planet.

The Food and Drug Administration (FDA) didn't use data to approve genetically modified (GM) food as safe, and they didn't use independent safety tests on these foods. The only safety testing done is by the very companies that stand to profit from selling their own GM seeds as well as the accompanying chemicals. Sixty percent of vegetables seeds worldwide are controlled by four large companies. In the United States, GMO foods include soy, corn, sugar, alfalfa, cotton seed oil and fabric, papaya, canola, zucchini, and yellow squash. In some areas, apples, potatoes, and salmon are also being genetically engineered. Wheat, rice, and flax are not GMO but have genetically modified cousins that can cross-pollinate with them. Unfortunately, the FDA hasn't conducted safety studies on GMOs. No studies so far have shown that genetically modified food can actually increase crop yield or even feed the world.

Artificial/Processed/Fake Food

When you give your child junk food, you are going to get junk kids back, as junk food can harm your child's brain and body. This is all the white stuff, like white flour, bread, cakes, cookies, and other baked goods. They contain lots of ingredients and have a very high glycemic index. They are full of partially hydrogenated oil (canola, soybean, corn, and other vegetable oils), food additives, artificial preservatives, artificial colors, and artificial flavors. A study in *Clinical Pediatrics* showed that in products that were marketed for kids (43 percent of all food), 96.3 percent of all candies and 94 percent of all fruit flavored snacks contained artificial dyes.[148] These foods are packed with additives, inflammatory oils, artificial sweeteners, GMOs, and sugar!

Junk food damages the gut flora, which leads to intestinal inflammation, leaky gut, and chronic illnesses. These artificial ingredients we feed our children can actually contribute to allergies, motor skill issues, hyperactivity, and even cancer.[149] Junk food consumption shapes adolescents' brains in many ways. It impairs their ability to think, learn, and remember, and they score lower on memory tests; junk food even interferes with an adolescent's ability to control impulsive behaviors, which increases the risk of teenage depression and anxiety.[150] In 2013, researchers recruited more than two thousand children between the ages of eleven and fourteen living in London; each answered questions about what they ate and how they felt. The study determined that adolescents who ate the most junk food were nearly 50 percent more likely to show signs of depression.[151]

Let's examine some of these artificial, processed, and fake foods:

Additives: These cause uncontrollable hunger and binge eating; they extend the shelf life of foods.

Artificial sweeteners: Sweeteners like aspartame and sucralose are synthetic chemicals that cause hunger (leading to leptin resistance, which prevents you from knowing when you're full),[152] gas, and bloating. They act as an excitotoxin, which damages neurons in the brain,[153] leading to neurological effects like headaches and migraines; alter frontal lobe activity;[154] lower the amount of serotonin, which increases anxiety and causes sleep issues;[155] contribute to cardiovascular disease and type 2 diabetes; can cause allergic reactions; alter the gut microbiome,[156] leading to insulin resistance, inflammation,[157] and cancer;[158] decrease nutrient absorption; and contribute to weight gain, worsening the obesity epidemic.[159] Sucralose especially has a detrimental effect on gut bacteria.[160]

Artificial colorings: These are associated with everything from cancer to hyperactivity in children.[161]

> Blue #1: The worst artificial color, it is linked to hyperactivity and the risk of kidney tumors; some research suggests it is a potential neurotoxin.[162]
>
> Red #3: This dye is an animal carcinogen.
>
> Red #1: This dye leads to liver cancer.
>
> Red #40: This dye is linked to hyperactivity in children and accelerating the appearance of tumors.[163]
>
> Yellow #5 and Yellow #6: These dyes are linked to hyperactivity in children and are found to be contaminated by carcinogens like benzidine. Yellow dyes are xenoestrogens that disrupt children's hormones.[164]
>
> Caramel-colored or brown food coloring: This dye is linked to cancer.[165]
>
> Green #1: This dye can lead to liver cancer.
>
> Orange #1 and #2: These dyes can lead to organ damage.

Aluminum additives: These are linked to neurotoxicity.

Azodicarbonamide: This is a dough conditioner. The World Health Organization (WHO) has linked this substance to respiratory issues, asthma, and allergies. When baked, it produces a breakdown product called semicarbazide (a carcinogen) and urethane (a suspected carcinogen).[166]

Butylated hydroxytoluene (BHT): Used as a preservative, it affects the signaling from our gut to our brain that tells us to stop eating;[167] it also caused cancer in animal tests. California lists butylated hydroxyanisole (BHA) as a carcinogen.[168] Anything sound familiar? Yup, butane is a toxic gas!

Calcium propionate: Found in all commercial bread, it produces a neurotoxin and affects the microbiome; it is linked to autism, ADHD,[169] and sleep disturbances in children.

Calcium and sodium caseinate: This is a toxic dairy extract.

Carrageenan: This causes leaky gut and inflammation, and it is a possible human carcinogen.[170]

Citric acid: A preservative and flavor, this additive used in packaged foods is typically derived from mold made with GMO corn—not from fruit.

Dextrose: A heavily processed form of sugar, it is usually made from GMO corn that produces its own insecticide.

High-fructose corn syrup: It has been shown to be associated with insulin resistance, hypertension, and impaired glucose tolerance. A diet full of processed sugar leads to inflammation and is responsible for the obesity, diabetes, heart disease, and dementia epidemics, leading to premature death.

Microwave popcorn: It contains PFOA, a synthetic chemical linked to cancer and hormone disruption, and diacetyl (the butter-flavoring chemical) is linked to lung damage.

Monosodium glutamate (MSG): This neurotoxin kills brain cells, causes headaches and allergies, and damages the gut. It increases food cravings and irresistibility to the food. Other names of MSG are yeast extract, glutamate, caseinate, natural flavor, autolyzed protein, hydrolysed yeast, disodium 5-inosinate, and disodium 5-guanylate.

Natural flavors: These come from a proprietary mixture of chemicals derived from anything in nature. Many flavors may have up to 100 ingredients, including synthetic chemicals, propylene glycol (used as a solvent), and the preservative BHA, as well as GMO-derived ingredients and MSG.

Nitrates and nitrites: Found in processed meats, these are "probable" carcinogens according to the WHO.[171]

Sodium phosphate: This preservative is linked to increased risk of heart disease, accelerated aging, kidney disease, and mortality.

Polysorbate-80 or lecithin: Commonly found in vitamins, chewing gum, and ice cream, these are linked to autoimmunity.

Potassium bromate: Linked to various cancers, it has been banned in the United Kingdom, Canada, and the European Union.

Propyl gallate: Used in food with animal fats, it is believed to be an endocrine disruptor, and it may be carcinogenic.

Propylparaben (E216) or methylparaben: This synthetic preservative is linked to breast cancer and reproductive problems.

Sodium benzoate (E211) or potassium benzoate (E212): These synthetic preservatives, when combined with vitamin C, produce benzene, a known carcinogen.

Soy protein isolate: Highly processed soy (most of which is made with GMO soy) causes hormone disruption and inhibits absorption of calcium and other vital minerals in the diet. Processed soy products can stimulate the immune system to produce antibodies and contribute to food sensitivities and inflammation.[172]

Sulfides: These cause allergies and inflammation.

Tert-Butylhydroquinone (TBHQ): This synthetic preservative is linked to behavior problems, stomach cancer, liver enlargement, and vision issues; it negatively affects T cells, promoting allergies.

Theobromine: In animal testing, it had a possible effect on reproduction and development.

Titanium dioxide: This food color used to brighten foods leads to inflammation.

Vegetable oils: Partially hydrogenated oils like corn, soybean, canola, safflower, sunflower, and trans-fats are found in shortening, margarine, and spreads or anything that is hydrogenated. They are commonly found in refined baked goods. These oils also contain pro-inflammatory omega-6 fats and result in gut dysfunction/leaky gut; they lead to immune dysfunction, interfere with normal cell metabolism, and are hazardous to health. They increase our chances of heart disease, promote obesity, and are linked to insulin resistance, prediabetes, type 2 diabetes,[173] and cancer.[174]

Sugar

Sugar is a legal drug. Refined sugar has now infiltrated our children's lives, as it is found in 74 percent of packaged foods. The National Health and Nutrition Examination Survey for 2011–2016 reported that 84.4 percent of infants and toddlers consumed added sugars every day. In the United States, toddlers between the ages of nineteen and twenty-three months consumed an average of more than 7 teaspoons of sugar each day, and older kids had about 19 teaspoons per day![175] That is three times more than the updated recommendations.

Sugar negatively affects a child's body. Bad "bugs" thrive on sugar, leading to overgrowth of pathogenic bacteria and yeast species, which then result in more sugar cravings. Sugar also drastically weakens your child's immune system. The oxidative stress and imbalance in the microbiome leads to inflammation, as it interferes with the ability of the white blood cells to destroy toxins and fight infection, making your child sick. All this occurs within minutes after eating sugar, and it can last for several hours! Refined sugar disrupts your child's blood sugar balance, increases insulin levels, causes higher cortisol levels, reduces HDL ("good" cholesterol), raises LDL ("bad" cholesterol), and causes high triglyceride levels. This leads to belly fat accumulation, cancer, diabetes, tooth decay, and fatty liver.[176]

Sugar negatively affects our brains and our behaviors. Studies have shown that there are alterations in the stratium, amygdala, cingulate cortex, prefrontal cortex, thalamus, and nucleus accumbens after sugar intake; after twelve days of sugar intake, there were major changes in the brain's dopamine and opioid systems.[177] Sugar weakens the prefrontal cortex and stimulates the brain reward centers, the same parts of the brain that are stimulated by addictive drugs (like heroin or cocaine) and withdrawals. Sugar intake triggers changes in the area of the brain called the hippocampus (memory and stress), which leads to cognitive declines and problems in memory and learning. When our children are inflamed, they are more impulsive and crave the wrong foods, which leads to fatigue, brain fog, anxiety, mood swings, ADHD, behavior issues, anxiety, and sleep issues.[178] Sugar increases food intake and appetite.[179]

Avoid sugar and all its other code names: bran sugar, dextrose, glucose, dextran, fructose, agave, barley malt, brown rice syrup, high-fructose corn syrup (HFCS), hydrogenated starch, maltodextrin, maltose, lactose, disaccharides, monosaccharides, sorghum, sucrose, and xylose. Avoid sugar-sweetened beverages, like soda, sports drinks, and iced tea; these have led to kidney failure, high blood pressure, diabetes, fatty liver, heart disease, and so much more. Avoid fruit juices as well, as they contain a lot of sugar.

Get the picture? Isn't this crazy? This is what we are giving kids for treats, for snacks, and for breakfast, lunch, and dinner . . . and then we wonder why they are getting sick! So we need to avoid anything on the label that says "artificial," "flavors," "spices," or even "natural" (it may be extracted from chemicals that aren't listed). These food companies are no longer food companies; they are actually chemical companies!

Time-Restricted Eating

Sugar, processed foods . . . we are currently living in a time where our hunger is manufactured, making us eat all the time. Modern science has now found so many physical benefits for fasting, though there have not been enough studies in children.

One study showed that when one group of mice was allowed to eat freely all the time, the mice became more obese and unhealthy. Another group ate the same number of daily calories as the first group but restricted it within an eight-hour window; these mice had less than 12 percent body fat compared to the other group, which had 40 percent body fat.[180]

We know in adults fasting activates the Nrf2 gene pathway that improves detoxification and stem cell activation, which triggers new cell formation and increases mitochondrial function and autophagy; autophagy is the body's natural cleaning process, which removes damaged proteins and clears damaged cellular parts that may lead to cancer, eliminates pathogens, and helps in cellular repair and regeneration. Fasting increases antioxidant function; increases production of beta-HBA, a super-fuel for the brain and body; stimulates the production of BDNF, the brain's growth hormone, which can support function of brain cells; accelerates weight loss; increases fat burning; lowers blood insulin and sugar levels; possibly leads to the reversal of type 2 diabetes; possibly improves mental clarity and concentration; increases energy; possibly increases growth hormone; improves the blood cholesterol profile; possibly increases the lifespan; and so much more. Intermittent fasting has been found to inhibit the development and progression of the most common type of childhood leukemia.[181]

Though more studies are warranted, what we know for sure is that humans are not meant to eat all day long, every hour of the day, so there should be periods of fasting—for example, when a child sleeps through the night. During a wake state, move toward giving the child breakfast and dinner around the same time and limit late-night eating to balance insulin levels. Once the child has removed the majority of "junk food" from the diet and has been taught to be mindful of his body, he will be able listen to his body and eat when his body needs food.

Now What Do I Feed My Kids?

Take a deep breath, and take it one day at a time. One meal at a time. When my kids get hungry, I have them focus on foods they can have by going down the list: What is my veggie, my clean protein source, my healthy fat, my fruit? And don't forget water, because dehydration can lead to cravings. Let me share what I do in my home:

1. Model good behaviors. You gotta do what you want your kids to do, as they follow what you do, not what you say. If it's not good for you, it's not good for them, either.

2. Educate and empower your child from the inside out. My kids know exactly what happens when the food enters their bodies—good and bad. Have them read food labels, so they have the knowledge; then they are more apt to make better decisions. In our house, we call fake food what it is: chemicals. Empower your children to go down the list and eat the rainbow to keep meal times fun, easy, and colorful!

3. Stock up for success. In my house, my pantry and fridge are stocked with healthy foods. There is nothing there that they can't eat. This takes away the constant negativity around food and empowers the child.

4. Be prepared for after school, lunch, and post-activity snacks. Planning ahead saves me so much undue stress. I always make extra dinner, and that is what the kids will have the day after. I will pack fruit, veggies, olives, cassava flour chips, almond flour crackers, nuts, seeds, hummus, guacamole, or salmon/sardine salad (canned salmon with avocado mayo) to take with me when we are out and about. I will also bake or buy almond or cassava flour cakes or cookies so they can have a treat.

5. Get the whole family involved. In our house, we have three generations who are prioritizing their food and health. Getting the kids involved with cooking, grocery shopping, and gardening helps them learn healthy habits from the beginning, and they are more apt to eat the foods they picked, grew, and cooked together. It also helps them develop social intelligence and self-esteem. Cooking food together lowers the risk of obesity and eating disorders for children and teens.

6. Eat meals together. Family meals lower stress, improve mental health, and support a child's development. Studies show that eating meals together can lower teen substance abuse, improve grades, and increase self-esteem.

7. Teach your child to say, "No, thank you." My kids know it's okay to say no to food when they know this food is not really food . . . it's chemicals . . . so they say no to chemicals.

8. Provide healthier options for parties and outings. In my house, I take food to most parties I go to—just because I really love to cook. No host has ever said no to lentil pasta and almond flour brownies sweetened with honey. I will make enough for the whole party; they taste delicious, and the dish becomes a conversation piece! I pick my friends and my parties wisely, so most have the same morals I do. Remember, just do the best you can.

9. Call and research restaurants ahead of time. In my house, we eat 100 percent non-GMO and 99 percent organic to the best of our ability. I *love* eating out, but I limit it for treats. We look for and support

restaurants that will provide non-GMO organic options, so I will call up and ask them.

10. Don't stress yourself out! Do the best you can! Take it one meal and one day at a time.

This is what our family meals look like (check out my Instagram @holistic mommd). Remember, I keep it super simple and nutritious:

Breakfast: veggies, clean protein, healthy fat, and some fruit. Examples include foods made with coconut, nut, cassava, and seed flours like pancakes, waffles, muffins, banana bread, eggs, quiche, no-nitrate sausages (chicken, beef, and turkey) or kabobs, no-grain cereal in almond milk with fresh or frozen berries, smoothies, greens, fruit or nut or seed butter, fresh fruit, chia pudding, fermented vegetables and fresh veggie juice.

Snacks: veggies, clean protein, and healthy fat and fruit. Examples include sugar snap peas and guacamole, nuts with blueberries, and veggie and protein rollups. I lay out a plate of rainbow fruit and veggies that the kids can snack on.

Lunch and dinner: veggies, clean protein and healthy fat. Examples include soups, egg/chicken/tuna salad, veggie and protein rollups, zucchini pasta with meat sauce, chili, lettuce wraps, stir fry, no-grain tortilla/naan, cauliflower rice, cassava flour tacos, burritos, chicken wings, curries, lentils, almond flour lasagna, lentil pasta, steamed veggies, blackened fish with sweet potato fries, and squash. The ideas are endless!

Eating real food can improve a child's brain, body, and behavior, but it also can address social justice issues, poverty, violence, and educational gaps in learning; it even can improve national security. Real food can help with restoring the soil, restoring our plant and animal species, and even fight against climate change. When we educate, empower, and nourish, our children start to become mindful of the foods they choose and how the foods make them feel, and they are able to use food as medicine to help them thrive. When we empower a generation of children who can listen to their own bodies, we can positively change the current status of humanity. It's so exciting!

DETOXING OUR CHILDREN'S BODIES WITH A PURE ENVIRONMENT

Our children are being exposed to and are more vulnerable to more and more chemicals, radiation, plastics, pesticides, and pharmaceutical drugs than ever before.[182] Children's bodies are closer to the ground and continuously developing, and because the blood-to-brain barrier is not fully developed, the developing brain is particularly vulnerable to environmental toxins.[183]

Our bodies are naturally designed to process and get rid of toxins or other compounds that could be damaging to the body. The more toxins our children are exposed to, the harder their cells have to work to get rid of them. The United States imports about 45 million pounds of synthetic chemicals daily, and about one thousand new chemicals are put into use every year; shockingly, only five chemicals have ever been banned in the United States. Most of the chemicals our children are exposed to daily actually lack safety testing before they end up in our food! Over the next twenty-five years, global chemical production is expected to double to more than a trillion pounds per year! Approximately ninety thousand compounds are approved for commercial use right now, but only a handful have been tested for toxicity! In 2004, the Environmental Working Group (EWG) analyzed the umbilical cord blood of ten random newborns. They found an average of two hundred industrial chemicals present in each newborn, along with persistent pesticide-breakdown products that had been banned thirty years prior to the study.[184] This is crazy! So why is this a problem?

The liver is important for detoxing the body; it takes all the stuff that doesn't belong—like toxins, old blood cells, and spent hormones—and ships them off to the kidney, large intestine, skin, and/or lungs to remove from the body. When these little bodies are constantly exposed to toxins, it forces the liver to work extra hard to get rid of them. If there is an overload all the time, then the toxins start to accumulate, which disrupts the ability to detoxify and forces the liver to hold on to the toxic chemicals it should have removed. Children have immature detoxification systems with reduced liver enzyme activity, which decreases their ability to break down chemicals, which leads to further accumulation. Toxins can actually affect three generations simultaneously and can affect the proteins that control gene expression as well as other mechanisms involved in controlling gene function. When toxins accumulate in the body, they can damage the mitochondria,[185] affect our epigenetics, and inflame the gut, which worsens inflammation and leads to autoimmunity and chronic conditions like autism, ADHD, allergies, and asthma. Toxins also make the body numb to insulin and leptin, which increases insulin resistance and leads to difficulty with losing weight, diabetes, metabolic syndrome, and even cancer.

New research shows that maternal exposure to a common and ubiquitous form of industrial pollution can harm the immune system of offspring and that this injury is passed along to subsequent generations, weakening the body's defenses against infections such as the influenza virus.[186] The effects of such an exposure during prenatal and/or childhood development are permanent. Many toxins can directly influence the prefrontal cortex.[187]

In order to deal with the toxic/impure overload our children are exposed to, we must try our hardest to avoid toxic exposures and support their bodies' natural ability to detoxify, thereby building resilience.

Oh Toxins, Oh Toxins, Where Are You, Toxins? Come Out, Come Out Wherever You Are

Toxins are located all around us, and some are out of our control. So we need to focus on what we can control: our home.[188] If you live in a typical house, your child's mattress and pajamas likely have chemicals, including flame retardants. Bedding has chemicals left from detergents and softeners; the floors' backing may have carcinogens like 4-phenylcyclohexene (4-PCH) or perchloroethylene (PERC); and the household furniture may be off-gassing chemicals like benzene into the air our children breathe. Our children's food and water are full of toxins. Their body products can be filled with chemicals like parabens or phthalates, which are endocrine disruptors. That is a lot of chemical exposure!

Hormone-Disrupting Chemicals

Xenoestrogens are readily absorbed and mimic the effects of our hormones, such as estrogen. They can send mixed messages to the endocrine system, disrupting the hormones' natural actions. Xenoestrogens build up in fatty tissues and lead to increased inflammation. They can be linked to early puberty, difficult and early periods, male infertility, low sex drive, obesity, and even cancer. Many toxins, like PCBs, BPA, mercury, and lead, disrupt dopamine or dopaminergic neurons in the prefrontal cortex.[189]

Xenoestrogens like phthalates can be found in toys, plastics, shower curtains, and nail polish. They can disrupt fetal development and impair fertility, and they are implicated in cancers, endocrine disruption, weight gain, asthma in children, birth defects, ADHD, diabetes, and obesity. Recent studies have shown that early exposure can adversely influence neurodevelopment by disrupting thyroid hormone homeostasis, altering brain lipid metabolism, lowering gonadal hormone concentrations, and lowering IQ; exposure also can be linked to problems with attention, hyperactivity, and poorer social communication,[190] which lead to children's problem behaviors.[191]

Triclosan is an antimicrobial agent often added to antibacterial soaps, toothpastes, body washes, deodorants, and hairsprays; it also can be found in kitchenware, toys, furniture, and clothing. The Environmental Protection Agency (EPA) has labeled this as a pesticide, and it is no more effective than plain soap. It is implicated in increased levels of allergies in children and the development of antibiotic-resistant superbugs, and it is being studied as a potential cancer-causing agent. Triclosan exposure may decrease circulating thyroxine levels or cause neuron apoptosis, which may adversely affect neuro-development, leading to behavior problems.[192]

Fluoride is an industrial waste by-product added to water supplies to attempt to minimize dental decay and is classified as a drug, administered without a specific dose for all to consume. All fluoride toothpastes have a warning to call Poison Control if swallowed. Any cavity prevention can be accomplished via topical fluoride and optimal nutrition. It is found in supplements, medications, toothpaste, black tea, red tea, and canned food items. It is a neurotoxin[193] that damages more than two hundred enzymes and causes developmental neurotoxicity that persists over generations.[194] Fluoride lowers IQ,[195] increases behavior issues,[196] disrupts the endocrine system, blocks iodine absorption, increases the likelihood of thyroid issues and cancers, increases oxidative stress, and interferes with cell signaling from neurotransmitters, growth factors, and other hormones.

BPA (bisphenol-A) is found in plastics such as containers, store receipts, and baby formula cans. BPA impairs brain development in newborn babies, stimulates autoantibody production, and causes problems in the small intestine and hormonal signaling by disrupting estrogen. It affects the thyroid, leptin levels, and androgen functions in the body, promoting weight gain, insulin resistance, and diabetes. Associations have been made between prenatal BPA exposure and differences in children's brain microstructure, which appeared to mediate the association between this exposure and children's behavior symptoms.[197]

Perfluoroalkyl and polyfluoroalkyl substances (PFAS)—for example, perfluorooctanoic acid (PFOA)—are human-made chemicals, also known as the "forever chemicals" because they remain in the soil and water for long periods of time. They are found in contaminated fish, food packaging to prevent it from sticking or leaking, cosmetics, water supplies, contaminated soil, and cookware; these chemicals are released when nonstick pans that contain Teflon or polytetrafluoroethylene (PTFE) are scratched and/or heated. EWG research estimated that PFAS contaminants may be in the drinking water of *110 million Americans*. In 2016, a Canadian study found PFAS chemicals in more than 90 percent of the nearly two thousand cord blood samples collected from pregnant women.[198] PFAS chemicals disrupt our hormonal and immune systems, decrease energy, decrease mental concentration, and lead to liver damage. They are linked with developmental problems in animals and are known carcinogens.

Dioxins and polychlorinated biphenyls (PCBs): These were banned in the 1970s, but they still persist in the environment and in our bodies. They are found in meat, dairy, fish, and other seafood. PCBs lead to inflammation, autoimmunity, cancer, diabetes, and heart problems.

Polybrominated diphenyl ethers (PBDEs) are found in flame retardants in furniture, upholstery, and mattresses; baked foods; plastics used in computers, appliances, and other electronics; tea and citrus-flavored drinks; and gluten-free products. They are associated with endocrine disruption and systemic and developmental effects in children.[199]

Volatile organic compounds (VOCs) found in perfumes, air fresheners, household cleaners, and shampoos are neurotoxic.

Heavy Metals

Heavy metals are also common toxins in our environment and can be very toxic in low concentrations. Examples of heavy metals include mercury, lead, and arsenic.

Mercury can be found in silver fillings for tooth cavities, cosmetics, pesticides, and certain fish (highest in tuna and swordfish). Sixteen percent of American women of child-bearing age have blood mercury levels high enough to increase the chance of harm to their fetus. Exposure in pregnancy can lead to problems in language development, cognitive function, and general intelligence;[200] dementia; developmental problems like intellectual disability; cerebellar ataxia, limb deformities, altered physical growth, and cerebral palsy; and sensory impairments.[201]

Mercury exposure can lead to altered cell migration, cell proliferation, and cell death, leading to lower scores for attention, hand-eye coordination, and other fine motor responses. In older children, mercury can lead to delay in transmission of auditory brain signals. Mercury can also cause developmental delays, behavior issues, and learning problems. Children, teens, and pregnant women should avoid mercury-containing fish.[202]

Lead can still be present in older homes, paint, older water pipes, and occasionally in certain cosmetics and pottery from China. In 2020, UNICEF and Pure Earth reported that every third child in the world has too much lead in the body, and roughly eight hundred million children are still exposed to lead.[203] Lead is stored in our bones for years. It is a neurotoxin, associated with developmental delays, neurotransmission disruption, synaptic trimming, and synaptogenesis, which leads to impaired IQ for the rapidly developing brains of exposed fetuses, lower cognitive function, attention deficits, poor executive function, learning disabilities, anemia, and possibly heart problems. Lead exposure is a potent predictor of behaviors linked with delinquency and criminality, such as impulsivity, hyperactivity, and aggressive behaviors.[204]

Arsenic is found in drinking water, apples, rice, chicken, cereal bars, rice pasta, and organic nondairy formula; on produce; and in household detergents, colored chalk, rat poison, and automobile exhaust. There is no federal limit on arsenic in rice and its products,[205] and it is associated with anemia, digestive issues, neurotoxicity, and weight loss.

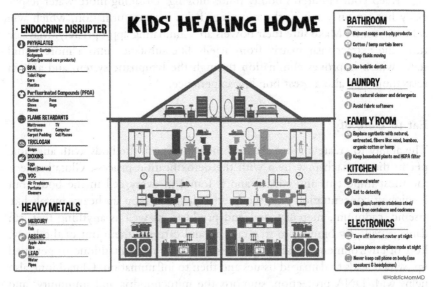

Figure 3.7.

Detoxing Kids Naturally

Move Fluids to Detoxify

The skin is a major elimination organ for toxins. Sweating and cleansing ourselves helps eliminate what is harmful to the body or what the body does not need. Examples include exercising, spending some time in a sauna, and brushing/exfoliating the skin. Taking a bath with Epsom salts, sodium bicarbonate, seaweed, or sea salt (preferably alternating them) may help eliminate toxins and is great for lowering any reactions from detoxing or die-off reactions (will discuss more later). Skin brushing can help eliminate toxins by removing all the dead cells from blocked pores. Use a natural soft bristle brush to scrub the skin from the extremities; also scrub the belly toward the heart. My kids take an Epsom salt bath weekly and try to dry brush before they shower. For older kids, oil-pulling with coconut oil and infrared saunas can also be helpful for pulling out the toxins, as it can boost circulation; it also relieves sore muscles, increases relaxation, and improves sleep. You can also alternate between hot and cold showers, as this also boosts circulation and improves detoxification. All you need to do is stand in the shower for one minute under cold water (as cold as you can tolerate) and then one minute under hot water (as hot as you can tolerate); repeat about five times. This gets the vessels to relax and dilate and helps the skin pump blood.

Keep your children's bodily fluids moving. Drinking more water (especially hot lemon water in the morning) helps increase urination, which will rid toxic waste. Make sure their bowels are eliminating appropriately. Massage turns the extracellular matrix from a jelly-like substance into a more liquid state, which improves elimination through the lymphatic system and aids in relaxation; it is also a great bonding experience.

Eat to Detoxify

The ability to create a more alkaline environment in the body with an acidic pH in the stomach may help with the detoxification process. Glutathione is the most important antioxidant and is found in every cell in the body, but its highest concentration is in the liver. It helps to mop up heavy metals like arsenic, cadmium, mercury, and end products, as well as anything that can damage cells, by binding to free radicals and carrying them out of the body. Lots of environmental toxin exposures can cause the glutathione to get used up, which leads to damaged tissues and then to inflammation. Glutathione also helps with DNA protection, supports the mitochondria and immunity, and protects against heart disease, cancer, dementia, and other chronic illnesses.

Raw fruits, vegetables, herbs, and spices have the most potent detoxifying effects, so get as many servings in as possible. Examples of foods that are packed with fiber and sulfur include asparagus, bok choy, celery, citrus, kale, mushrooms, onions, garlic, green apples, kiefer, kimchi, sauerkraut, olives, plums, and cruciferous vegetables such as broccoli, Brussels sprouts, beets, cauliflower, watercress, cabbage, Swiss chard, and collard greens. Other foods that are great for liver support are salmon, berries, pumpkin seeds, olive oil, lentils, Brazil nuts, wheatgrass, and grapes. These are full of enzymes that support the liver and gallbladder. Some kids have handicapped enzymes; however, genetics aren't their destiny, and eating the right foods can help give the body the raw materials required for making its own glutathione. Help your child's body make its own glutathione by eating plenty of garlic, onions, cilantro, and cruciferous veggies like broccoli, kale, cauliflower, and cabbage.

Top beverages are apple cider vinegar, dandelion tea, milk thistle tea, and chamomile tea, as they all cleanse the liver and gallbladder. Herbs that can help in detoxification include caraway, dill seeds, curcumin (turmeric), rosemary, thyme, cumin, basil, poppy seeds, oregano, black pepper, and cilantro (a natural chelator).

Swap Out Toxic for Clean

Unfortunately, our food, water, air, homes, and body care products are often the source of hidden toxins that our children are interacting with daily. With all the things you can't control, let's focus on what we can control—the home. Start with one thing and switch out toxic for clean. The following sections offer some strategies.

Air

We breathe the air in our homes more that we breathe the outside air, and according to the EWG, the air inside our house is about two to three times more polluted than outside. All the chemicals in the house are still likely off-gassing, and inhaling chemicals may be as dangerous as consuming them. Filtering the air from toxins can optimize detoxification. Turn on an air filter, so you are breathing clean air all day and night, which lowers the body burden of toxins and optimizes detoxification and healing while you sleep. Decorate the home and kids' rooms with house plants, which can help detoxify the air they breathe. Choose plants like spider plants, aloe vera, weeping fig, Chinese evergreen, bamboo, Gerber daisies, English ivies, and chrysanthemums.

   Over time, replace synthetic carpets, rugs, window treatments, furniture cloth, or bedding (as they can gradually release synthetic materials into the air you breathe) with natural, untreated fibers like wool, organic cotton, hemp, or bamboo. Avoid flame retardants. Paint with low or no volatile organic compounds (VOCs) for indoor surfaces, and say no to air fresheners. Don't spray pesticides around or in the home. Avoid plug-ins, sprays, and candle air fresheners. Open windows to help the air circulate. Carbon monoxide detectors and fire alarms are important for your home, and make sure they are checked every six months. Change vinyl shower curtains to PVC-free materials.

Water

The toxins in our water can disrupt the gut microbiome and lead to inflammation. To reduce the amount of toxins or even drugs in the tap water, use purified water, with a reverse osmosis unit that has a triple filtration process. It is important to reduce the amount of toxins/drugs, heavy metals, bacteria/viruses/parasites, nitrates, VOCs, sediment, medications, and copper in tap water, so even consider eventually buying a purification system for the entire house that also includes a fluoride filtration system. Trace minerals are necessary, so these can be added back to the water. Avoid BPA-containing and "BPA-free" plastics, as the alternatives are really no better.

Kitchen

Minimize the use of the microwave, and never put plastic in the microwave. Change the cookware to pots and pans made of glass, ceramic, non-coated stainless steel, or cast iron. If you use ceramic pots, look for ones that are lead free, unglazed, and unvarnished. Eliminate all plastics and replace with glass, stainless steel, bamboo, or ceramic. Store food in ceramic or glass containers; replace plastic kitchen tools with wooden utensils and cutting boards; use a glass teapot and steel or glass water bottles. Avoid cling wrap, use unbleached parchment paper, and look for BPA-free cans. Transfer frozen food to glassware when you heat. If you need to use aluminum foil, lay unbleached parchment paper between the food and the foil to limit contact.

Cleaners

Switch out chemical cleaners, laundry detergents, and such with natural nontoxic or "green" household cleaners. Vinegar, baking soda, and hydrogen peroxide can take care of most of what you need done. Avoid artificial hand sanitizers.

Personal Care Products

What you put on your child's skin is as important as what you eat, as the skin is an excellent delivery system for chemicals. Look for a natural brand of deodorant that doesn't contain aluminum. Choose organic, gluten-free, and nonallergenic soaps, shampoos, skin care, cosmetics, and feminine hygiene products, as well as cosmetics with no preservatives. Check out products on the EWG website (https://www.ewg.org/skindeep/) to see how safe it is for you and your family.

Oral Health

The health of our mouths determines the health of our bodies. Brushing with non-fluoride, all natural, organic toothpaste and flossing are important for oral health. Tongue scraping can help remove leftover toxins, bacteria, and dead cells from the tongue to prevent bad breath.

Studies have shown that the milk a baby drinks all night long in a bottle can lead to cavities. Most procedures done by regular dentists can pose a threat for toxin exposure, so be sure to see a holistic or biological dentist who will make sure the biocompatible materials are safe and right for your child. Say no to amalgam fillings and replace all metal fillings with white resin (though it is plastic, it's better than mercury) or zirconium.

Electronics and EMF Exposure

Electromagnetic fields (EMFs) are gaining new attention. We are literally swimming in a sea of EMFs all day long from cell towers, computers, microwaves, Bluetooth devices, and most important, from cell phones. A study involving seven hundred adolescents showed that electromagnetic fields may have adverse effects on the development of memory performance of specific brain regions exposed during mobile phone use.[206] A study by Yale University researchers showed that exposure to radiation from cell phones during pregnancy affects the brain development of offspring, potentially leading to hyperactivity.[207] Negative health effects of EMF exposure include cellular dysfunction and increased intracellular calcium, which is responsible for generating oxidative stress that causes DNA damage, increases the levels of nitric oxide (NO) (excessive amounts are dangerous), and causes superoxide genetic mutations and disease.[208]

Limiting exposure to EMFs can optimize health and healing. EMFs can be present in electric power lines, cell phone towers, Bluetooth headsets, Wi-Fi routers, Wi-Fi hot spots, computers, laptops, cell phones, radio and television towers, microwaves, and florescent and compact florescent lighting, among others. To reduce exposure, turn off the TV router at night and never carry a cell phone on the body; use a speaker or non–Bluetooth headset at all times; and switch cell phones to airplane mode anytime you can (especially at night). Don't place laptops or phones near your child's lap area. Don't rest cell phones or laptops on a pregnant belly. Children should not sleep with phones or have phones near their heads. Do not use sleep monitors or Wi-Fi-linked stuffed animals, tablets, or iPads. Keep the Wi-Fi routers away from your children, and purchase EMF protection devices.

Detoxing from technology can also be important, as we are just beginning to understand how these devices affect us. Have your teens turn off notifications and unfollow people who don't benefit them. It is important to model this behavior.

Outdoors

To reduce exposure to pesticides, make sure to eat as much organic produce as possible, wash fruits and veggies under running water to reduce traces of pesticides that remain on the surface, never use bug bombs or broad-spraying pesticides, and focus on chemical-free pest control products, like boric acid.

Use organic lawn fertilizer companies. Have children stay off of the lawn if it has been sprayed with a chemical fertilizer until it has been exposed to at least a quarter-inch of rain or a good watering. Wait at least twenty-four hours before you allow kids to play on that chemically fertilized lawn. Use food scraps as compost (e.g., egg shells).

Limit noise pollution when possible, and if you are in an area with a lot of noise pollution, white noise machines, air plugs, and noise-canceling headphones can be used. The WHO reports that children who live in areas of high aircraft noise have higher stress levels, poor attention, and even delayed reading ages.

Detoxify the Whole Child

Detoxifying isn't a separate entity but a combination of the whole. Optimize digestive health, eat anti-inflammatory nutritious food, and reduce stress with relaxation. Improve sleep, our social lives, and our soul by practicing forgiveness and meditation. These actions are all key in optimizing your child's overall health and well-being.

Again, knowledge is power. The knowledge about what is lurking in your children's environment allows you to take control and get back in the driver's seat of your family's health and decisions. Slowly start to make these changes with your children, reading labels of the foods and products they use. Incorporate these detox methods into their daily routine, and tell them why they are doing it. Don't spend time worrying about what you can't control; take it one step at a time, one day at a time, and one product at a time. By limiting these toxic exposures and educating and empowering your child, you build a mindful child who is in tune with nature and makes environmentally safe choices, which lowers the overall toxic burden and improves the brain, body, and behavior.

FOUNDATIONS OF HOLISTIC PARENTING: DIGESTIVE HEALTH AND DETOXIFICATION

1. Digestive Health
    a. Focus on real rainbow food.
    b. Incorporate veggies, clean protein, and healthy fat.
    c. Hydrate.
    d. Add bone broth, prebiotics, and probiotics.
    e. Eliminate fake food.
2. Detoxification
    a. Locate the toxins.
    b. Keep fluids moving.
    c. Eat to detoxify.
    d. Swap out toxic for clean.

• 4 •

The Four S's

KIDS BUSTING STRESS

Overworked parents, overscheduling, unrealistic expectations, lack of real human connection, war, school shootings, pandemic fears, politics, social media, and the list goes on. Our children are growing up in a world filled with negativity, lack of control, fear, hopelessness, and stress. A recent study of one million children reported that those who suffered from social (financial poverty or long-term unemployment in the family) or stressful adversity (death of a parent, divorce, alcohol/drug abuse among the parents) in childhood had an increased risk of premature death in early adulthood (sixteen to thirty-six years of age).[1] Stress has a toll on the child (and subsequently adult) brain, body, and behavior, which influences a child's entire life.

Stress activates the panic systems in a child's brain, leading to an overactive stress response system and leaving impacts on his spiritual, physical, and emotional well-being.

What Is Stress?

The stress response, also known as the "fight or flight" mechanism, occurs when the body feels threatened. When the amygdala senses a threat, the hippocampus links the fear response to the context in which the threatening stimulus or event occurred; it then sends signals to the hypothalamus and pituitary gland, activating the stress pathways and impairing the prefrontal cortex. To deal with the stressor and protect the body, it releases cortisol, which then triggers a cascade of events in the body, including releasing adrenaline and noradrenaline. Cortisol continues to be secreted until the stressor resolves, the adrenal glands tire out (a state normally referred to as adrenal fatigue), or you learn to manage stress effectively.

This response can be lifesaving in emergency situations, where you need to act immediately, but with constant bombardment and little down time, it starts to wear the body down. During this state of imbalance, it leads to suppression of the immune system, inflammation, and chronic illnesses, and it can affect every organ, including the brain, as it sabotages the relationship between the prefrontal cortex and the amygdala.[2] This promotes new neuronal growth in the amygdala, which leads to bad decision making and impulsivity.

Signs of stress are different in each child, depending on the age of the child/teen. Preschoolers may have nightmares, lose weight and/or appetite, fear being separated, or scream or cry a lot. Elementary school children become anxious or fearful and have difficulty sleeping and concentrating. Teens feel depressed, begin abusing drugs/alcohol, take sexual risks, develop eating disorders, or engage in self-harming behaviors. Children who have experienced trauma may struggle with getting help.

Effects of Stress on a Child

Let's briefly discuss how stress can influence your child's body, brain, and behavior. Research has shown that stressful events can trigger emotional and even physical reactions that can make your child more prone to a number of different health conditions, including heart attack, obesity, diabetes, cancer, and stroke.[3]

Stress and the Child's Brain

Cortisol is linked to the development of the baby's amygdala,[4] so prenatal maternal stress can affect the critical regulatory circuitry,[5] influencing the development of the child's behavior and social and emotional development.[6] An infant's brain is literally shaped by the mother's experiences.[7]

As a child grows, chronic stress acts like fuel for the amygdala, promoting new neuronal growth[8] and making the child more vulnerable to developing bad habits and addictions. Elevated levels of cortisol have been shown to inhibit the neurogenesis in the hippocampus, diminishing its functional capacity, leading to the inability to create, store, or retrieve memories. When this happens, the child has difficulty contextualizing new information and assessing new situations. The experience of more stressful and traumatic life events predicted weakened amygdala–anterior cingulate cortex connectivity, leading to complex decision making, impulsivity, and difficulty focusing; additionally, the limbic system can go into overdrive, where small triggers can create an emotional reaction, surfacing unwanted memories.[9]

A 2020 study from the Stanford University School of Medicine showed that in chronically stressed or anxious children, the brain's fear centers from the right amygdala and sends signals to the decision-making prefrontal cortex, which makes it harder to regulate negative emotions.[10] High stress turns thoughtful decisions to reflective, impulsive, irrational, and emotional decisions; increases anxiety; and leads to aggressive behavior, attention problems, mental health difficulties,[11] and poor memory. Stress blocks the capacity to build higher-level thinking and reasoning skills that your child requires to thrive. Adolescents can make more risky decisions with increased perceived stress and heightened reactivity to acute stress.[12]

Stress and the Immune System

Stress releases substances like adrenaline and norepinephrine into the gut, making the lining of the digestive system more permeable and inflammatory.[13] Stress suppresses secretory immunoglobulin A (IgA), an immune molecule;[14] decreases natural killer cells and anticancer proteins; increases inflammatory markers; and makes one susceptible to the reactivation of infections (specifically Epstein-Barr virus), which may lead to autoimmunity.

Stress and the Gut

The brain and the gut[15] (also known as the second brain) are connected via the vagus nerve, a thick bundle of nerves that runs all along the spinal column; this is known as the gut-microbiota-brain axis. The gut contains its own receptors that react to the gut bacteria and its metabolites and produce neurotransmitters. Stress can lower the release of hydrochloric acid, affect the activity of digestive enzymes, lower the absorption of nutrients,[16] promote overgrowth of bad bacteria, and affect good bacteria negatively (which lowers our level of probiotics)[17]—even in acute stress like childhood trauma. These pathogenic bacteria interfere with the production of vital neurotransmitters. Stress increases food cravings to allow the bad bacteria to thrive further. Studies have shown that adding good bacteria, such as *Bifidobacterium longum* and *Lactobacillus rhamnosus*, back into the body, along with the use of prebiotics, can relieve stress, lowering cortisol.[18]

Stress and Hormones

Stress leads to high cortisol levels, which raises blood sugar levels; creates imbalances in reproductive hormones, leading to increased polycystic ovarian syndrome; and triggers leptin and insulin resistance, leading to weight gain around the middle. Ultimately, stress may cause full-blown diabetes and further inflammation.[19]

Causes of Childhood Stress

Stress could be a response to a negative change in a child's life—for example, helicopter or harsh parenting, negativity, illness, injury, changes in lifestyle, problems with friends, bullying, peer pressure, body changes, parental divorce or separation, worrying about grades, money issues, violence, unrealistic expectations, an overbooked schedule, even trauma or any adverse childhood experience.

Adverse childhood experiences (ACEs) are common. Roughly 61 percent of adults surveyed across twenty-five states reported that they had experienced one type of ACE, and one in six reported they had experienced four or more types of ACEs.[20] These events can be abuse, sudden or violent loss of a loved one, neglect, serious accidents, life-threatening illnesses, military-related stressors, violence, divorce/separation, physical or sexual assault, and even natural disasters or terrorism.

But stress in children is not the only problem; a parent's stress can lead to problems, starting from before birth, as we discussed above. New research finds that children actually had a physical response when parents tried to hide their stresses and emotions.[21] College students whose parents lay on the guilt or try to manipulate them may translate feelings of stress into similar mean behavior with their own friends.[22]

When we overprotect our children, their threshold for registering potential danger gets lower and lower. If we instill fear into our children, they start to lack confidence, which leads to anxiety. As a result, when it is time for them to fly, they can't. Instead of overprotecting or controlling them, we need to give them the tools they need to fly!

Stress Management in Children/Teens

Chronic stress and chronic inflammation take us all down the path to needing a quick dopamine hit, like internet surfing, seeing how many views or likes a post has received, shopping online, or eating junk "comfort" food, which increases the chances of addictions[23] or chronic use of short-term fixes. Just like we can teach a child to wash his hands after using the bathroom, we can empower and educate our children with stress management routines that can lower inflammation, increase prefrontal cortex functioning, and help them develop strong self-regulation skills to increase resilience in a changing world. Every child is different, so work *with* your child to create a routine that integrates these fundamental foundations into his daily life.

Balanced Routine = Balanced Body, Brain, and Behavior

Safe, Secure Environment

Offering our child an encouraging, safe, loving, serene, and well-structured environment, keeping the lines of communication open, being careful not to judge or negate feelings, and disciplining in ways to preserve dignity can deepen the emotional bond between you and your child. A child who knows she is loved regardless of her flaws, imperfections, or mistakes is able to create a foundation for growing, learning and correcting herself into who she really is.

Clear Rules and Structure

In childhood, the prefrontal cortex isn't developed fully yet, so children need order in their lives, otherwise the amygdala can easily take over. Using harshness can shut them down and lead to more resentment, which can trigger an exaggerated response next time around. Work together and establish realistic family rules, clear boundaries, and your family's "nonnegotiables," which will help your child develop the ability to visualize an action plan, foresee any problems that could occur, and come up with a plan to deal with them. In my house, we have clear instructions for the children, from what to do when they wake up to what they are supposed to do after school and what to do before bedtime. The rest of the time, they are able to decide for themselves what they want to do and how they want to structure the rest of their day. We don't have to keep them "entertained" all the time; they are fully capable of keeping themselves entertained. Sometimes a child needs "alone" time, a personal space for inner-reflection, dreaming, creating, thinking, and growing. I have decreased the number of playdates, and I allow the children to choose the activity they want to participate in. I also avoid overscheduling them. Be mindful of how much you "command" your child, and limit it to their character and responsibilities.

I also use this method to prepare them for other events (such as going into stores, parties, playdates, school drop-off, and such). When we go into a store, for example, I tell them exactly what we are looking for, what happens if they see something they want, how long we will be in the store, and such. Help their brains map out and visualize what is going on and what your house rules are regarding each different situation. As the child grows, we will work together to come up with an action plan to handle certain situations.

Clear Rules around Technology and Screens

With the pandemic and online school, children and teens are spending more time on screens than ever before. In a 2021 study, researchers found that kindergarteners from low-income families spend more than six hours a day in front of the screens, nearly double the amount before the pandemic.[24] Children's eyes are much more sensitive to the blue light, as their eyes are not fully developed. Constant overexposure to screen time/blue light, especially at night, can disrupt sleep, which can lead to learning problems,[25] weight gain,[26] depression, and suicide.[27] Young adults who used more than three hundred minutes of screen time per day were 2.8 times more likely to develop depression within six months.[28] In a 2019 study published in *JAMA Pediatrics*, brain scans revealed that toddlers who spent more time in front of screens had lower myelination, or "white matter integrity," in their brains.[29] Further testing showed that they had lower literacy and language skills. Another study, this time of 180 parent couples with children under five, measured the interference that technology causes in parent-child interactions; the researchers found that technology led to more behavioral and emotional problems in children.[30] In 2018, WHO added gaming disorder to its international classification of disease. Internet porn is an uncomfortable topic, but it is reaching kids at a younger age and more profoundly than most parents realize.

Technology use carries with it myriad other potential consequences, among them cyberbullying, sleep deprivation, poor posture, back and neck pain, obesity, loneliness, diminished eyesight, anxiety, depression, body image disturbance, and addiction. Studies show that too much screen time can literally negatively rewire a child's brain. It is important to set clear rules around screens and technology. Technology can add so much extra stress to a parent's life, so delay it as long as possible.

A good indicator to know when to allow children to use technology is when they are able to regulate their own emotions and manage their time, and when you know their prefrontal cortex is heading in the right direction. It is important to model these healthy habits, choosing healthy stress management alternatives to tech time, such as reading, nature, and hands-on activities. I always have open communication with my children about what I am doing on my screens—for example, researching, writing my book, working, or paying the bills.

First, do your own research. Just because a certain piece of technology is available doesn't mean that it's a good fit for your family. Help your children be mindful consumers of tech. Have conversations about tech use, be present and engaged when screens are in use, co-view when possible, and help your child recognize stereotypes and advertising messages, as well as other problematic content. Set expectations of limits, always check in, ask questions, monitor use, and encourage independent analysis and decision making. If your child wants more time online, ask him how he plans to manage his time and self-regulate his tech use. Check in by asking your child to print out and report his browser history, and then discuss what he is seeing; work together to set software for filters or for restricting access to inappropriate content. As the child grows, you can come up with these rules and consequences together, being crystal clear with boundaries and expectations. Come up with tangible consequences, such as repaying someone or writing out an apology when these rules and expectations are broken.

Working as a Team

We have a rule in my house: I am not going to do something if you can do it yourself. We work together as a family, as a team. Giving children responsibilities at an early age with age-appropriate tasks helps them realize that they can help the family, be leaders, and accomplish anything they want. Start to "train" your children at a very young age, letting them know they are a critical part of the family dynamic. Give them lots of practice with simple real tasks throughout the day and work up to more complicated tasks. Model the behavior regularly, never criticize or push them away, acknowledge whatever they are able to contribute, and connect their actions to their maturity.

Simply asking them to clean their rooms before coming downstairs, to do the laundry, or to do the dishes makes them feel like part of the family and gives them a sense of accomplishment. Studies have shown that giving a child responsibility, even in early elementary school, is associated with later development of self-competence, prosocial behavior, and self-efficacy.[31] Responsibilities can help to decrease stress in everyone, and the home's physical environment can actually have an effect on a person's subjective well-being, decision-making skills, and inflammation.[32] Let them do certain activities completely on their own, like schoolwork and chores, as the ability to make their own decisions strengthens the prefrontal cortex/executive function and gives them a sense of freedom. Kids love games and play, so teach them in a fun way. We clean the floors looking for treasure! They all love it!

If we are constantly helping them, we are effectively saying, "You can't succeed unless I'm looking over your shoulder." This actually lowers a child's self-confidence.

Increase Nature

Children spend four to seven minutes a day in unstructured play outdoors and more than seven hours a day in front of a screen, and screen time is increasing so much more due to the pandemic. Nature heals our children's bodies from the inside out, as we have evolved from nature. By moving away from nature, we have had an increase in asthma, autoimmune disorders, food allergies, and lower activation of the prefrontal cortex. Spending some time in nature can actually de-stress us and lower inflammation,[33] boost the immune system, restore brain connections, increase higher prefrontal cortex activity, and improve overall brain health. It also boosts serotonin, leading to better mood and improved ability to focus; improves sleep, mindfulness, and our ability to cope with whatever stresses may be in our path; improves test scores[34] and facilitates cooperation and sustainable behavior.[35] Experiencing nature also lowers cortisol, enhances positive emotions, improves cognition, helps with focus, improves attention, and even increases energy. Despite the overall benefits, race-based inequity does occur,[36] as economically disadvantaged and minority youth are less likely than their white and wealthier counterparts to spend time in green natural spaces.

Nature is free and so beneficial. We should try to get our families to spend at least thirty minutes a week in nature, if not more. Wake up to natural sunlight and spend some time outdoors when you get up, and have your children play outdoors when possible. The sun helps balance hormones—for example, melatonin, which helps us fall asleep and regulates stress. So help them build a garden, build a fort, hug a tree, and go on a hike. Grounding (or earthing) helps put our body back into balance by transferring electrons from the ground into our body; it helps us sleep better, lowers pain, and balances the nervous system.[37] Spending time in nature and observing and contemplating creations are important ways to lower stress. Outdoor time will also help children digitally detox, which will increase their sense of peace.

Mindfulness and Meditation

Mindfulness is how your child is feeling right now, in *this* moment, internally and externally. Staying calm and present in the current moment will help bring the nervous system back into balance and decrease stress. Being present helps you not worry about the past and future, and it limits stress; it can be applied to almost any activity you are engaging in (e.g., eating, exercising, walking, meditation, and/or working).[38]

Mindfulness calms the amygdala and helps our children reconnect to our calm.[39] As we discussed earlier, mindfulness meditation has so many benefits, specifically when it comes to making better decisions. It decreases emotional reactivity, aids in gaining empathy, and improves concentration. Mindfulness meditation improves children's cognitive, emotional, and social abilities.[40] Mindful parenting techniques can augment traditional behavioral approaches to improve children's behavior through specific parent-child interactions.[41] Research on the impact of mindfulness on children is still in its early stages, but studies have shown that in schoolchildren these practices can lower levels of stress, aggression, and social anxiety; improve executive function, such as inhibition and working memory; and contribute to better school performance.

Meditation improves overall quality of life[42] and health by changing the body and mind. When a person practices daily meditation and positivity, it not only intensifies calmness but also cultivates optimal physical health. When the spiritual energy begins to flow, blood circulation improves[43] and blood pressure decreases,[44] cortisol and stress levels go down, digestion improves[45] and the body detoxes, decision making improves because of smaller amygdalas,[46] and cardiovascular health, sleep, memory, attention, and focus[47] improve. Additionally, unhealthy genes are switched off,[48] and the overall immune system is enhanced.[49] Meditation also helps control stress and emotions.[50] Overall meditation helps us empathize with others and take care of our health and our planet.

Through meditation and mindfulness techniques, one can improve the connection in the brain between the amygdala and prefrontal cortex, strengthening the areas of the brain that can keep us present and focused. My children have taken courses and watched videos online to learn mindful meditation for kids, and during their lunch hour, they are able to practice it to refresh their minds. We incorporate belly breathing along with our meditation to help keep us in a parasympathetic mind-set; this gives time for the amygdala to allow the information to flow to the prefrontal cortex, overriding the fight or flight response and enabling mindful behavior. Diaphragmatic breathing has an impact on the brain, gastrointestinal tract, and respiratory and cardiovascular systems.[51] Heart rate variability (HRV) is a measure of the vagus nerve function, and when HRV is optimal, it lowers cortisol and improves the immune function. Mindfulness, meditation, laughter, belly breathing, emotional freedom technique (EFT; also known as tapping or psychological acupressure), and HeartMath (a form of biofeedback that focuses on heart wave variability and coherence) can improve overall HRV.

The Power of Play and Exercise

We are living in a world of structured learning, leaving less time for unstructured play. Play can help children's brains grow and mature in the frontal lobe as they use their imagination. Play builds cognitive skills, improves language development and problem-solving abilities, and advances other executive functions like planning and predicting. Play with others teaches fairness, cooperation, and empathy. Play shows children how to deal with consequences and how to be ethical. It also reduces stress and builds emotional resilience. Play can also improve immune function; lower blood pressure; build new growth in the hippocampus; improve self-esteem; and increase the brain-derived neurotrophic factor (BDNF, a key molecule involved in plastic changes related to learning and memory), which enhances the development of noradrenaline and dopamine systems in the child's brain systems that are vital for a child to be able to focus on learning.[52] Similarly, preschoolers who played after being dropped off at school were less distraught and tolerated the separation with more balance than their peers. Interactive play can enhance the emotional regulatory functions in the frontal lobes, helping children manage their feelings better. Playing alone also develops a sense of independence in children; it allows them to be comfortable in any situation, helps develop their preferences and interests, and develops imagination and powers of concentration.

Regular exercise is crucial for the overall health and wellness of our children's brains and bodies. Exercise lowers markers of systemic inflammation;[53] enhances brain health;[54] enhances learning and cognition;[55] builds the prefrontal cortex, which helps children regain control of their bodies; and even changes our children's thoughts and emotional states. Exercise can manipulate DNA expression, reduce cravings, regulate appetite, improve insulin sensitivity, balance cortisol, improve digestive function by increasing microbial diversity, improve detoxification, boost happy chemicals in the brain, sharpen memory, strengthen our bones and muscles, help build healthy bones, increase self-confidence, and keep chronic diseases at bay. Getting kids moving and playing daily is important for better brains, bodies, and behavior.

Stress is inevitable, but it doesn't have to take control of our children's health or their everyday decisions, so the foundations of holistic parenting can help lower overall stress. Providing real food; lowering toxins and optimizing detoxification; surrounding our children with love, responsibilities, support, structure, mindfulness, play, and nature; and optimizing their sleep and positivity can all be incorporated to manage their stress appropriately. Mindful children reflect on their emotions, are able to sense their stress levels, figure out where the stress is coming from and decide which stress management technique to incorporate into their daily lives, and work toward bringing their internal and external world back into balance.

KIDS VERSUS SLEEP

Bedtime! Does that word make you smile from ear to ear? Sleep is so important for adults and children because it allows their bodies to recharge for the next day. But unfortunately, according to the Centers for Disease Control and Prevention (CDC), six in ten middle schoolers and seven in ten high schoolers are not getting enough sleep.[56] Studies show that more than half of children (52 percent) in the United States don't get the recommended nine hours of sleep they need.

Infants (four to twelve months) need to sleep twelve to sixteen hours daily; children between the ages of one and two need eleven to fourteen hours; children between three and five need ten to thirteen hours; children between six and twelve need nine to twelve hours; adolescents between thirteen and eighteen need eight to ten hours; and adults need seven to nine hours of sleep.

A major cause of lack of sleep is the increased use of blue light (the wavelength of light on the spectrum of visible light), which is especially emitted from our electronic devices. Blue wavelengths can help boost our attention and mood during the day, but at night they can lead to problems.[57] Nearly half of all children are using screens the hour before bed,[58] which can lead to problems, including a lower expression of BDNF and an increase in mood disorders.

Children's and teens' brains are developing at a rate of eight hundred synapses per second, and when the child sleeps, the brain continues to form and strengthen these connections. Deep sleep correlates with the myelin content of the brain.[59] Getting enough sleep normalizes cortisol levels, improves memory, cleans your brain, and helps control weight and overall inflammation. Our body doesn't consume much energy while we sleep, so it leaves more energy available over eight or nine hours per night for the body to remove toxins, make hormones, activate cellular repair, boost the secretion of growth hormone, mend injuries, and fight infections. Sleep is important to prevent type 2 diabetes, obesity, poor mental health,[60] injuries, and even attention or behavior problems or poor emotional and social function.[61] A recent study found that 48 percent of kids who did sleep enough had a 44 percent higher likelihood of demonstrating curiosity in learning new information and skills. They were also 33 percent more likely to complete all their homework and 28 percent more likely to care about doing well in school.

Studies show that even missing an hour of sleep can reduce the cognitive maturation process by the equivalent of two years, even dropping IQs by 7 percent with a single missed hour.[62] Children who experience poor sleep during preschool and early school years have an increased risk of developing cognitive and behavioral problems in mid-childhood. Sleep restrictions were also found to increase irritability, acting out, and restlessness; lead to depression in adolescents;[63] and lead to significant impairments in daytime neurobehavioral functioning in children, which can be due to the impact on the prefrontal cortex, basal ganglia, and amygdala. Sleep deprivation results in difficulties with executive functioning, reward anticipation, and emotional reactivity.[64] It impairs frontal lobe function;[65] affects leptin and ghrelin hormones; causes increases in body mass index and waist circumference; increases insulin levels and insulin insensitivity; and causes weight gain, especially when children stay up past 9:00 p.m. or later, as found in a 2020 study in *Pediatrics*.[66] All these factors can contribute to challenging behaviors, hyperactivity, reduced academic performance, substance abuse, suicide, and other behavioral challenges. Young people who prefer to stay up late are more impulsive than their peers who go to bed early, which makes them more likely to drink alcohol and smoke.[67]

A bedtime routine is the best way to get children to develop healthy sleep hygiene habits. A good bedtime routine promotes our children's well-being. Any activity that families undertake as part of their sleep routine can enhance parent–child relationships and create a stronger bond to promote children's physical and prosocial development.

Optimizing Sleep

Sleep hygiene[68] includes practices that, when implemented, promote better quality of sleep, and bedtime routines are an important part of that. Develop a sleep routine with your child. Every child is different, so let her lead. This limits control and keeps cortisol low before bedtime.

Your child's sleep routine starts with the moment she wakes up. Wake up with prayer and gratitude. Focus on real foods and limit daytime sleep disrupters like caffeine, sugar, stress, lack of movement, and too much artificial light or evening exposure to fluorescent light. Foods to help your sleep include walnuts, avocados, and green leafy vegetables. Stay well hydrated and replace caffeine with relaxing teas like chamomile. If your teen needs caffeine, limit it to the morning hours only.

Increasing the bright light exposure for at least thirty minutes between 6:00 a.m. and 8:30 a.m. provides natural light cues for circadian rhythms and keeps children alert. Exercise regularly in the morning or afternoon. Periods of time with direct contact with the ground can help create an internal balance to optimize sleep.

Start preparing your child for sleep. Start winding down about two hours before bedtime by taking time to relax, using either mindful meditation or other stress-relieving strategies. Give her a warm bath with Epsom salts and lavender oil. Have your child set aside time to write down her worries and talk about them. Turn off electronics at least ninety minutes before bedtime, as this will allow her melatonin and cortisol levels to normalize; minimize blue lights from electronics, and use amber lights or glasses to filter the blue light.

Digital programs can be used for the computer and other electronic screens to change the screen color from blue to orange as the sun sets. Flip switches to turn off the Wi-Fi routers, put her phone six feet away or in another room on airplane mode, and turn off notifications to limit electromagnetic fields (EMFs). Have your child stop eating at least ninety minutes before sleep. If she does get hungry, she can eat a meal high in fat and lower in carbohydrates, as elevated insulin will disrupt your child's sleep.

In order to get your child to have an amazing, restful, and deep sleep, you need to prepare for success by creating an environment that is conducive to optimal sleep. Play soft music or scripture in the background. Clear out the clutter, hang blackout curtains on the windows, set the night room temperature to about 68 degrees Fahrenheit, and limit noise (or use a white-noise fan to block background noise). Socks can help keep extremities warm. Adding a household plant to the room can improve the air quality and inhibit EMFs.

Sleep Training

When we take into consideration the child's brain and body, we as parents can use logic to figure out what works for our family. Obviously, sleep is important, but leaving a screaming child alone in a bedroom can lead to increased stress hormones that wash over her brain and stimulate the same parts of the brain that are activated during pain. Comforting a child helps turn off the stress cycle. Some studies have shown that these times of early stress can lead to death of cells and other important structures in a child's brain.

Letting children "cry it out" is an idea that has been around since at least the 1880s, but now recent studies show that letting a child become distressed can actually harm the child and her relational capacities in the long term. Crying actually kills neuronal connections, especially when the child is distressed. Too much stress actually suppresses the glial cell division, and the glial cells take care of myelination.[69] The brain is developing quickly at this stage, and great distress can damage the synapses in a child's brain. Babies don't self-regulate or self-comfort in isolation, and they can learn to stop trusting.[70]

Sleep training doesn't have to involve allowing the child to cry hours on end. It is important to help the child calm the brain at bedtime.

1. *Create a soothing routine.* Because the prefrontal cortex is still developing, the brain needs a routine. When they are a newborns, it might be a little difficult, but the earlier you can start, the better. For example, a calming bath and then a story can help regulate your child's bodily arousal system. My children to this day have their bedtime routine that was set when they were newborns: a calming activity, a shower or

a bath, and then a book. I would put them to bed when they started to get drowsy, and then I would put on calming scripture as they began to fall asleep. The routine became a signal for their brains to start falling asleep. Remember, consistency matters.

2. *Gentle, mindful sleep training.* Not all sleep training is bad for the brain. Doing things like holding your child; playing a recording of your voice; hugging your child every time he tries to get out of bed; and letting your child know you love him, that he is safe, and that you are there for him will help calm your child's immature brain systems. When my children were babies, I would hold their hands while singing to them in their beds, while showing them that I was there for them. They would cry, but I would comfort them the entire time, letting them know I would not be taking them out of the crib. When they understood, they realized that it was time to sleep. I would let them hold my hand through the crib, and I would let them hold a scarf of mine that would smell like me. This way sleep training involves as few tears as possible (for both of us), doesn't have any long-term effects, and is more of a bonding activity than a stressful one.

3. *Any learned behavior takes time.* Listen to your gut; every situation is different. What works for one family may not work with another. Talk to your primary care physician to determine what will work best with your individual situation.

Sleep heals. Holistic parenting can help mold a mindful child who is able to prioritize sleep, learn the signs of insufficient sleep, know when his sleep quality is lacking, and know how to fix any imbalances.

SOCIAL HEALTH: LOVE HEALS

The one most important ingredient for children with healthy brains and bodies is unconditional *love*. Starting from a very young age, we have learned to depend on each other; we depend on parents, siblings, teachers, coworkers, spouses, and friends to survive. Our children need positive experiences for pathways in their brains and bodies to work.[71] That secure attachment releases oxytocin (also known as the "love hormone"), which significantly strengthens our immune system, develops empathy for yourself and others, and promotes emotional strength and self-regulation in children.[72]

Empathy is the ability to feel and understand emotions of others. Cognitive empathy involves understanding another person's emotions on an intellectual level, taking into consideration someone's situation and how that person would react. Affective empathy is feeling someone else's emotions after observing their expression or other mood indicators. One study helped to clarify the link between oxytocin gene methylation and parental empathy.[73] Secure attachment equips children to regulate their emotions, gives them the sense of who they are and the confidence to try new things, and protects them from major mental and physical health problems later in life, as it trains the nervous system to run smoothly.[74] Children with secure attachment relationships tend to grow into adults who can experience a broad range of emotions without shutting down or becoming overwhelmed. In other words, giving and receiving love inspires healing—physical, emotional, and spiritual—in children and adults.

Since the 1990s, scientists have been researching mirror neurons. Mirror neurons show activity when someone observes an act being done or when they actually perform the act themselves, and these neurons play a large role in speech, language evolution, emotional intelligence, empathy, and even learning and understanding.[75] Positive company can increase a person's sense of belonging and purpose, boost happiness and reduce stress, improve self-confidence and self-worth, and help a person cope with any traumas. Based on the results of brain MRIs and blood and saliva tests, we know that feeling loved and supported releases hormones into our bloodstream; such hormones include serotonin, relaxin, endorphins, and oxytocin, which keep us happy and healthy. These hormones lower cortisol, improve blood circulation, lower blood pressure and heart rate, improve digestion, clear out toxins, increase natural killer cells and a number of white blood cells, and increase red blood cells, IgA, and helper T cells, activity that helps the immune system clear out infections and renew energy to repair cells and fight cancer. This helps lower inflammation overall, which improves sleep, relieves feelings of restlessness, and decreases chronic pain as muscle tension and pain perception lower. Studies have shown that having pets releases the same hormones, and pet owners live longer than people who don't have pets.

Recent studies in *JAMA Network Open* reassessed the impact of the presence and awareness of social support. The researchers found that young adults who perceived higher levels of social support (the feeling that there is someone who they can depend on for help should they need it) at the age of nineteen showed lower levels of depression and anxiety symptoms and fewer mental health problems one year later.[76] The study also found that even in cases where people previously experienced mental health problems, social support was beneficial for mental health later on. They found that people who experienced greater levels of social support experienced 47 percent less depression and 22 percent less anxiety than those with less social support. The team found that those who reported higher level of perceived social support were at a 40 percent decreased risk of experiencing suicidal ideations and attempts. Love and secure attachments strengthen the body and help regulate emotions, attention, and behavior, which mitigate the effects of stress and promote a lifelong healthy development.

Negative Impacts

But is this the case today? The problem with today's world is that our children are growing up with negativity, judgment, criticism, and bullying, and they are surrounded by so many people, virtually or in person, who are pushing them down and not lifting them up. Children with insecure attachment are more vulnerable to mental health problems and have difficulty managing emotions.[77] Severe childhood deprivation and neglect can have lasting and deep-seated social, emotional, and cognitive problems[78] as well as severe lack of language, which lead to increased risk of depression and reduced growth in the hippocampus that can contribute to learning and memory impairment.[79] Negative relationships and loneliness can lead to increased cortisol levels (which deplete our immune system) and an earlier death.

Parental involvement is consistently linked with positive childhood outcomes throughout development. The opposite of neglect is helicopter parenting, which can be particularly harmful during emerging adulthood when young adults are working toward developmental goals of self-reliance and autonomy. Research has shown that children with hyper-involved parents have more anxiety and less satisfaction with life.[80]

It also is very difficult to control what a child experiences with social media and smartphones. Tech companies have spent years studying how to hijack our behaviors that lead to dopamine surges in our brains in order to infuse their products with techniques that trigger their release, which lead to addictions. They have turned notifications red; they play with our need to be liked and feel connected; and they added autoplay so we can mindlessly scroll through social media, which feeds our fears of missing out. Children's frontal lobes are not fully developed, so they are more likely to become addicted. Teen brains are biologically driven toward dopamine-producing behaviors like taking risks, trying new things, and being admired by friends. A 2018 study showed that having a smartphone present during a conversation between two strangers was linked to more distraction[81] and lower levels of perceived empathy.[82]

This can even start prenatally, as studies from Harvard School of Public Health have shown that poor family functioning during pregnancy leads to smaller hippocampus and capital lobe sizes in childhood, which contributes to a difficulty in regulating emotions and performing in academic settings.[83]

Our environment can influence our behavioral intentions and our emotional states, helping us imitate others and their emotional states. Not only do our experiences determine our brains, but our everyday discussions, jokes, hugs, and arguments can also literally change our children's brains, bodies, and behavior.

Creating a Secure Attachment

Unconditional Love Builds a Better Brain and Body

Love heals. When your child learns that you will love and honor her despite her mistakes, flaws, failures, and imperfections, love will mold that child to be the best she can be. There is also so much more we can do to optimize our children's social experiences. We can optimize our children's secure attachment with unconditional love, proper communication, empathy, and family time, and we also can do this by educating them about mindful awareness and how to deal with social dilemmas properly. Surround your child with as much unconditional love as you can find, including from grandparents, aunts, and uncles. Limit harsh, negative interactions as best as you can.

Eye-to-Eye Communication

All children want to be seen, want to be loved, and want to be valued. Communicate with your child down at her level. Proper communication is key to integrating the whole brain of the child and the teen. Because your child's prefrontal cortex is not developed fully yet, our job is to give our child the opportunities to build the prefrontal cortex, so it can grow stronger every day. Remember, a child can easily get overloaded with an emotion, so help her connect the prefrontal cortex by getting down at her level. You can lessen the emotional load from the amygdala; this leads to a more rational brain, where the prefrontal cortex can help take some charge back, which allows your child to bring some balance back to the brain.

When your child is hurt, don't just shrug it off; instead, help him name it (to try to engage the prefrontal cortex), try to understand what he may be going through, and validate him. When your child approaches you, make sure to make eye contact and be emotionally present. Especially nowadays it is important to put your screens away and to make sure you maintain eye-to-eye contact and validate what your child is saying and feeling. Listening and validating are the most valuable gifts we can give to our children. This will help them create meaningful friendships, as we can model social rules and understanding, and we can show them how to treat their friends.

Empathy

I have one big rule in my house: "Don't treat others the way you don't want to be treated." Helping the children understand others' feelings will help them build their prefrontal cortex. Teach your child to recognize what the other child might be feeling; teach them nonverbal communication and tuning into others. Teach the child/teen how to make things right after a conflict. I use every opportunity to teach our children about empathy, but it really starts with being a great role model. As your child goes about her day, guide and educate her, and when she is disrespectful, let her know right away that what she said or did was rude and might hurt the other person's feelings. I usually ask, "Would you like to be treated the same way you treated him?" That simple question gets a child thinking and develops empathy and makes him more mindful of others.

Family Time

Family (and extended family) time can help your child build fun, memorable, and enjoyable experiences with positive reinforcements; this releases dopamine, which allows your child's brain to communicate better between cells and lowers stress. When you see your child, enjoy him and spend time with him; this floods the brain with oxytocin, which makes him feel safe and bonded. Teach the older children to take care of the younger children and be their support system. Find an activity that the whole family loves to participate in and schedule it into your routines. We love to ride bikes, go on hikes, and even play games together. Allow your children to choose the activity they wish to do with you.

Educate and Empower: Mindful Awareness

Educating and empowering our children will help them build their prefrontal cortex. Living mindful lives can help children not only name their emotions and find out what is out of balance but also figure out whether their social environments are out of balance. Most of the time kids misbehave when they can't control their emotions and bodies. Helping children understand their emotions/feelings and their bodies allows them to take control of their brains and bodies so much better. And when a child feels empowered, he is receptive to growth, instead of shutting down, which makes it easier for him to put his brain and body back into balance.

Help your child live a more mindful life. Teach her to listen to her body and emotions at that moment, and help her name the emotion she is feeling. If she is feeling sad, have her look into her life to find out what is leading to that emotion. Is it stresses in the environment? Friends? Bullies? Trauma? Food? Lack of sleep? The more a child thinks about what is going on with herself and why she feels off balance, the more she will develop the ability to quickly solve the underlying cause of the imbalance. This will help her get back into balance and help her make better life choices.

This process also works with finding good friendships. Help your child use his own mental ruler to determine which friends might be worth investing in and which ones would be better as acquaintances; help you child choose friends who will help lift each other up and not drag each other down. Provide your child with situations and settings for potential friendships to bloom. A child's preference for friendships varies as he grows, so be mindful of your child's desires. If your child is satisfied with his social life, then there is no need to force friendships. If your child gets rejected or shows concern about a strained relationship or a lack of friendships, then he might need help addressing the reasons why he is having problems.

Social Dilemmas

Discipline

When I talk discipline, I don't mean punishment, as they are two completely different things. A punishment is an approach that makes a child regret a misbehavior; it is an adult's fear-based reaction (often brought out by the adult's amygdala) to something that has occurred and an attempt to stop an unwanted behavior. Because it usually isn't thought out, a punishment doesn't really take the child's brain and body into consideration. The problem with punishment also is that if the parent is trying to teach the child about consequences and responsibilities and how to control his emotions, the child might not fully understand all that is happening because the prefrontal cortex isn't formed yet. Examples of punishments include such things as reduced (or zero) screen time if he doesn't complete his chores or grounding if he gets bad grades. Physical punishment is never okay. Studies have shown that those who were regularly spanked (once a month for more than three years with a belt or paddle) were found to have less gray matter in certain areas of the prefrontal cortex, which has been linked to mental health disorders like depression and addiction. Spanking when a child was three was linked to an increased risk of child aggression when the child was five,[84] and spanking has detrimental effects on brain development.[85]

Discipline, however, which comes from the Latin root "to teach," is the range of methods parents can use to teach their children to understand what is expected of them, so that they will make well-thought-out decisions. Discipline is a set of tools and guidelines that helps set a child up to allow her prefrontal cortex to take full change over the amygdala; this means explaining to a child what you expect from her, why you expect her to act this way, and what the outcomes and real-life consequences would be if she doesn't cooperate. Discipline is a thought-out plan that is not intended to hurt a child; it is intended to shape a child's future. Real discipline focuses on the misbehavior, not the child, and offers real-life consequences.

When it comes to younger children, figure out where the tantrum is coming from—the prefrontal cortex tantrum versus one that is coming from the amygdala. In a prefrontal cortex tantrum, the child is able to control her emotions and pushes buttons and terrorizes you until she gets what she wants. For this type of tantrum, it is important to make sure you keep clear boundaries and discuss inappropriate versus appropriate responses and behaviors. Refuse to give into your child's prefrontal cortex tantrum. In a downstairs amygdala tantrum, your child is so upset that she can't use her prefrontal cortex. For this type of tantrum, your child's brain is being hijacked by the amygdala. In these cases, it is best not to correct or control but, instead, distract, connect with, and comfort your child, and after the child calms down, you can start to talk to her about what was appropriate and what wasn't to engage her prefrontal cortex.

How are we going to discipline for good behavior?

1. *Model good behavior.* Connection and empathy are key to getting the good behavior you are looking for, and if there is misbehavior, it is important to find out why the child is out of balance. When children get empathy or comfort from a trusted adult, they are able to self-calm and self-regulate their bodies and brains. Relationships are critical to good behavior. Replace your anger and control with calmness and empowerment. If you yell and get angry, this response will model the wrong message to your child.

2. *Treat them like adults.* I treat my children like adults. We need to give them enough credit. I talk to them, set rules, take them to all my adult gatherings, and make sure they have real-life consequences, the way adults have. We need to give kids more credit. Kids will rise to your expectations.

3. *Set family rules.* From the beginning, set your rules. For example, in my family, when you wake up, say ten things you are grateful for, get up and make your bed, and brush your teeth. When you come downstairs, fix yourself breakfast and help with chores so everything is done before school starts. Make sure you communicate your house rules clearly, and be certain to enforce these rules consistently. Sit together as a family and create these house rules together, along with

their consequences. Stay consistent and say what you mean and mean what you say.

4. *Use choices and set "real-life consequences."* In my house, if the chores aren't done, then my children can't play because work comes before play. This simple rule has helped them finish their chores and even their school assignments before they start to play or get screen time. Make sure you set your consequences and then actually follow through with them. Once a child knows that your words are just meaningless, he will start to take everything else you say with a grain of salt. Teach your child that every person is responsible for their own choices. When your child suffers a consequence, it is a lesson he will not soon forget. So let reality be the teacher and don't back down. It is important to hold children accountable, and not to negotiate on your nonnegotiables.

5. *Appreciate good behavior.* Sticker charts, point systems, or just words of appreciation all engage and develop a child's prefrontal cortex. If a family doesn't appreciate, they can easily start to criticize a child's every decision, which continues to feed the amygdala and, consequently, feeds the bad behavior. Lots of attention to good behavior leads to more good behavior. Use your words very carefully; harsh words can activate the amygdala and lead to further disobedience and defiance. Just remember not to overpraise.

6. *When there is a problem, look for where your child could be "out of balance."* A child who is difficult to "train" usually has something off balance. Loneliness? Nutrition? Stress? Sleep? Gratitude? Does she feel isolated? Does she need more attention? Spending time together, looking for opportunities to praise the child, and making sure you are giving good direction are important for a child's overall health and balance. Remember to validate your child's feelings and then work together to find out what is out of balance. As a child gets older, she will be able to look within herself and figure out what is going on and correct it before the problem gets out of control.

7. *Start slow and build over time.* Decide what battle is worth it after taking into consideration the whole child and what kind of child you are trying to create.

8. *Foundations of holistic parenting.* These are super important to build healthy brains and bodies for optimal behavior.

Bullying

Bullying is the systemic abuse of power and is defined as aggressive behavior or intentional harm by peers that is carried out repeatedly and involves an imbalance of power. Today kids are bullied more than ever before, especially with more and more avenues that bullies can hide behind and still bully. According to the National Center for Education Statistics and the Bureau of Justice Statistics, between one and three students in the United States report being bullied at school. Bullying is usually an ongoing cycle, as the child who bullies has often been bullied either by a caregiver or by other children. Bullying can take many forms: verbal bullying, physical bullying, psychological or social bullying, and even cyberbullying. Bullying is a major risk factor for poor physical and mental health and reduced adaptation to adult roles, including integrating into work, being economically independent, or even forming lasting relationships.[86] Take each bullying situation seriously.

Bullying alters brain structure and raises the risk of mental health problems.[87] Researchers analyzed six hundred young people between the ages of fourteen and nineteen from different countries in Europe using questionnaires and brain scans. The analysis showed that severe bullying was linked to changes in brain volume in the caudate and putamen as well as levels of anxiety at the age of nineteen. Bullying can also lead to mental health problems, self-harm, depression, sleep problems, and even suicide in teens, with effects lingering into adulthood—for example, mental health issues, elevated C-reactive protein (CRP), suicidality, anxiety, smoking, less income, poor performance in school, difficulty managing finances, and poor relationships.[88]

When we recognize that a child is "off balance," we want to take a look at the entire situation. Learn the signs of a child who is bullied. The child, out of the blue, may have headaches, stomachaches, or trouble sleeping. His habits may change—for example, the child doesn't want to go to school or to a specific event he previously enjoyed. The child has feelings of helplessness or even low self-esteem, loses friends abruptly, or shows distress after spending time with friends at an in-person gathering or even online. Come up with a plan for how you can improve the situation; think about the child's strengths, focus on the positive, and determine who you can involve to try to improve the situation.

Let's be realistic: real life is filled with bullies. Dealing with bullies is a life skill children need to learn. I teach my children not to take bullying personally because the bullied child is more inflamed and "out of balance" or doesn't know how to treat someone any different. A bully actually can lack empathy; desires to be in control; feels frustrated, angry, or depressed; tries to fit in with a peer group that is perceived as bullying; and lacks social skills. If your child is the one bullying, again find out what is out of balance with the child, clarify expectations and consequences, make a plan, and help her focus on the positives. Everything we discussed in this book will help a child's brain and body work better so she can empathize with others, instead of fostering a "me versus them" mentality. Talk to your child about how to cope with peer pressure, and talk regularly about how they are feeling physically, emotionally, and spiritually. Inquire about peer pressure, and help your child with rising above it all.

Social Curve Balls

Life has its ups and downs, and resilience is key in optimizing a child's overall health and happiness. In difficult situations—for example, divorce, a move, loss, grief, a serious illness, or mass tragedies (including pandemics)—it is better to help build a child's prefrontal cortex to help him understand the current situation without the amygdala taking over due to acute stress. Children grieve differently than adults. Younger children may throw tantrums, become irritable, lose their appetites, have feelings of shame and guilt, have poor bladder and bowel control, and have difficulty sleeping. Older children may show signs of aggression, fear abandonment or rejection, have trouble sleeping, exhibit increased impulsivity, lose interest in hobbies/activities, change eating habits, and fear going to school.

Prepare your child for the new transitions in life. Educate her about the situation, come up with a plan to help prepare your child with the least disturbance, encourage open communication about what is going on, and find a way to maintain stability. Continue to work on brain and body as discussed in this book to optimize overall health and resilience no matter what life decides to throw at her. Teach her how to take a social curve ball and grow from it.

Parenting Teens: Drugs and Sex

There are many forms of addiction that plague our children. There's substance abuse, and now more and more of our youth are becoming addicted to other behaviors like gambling, eating, porn, internet usage, shopping, video gaming, and sex. Recent studies suggest that more than 80 percent of adolescents experiment with drugs or alcohol before adulthood.[89]

Set clear and firm rules, but take your foot off the control and judgment gas pedal. Hold them accountable with real-life consequences when they violate your nonnegotiables. You won't always see eye to eye with your teen. If your teen does storm off and slam the door, let him have his moment. Once the amygdala is in full control, there is no way to reason with him. Once he cools off, then you can sit down and listen to what he is feeling. Figure out why he is doing what he is doing, and find out what is "out of balance" in his life. Just like with anyone else, teens need respect, and they want to know they are valued and heard. Though teens are older, they actually need more time from you to listen to what is going on in their lives. Let them know you are there for them, and love them despite their "slips." It is important to empower them to turn their pain into their power.

Disciplining our teens takes extra caution because it can spiral out of control fast. A University of Pittsburgh psychology professor led a study of nearly one thousand families with teenage children to measure the effects of harsh verbal discipline (defined as yelling, cursing, or insulting after misbehavior) on children. In a 2014 paper, he reported that nearly half of the parents used harsh verbal discipline, but it wasn't effective in stopping the misconduct. Actually, the children who had been disciplined harshly were more likely to act out or show symptoms of depression when questioned the following year. The same effects were seen with parents who yelled at their children but who generally had a warm relationship with them, showing that parental warmth didn't lessen the negative impact of yelling or insults. When a parent uses harsh punishments, the child goes into a fight or flight state that can disconnect the prefrontal cortex. They are going to make mistakes. We all were there once, so treat teens with empathy. Treat them like adults, with respect, love, and positivity; work with them to come up with a set of rules and "real-life" consequences.

Love and Sex

We are living in a world where our children are becoming adults younger and younger. When it comes to love and sex, it becomes a confusing world. So let me be blunt—if you want to find the right person, hold off on sex until there is a real commitment.

There are a lot of people in the world who are not looking for any real connections and are only looking to get their joy by taking it from others. In order to know whether a person is worth sticking around for, in the beginning it is best to hold off on any intimacy, not to cloud the water, and to bless the relationship. If the other person really wants to be with you and truly loves you for your heart, that person will respect your decision and wait. This will test to make sure the person has the self-control and loyalty you desire in a spouse. You are a gem and deserve someone who will kiss the ground you walk on; you deserve someone who really loves you for you—all of you—not just your privates. Holding off of any intimacy and sex can help find the right person for you, who will support you, love you, and treat you like a king or queen.

Focus on building loving, pure relationships, as pure relationships will heal from the inside out. It is never too late to either build a new friendship or reconnect with old friends, as maintaining a healthy friendship or relationship is always an equal give and take. Spending time with family, dealing with imbalances in life, making eye-to-eye contact, and educating about mindful awareness of internal and external surroundings can help your children develop a strong sense of self-esteem, self-confidence, and belonging. When we use holistic parenting to raise mindful children, they will be able to examine their feelings and social environments and adjust their lifestyles and social environments to their benefit. Always let them know they are appreciated. Explain that investing time in finding high-quality friends will keep the body balanced, lower inflammation, and heal and prevent chronic disease, and they will be able to handle whatever social and physical problems come their way.

SPIRITUALITY: THE HEALING POWER OF GRATITUDE

Gratitude is an emotion expressing appreciation for what one has; it is a universal concept in nearly all of the world's spiritual traditions. When we have feelings of gratitude, we experience the spiritual. Expressing gratitude is a practice that positively affects our children's brains, bodies, and behavior because children's brains are "plastic," meaning that the nervous system is able to change its connections or "rewire" in response to different stimuli (intrinsic or extrinsic), and the inner circuitry can be changed.[90] Giving thanks to a supernatural power, benefactors, or others is one of the most effective ways to get in touch with our souls.

Being thankful helps create a subconscious world of positivity that governs 90 percent of our thoughts and actions. The positive energy boosts optimism, which in turn helps prevent disease and improves our immune system, well-being, and sense of happiness. Gratitude has the power to improve genetics, traumatic experiences, and years of learned behaviors. When our children start to focus on all the good they have, they shift their internal world with positivity, which leads to positive behaviors. This practice lowers the threshold for feel-good circuits to discharge in our brain and raises happiness indexes. Along with yoga, meditation, and prayer, mindfulness can slow brain activity and lessen the negative thoughts that permeate our lives.

Gratitude also affects heart rate variability. "Heart-felt" emotions—like gratitude, love, and caring—produce sine waves, or coherent waves, radiating to every cell of the body, which can be detected using technology that measures changes in heart-rhythm variation and measurements of coherence. Research shows that with "depleted" emotions—like frustration, anger, anxiety, and insecurity—the heart-rhythm pattern becomes more erratic, and the brain recognizes this as stress. This in turn creates a desynchronized state, which raises the risk of developing heart disease, increases blood pressure, weakens the immune system, impairs cognitive function, and blocks our ability to think clearly. Studies that extend this line of research on gratitude from adults to adolescents suggest that gratitude may hold similar benefits for youth and has a positive effect, including optimism, academic motivation, satisfaction with social relationships, and lower levels of symptomatology.[91]

We live in a world with negativity. The world is telling us we are never good enough. No matter who we are, we are "trained" to think negatively, and this negativity is also affecting our children. Negativity and criticism stimulate the amygdala, which impairs the hippocampus, increases stress, and overrides the prefrontal cortex. Depending on the environment, the brain will start to adapt with changes in the brain chemistry systems and brain structures specific to that experience. With all this bombardment of negativity, we need to make sure to consciously change our children's subconscious, which governs 90 percent of their thoughts and actions and shapes their every behavior.

Gratitude: Training Your Child's Subconscious

The subconscious mind is nothing but the "neural pathways" that have been established in the brain as a result of past beliefs and conditioning. Your child's subconscious does no thinking of its own; rather, it relies on your child's perception of the world around him and listening to verbal and nonverbal cues. When you consciously turn negativity to positivity, from the inside out, the neural pathway associated with negativity will take time to come down fully, so it is critical to continue gratitude regularly. Your child's thoughts and subconscious are powerful because subconscious negative thoughts can undermine health, while positive thoughts can boost the immune system and heal disease.

Practicing morning gratitude helps change your child's subconscious to immediately think positive. I also recommend you place sticky notes that say "I am grateful for this" all around the house on the objects you are thankful for, creating a zone of positivity to subliminally train your child's subconscious. You can place sticky notes on photos of people you love, your child's shoes, the bathroom mirror, lights, and so forth. Be thankful for simple things, things you take for granted in your internal and external world, things that go well, and people (or events) from the past who have helped you become who you are today. Older children can write in a gratitude journal.

Focus on happy memories. I have my children take all negative situations and use gratitude to improve them. A positive perspective can be a power, but a negative perspective can be a prison. With the 1 percent of hate in the world, concentrate on the love. Everyone is dealing with something; we need to take our children's pain and turn it into their power.

Words of Appreciation and Encouragement

Showing appreciation to those who have helped you in your daily life helps you and motivates others, which creates a peaceful environment. You can easily incorporate gratitude in any situation. Some parents may believe that their criticism is a form of love, but that criticism immediately shuts off the child's prefrontal cortex, as if in a state of stress. It is important to focus not on what a child is doing wrong but on what a child is doing right, and give positive, realistic feedback. Don't overpraise, but give acknowledgment and realistic support and encouragement. Remember, overpraising actually can backfire and can generate a lot of competition between siblings or can teach the child to always look to us on how feel about their actions. Ways to encourage a child include giving a gentle smile or rooting them on. Find ways for your child to feel successful. Extracurricular activities are great, so find something she loves and allow her to thrive, as this will help her develop self-confidence and feel connected and in control.

Teach Children to Forgive

Acts that have offended or hurt our children can always remain a part of their lives, attacking their health insidiously and increasing inflammation. Forgiveness involves a decision to let go of resentment and thoughts of revenge, lessening the hurt. Forgiveness helps them focus on other, positive parts of their lives; it can lead to feelings of understanding, empathy, and compassion for the one who hurt them. Learning to forgive is essential to spiritual health and allows peace to emerge from within.

How do we teach our children to forgive? We first need to know how to forgive. In order to forgive, try to understand others' actions; bring compassion and passion into the situation. This trauma is part of life, and most of us have dealt with trauma in some form. It is part of our story; it happened. This trauma came to us in ugly "gift wrap," and it made us angry. We walk around the world holding this "present" with this ugly gift wrap in shame, and we hide it from the world, which drags us down; we are unable to reach our maximum potential because of this "ugly" gift from the universe.

To learn to forgive, we must address the "gift," acknowledge that it existed, and change the gift wrapping. We must change it to a prettier gift wrap, to show that this "gift" is not something that we are ashamed of but, instead, something that made us better. This helps us assign a new meaning and a new positive label to the hurt. As crazy as it sounds, we need to be grateful for every person who may have hurt us because they have made us who we are today. We need to teach our children that pain is just a perfectly crafted chapter in their unique journey. This didn't happen to your child; it happened for your child. Help him again turn that pain into power.

When you change the gift wrapping, you will eventually resolve the negative charge attached to the event; it will allow you to forgive yourself and others as you surrender the pain. It will take time, maybe even years, but it will be the largest burden that was lifted from your child's shoulders and will allow them to truly fly.

Find Purpose

Help your children find their higher purpose. Teach your children that they have been put on this planet for a unique purpose, and that purpose is different for everyone. Mindfulness and gratitude will help them develop a positive attitude and reframe their stress and allow them to tackle it better. When you help your children clear out the clutter in their brains, they can start to think beyond themselves and find a higher purpose.

Research has shown that a strong "purpose in life" also reduces chances that your child's self-esteem will fluctuate with the number of likes he gets on social media.[92] Kids with purpose have stronger self-awareness, are more resilient, do better in school, and have a healthier, mind, body, and soul. Activities driven with purpose decrease emptiness and increase self-confidence, and these activities don't need trophies or huge acknowledgments. A lack of purpose has been linked to higher levels of the stress hormone cortisol, more abdominal fat, and other negative health markers.

We can help children create meaning by asking questions such as "Why is the world a better place because I am here?" or "What can I contribute?" Examine what gives your child joy and what his strengths are. Offer a variety of options and find potential mentors, observerships, or volunteer positions to help him find what makes him shine and sparkle!

Gratitude can help children build self-esteem and self-compassion as it can lead to having more positive feelings about themselves. Self-esteem is based on social comparison. When children believe that others think badly of them, they feel bad about themselves. If we can keep a child's subconscious positive, and have the child focus on her positives, it helps build connection through strong and satisfying relationships. Providing the child with the tools to be able to let go of subconscious negativity also builds competence. A child's subconscious immediately thinks positively; the brain is now free to make its own decisions and figure out personal values. When I see that my children are starting to be critical, judgmental, or negative, I have them increase the gratitude prescription.

Start with yourself. Model healthy self-esteem and self-compassion by taking care of yourself. Watch the words that come out of your mouth, and model behaviors you want your child to exhibit. Real self-esteem happens when children are able to let go of the question "Am I good enough?" With gratitude, they are always good enough. Creating a positive child in a world of negativity will take a daily conscious training to change her subconscious. Self-love or self-compassion means treating your own thoughts, actions, and needs with gentleness and caring consideration, instead of criticism, which comes from deep within. Stress the importance of effort and completion of a task rather than how the child performed. Let children know that their

The Four S's to Reinstate Hope and Healing

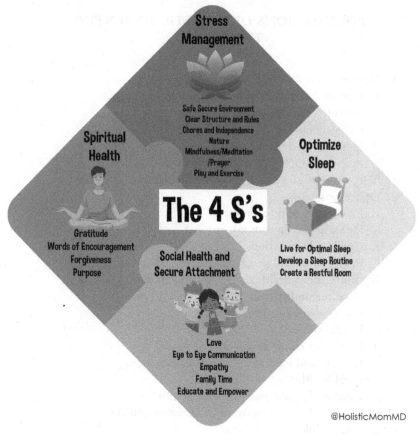

Figure 4.1.

failures don't define them and that setbacks are actually steps forward. Let your children take some risks and make choices on their own. Holistic parenting will create mindful children in control of their subconscious, their thoughts (which are filled with self-compassion and positivity), and their souls; it will foster children who are able to identify their pain and work on converting it into their power and purpose.

There is so much we can do! And I know it can get overwhelming. But no matter who you have in your home, from newborns to teenagers, all these techniques will help improve your parenting efforts. I try to find a way to incorporate these foundations of holistic parenting into my daily life. Once I have a routine, it makes life so much easier. This is so empowering! There is so much we as parents can do for our children and our families. Take it one day at a time, one meal at a time! You've got this!

FOUNDATIONS OF HOLISTIC PARENTING: THE FOUR *S*'s

1. Manage stress
   a. Provide a safe, loving and secure environment.
   b. Provide clear structures and rules.
   c. Delegate chores and responsibilities.
   d. Increase exposure to nature.
   e. Practice mindfulness and meditation.
   f. Recognize the power of play and exercise.
2. Optimize sleep
   a. Live for an optimal snooze.
   b. Develop a sleep routine.
   c. Create a restful room.
   d. Practice mindful sleep training.
3. Optimize social health and secure attachment
   a. Love unconditionally.
   b. Use eye-to-eye communication.
   c. Practice empathy.
   d. Engage in family time.
   e. Educate and empower—mindful awareness.
4. Spiritual health
   a. Change the subconscious with gratitude.
   b. Use words of appreciation and encouragement.
   c. Teach children to forgive.
   d. Help children find purpose.

Part III

THE HOLISTICMOM, MD'S RX: HOLISTIC, FUNCTIONAL, AND INTEGRATIVE APPROACHES TO SICKNESS

Helping Your Child's Body
with Sickness

*A*re you sick and tired of your child being sick and tired? When your child is sick, is not feeling well, or has a chronic illness, it can destroy your world. These symptoms are not something we are "fighting against" because in a war someone has to lose. Instead, these illnesses/symptoms are teachers, educating and nudging us that there is something off balance. Soft signs and symptoms— for example, colic, gas, spitting up, indigestion, congestion, rashes, cough, difficulty breathing, abdominal pain, diarrhea, bloating, constipation or other digestive issues, chronic ear infections, cradle cap, projectile vomiting, fits, tics,

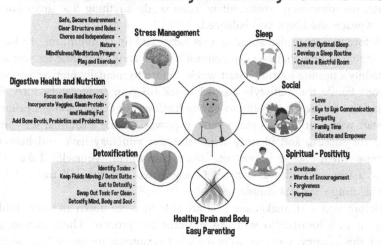

The Holistic Rx for Kids: Healthy Brain and Body to Save Our Future

Safe, Secure Environment ·
Clear Structure and Rules ·
Chores and Independence ·
Nature ·
Mindfulness/Meditation/Prayer ·
Play and Exercise ·

Stress Management

Sleep
· Live for Optimal Sleep
· Develop a Sleep Routine
· Create a Restful Room

Digestive Health and Nutrition
Focus on Real Rainbow Food ·
Incorporate Veggies, Clean Protein ·
and Healthy Fat
Add Bone Broth, Prebiotics and Probiotics ·

Social
· Love
· Eye to Eye Communication
· Empathy
· Family Time
· Educate and Empower

Detoxification
Identify Toxins ·
Keep Fluids Moving / Detox Baths ·
Eat to Detoxify ·
Swap Out Toxic For Clean ·
Detoxify Mind, Body and Soul ·

Spiritual - Positivity
· Gratitude
· Words of Encouragement
· Forgiveness
· Purpose

**Healthy Brain and Body
Easy Parenting**

@HolisticMomMD

Figure 5.1.

sinus issues, or adenoid issues—may be risk factors for development of bigger health problems down the road like autism, autoimmune diseases, or mood disorders. We should be so thankful for these symptoms, as they are our children's bodies talking to us. The body is letting us know to look a little deeper and not to continue business as usual. We just have to listen.

Alongside conventional medical care, when our children's bodies start talking to us, we need to take a deeper look at our lifestyle and environment. What is off balance? The foods? Vitamin deficiencies? Increase in detoxification? The environment? Stress? Sleep? Social health? Negativity? If we work to find out why our children are out of balance, we can help put their little bodies back into balance, thereby working toward healing/improving and preventing acute and chronic symptoms to the best of our ability.

Pure Food, Pure Environment, Pure Thoughts, Pure Words, Pure Friends, Pure Sleep, Positive Thoughts, a Pure Lifestyle = Healthy Mindful Brains and Bodies

---

Keep in Mind

You need to start by first taking care of yourself. You—not just the kids—can do everything we have talked about in this book, and you can do it together as a family. Make sure to always prioritize yourself first, as you can't give from an empty vessel. Make sure to protect your peace. Eat well, meditate, pray, exercise, do something artistic, sit in a sauna: do anything that gives you a sense of peace and keeps you balanced.

Before you start, plan ahead and set a date and find a minimum of a four-week stretch of time that you can commit to dedicating your time for you and your family's healing journey. Start weeks before to mentally prepare yourself and your family for a lifestyle change; stock up your fridge and pantry for success. The first week is going to be the hardest, but then it will get easier.

Start with gratitude, as perspective is power. Create a routine, set yourself up for success, and identify what obstacles you may have and how to overcome them. Most important, don't overwhelm yourself. Take one meal at a time, one day at a time. Going down that list will make it less overwhelming—it's that simple.

Before you start, make sure you are able to write down all your child's symptoms in a journal, so you can monitor the process. Then, as you go through this journey, you can really see what symptoms are improving, which ones are not improving, and which ones are getting worse. Any little step in the right direction is a step in the right direction.

Remember: Your child's symptoms may worsen *first* before they get better.

When your child starts to live a healthier lifestyle by introducing good food/products and removing the bad food/products, the body begins to destroy the pathogenic bacteria and viruses, which release toxins. This leads to worsening of symptoms, which is called die-off reaction. While symptoms can be different for each child, common symptoms of die-off reactions include fatigue, digestive reactions, low-grade nausea, mild headaches, and emotional irritability; these symptoms may last a few days to a few weeks. Epsom salt baths, sea salt, seaweed, and/or sodium bicarbonate (baking soda) and oral vitamin C can help with the die-off reaction and speed up recovery. Add half a cup of Epsom salts, sea salt, or baking soda to the bath water and soak for twenty or thirty minutes. Again, do what you can do easily. If daily is too much, start with whatever you feel comfortable.

Let's start putting your child's body back into balance. Listen to your gut, and start where you think your child needs the most help.

- Optimize digestive health and detoxification—purify your child's food and environment.
- Optimize stress management, sleep, social health, and spiritual health—purify the mind and heart.

OPTIMIZE DIGESTIVE HEALTH AND NUTRITION FOR HEALING

In order to optimize digestion, balance hormones and glucose levels to lower inflammation! Whenever we feed our children, we want to make sure the food we choose will heal our children, not hurt them. We want to make sure that it will lower chronic inflammation, not increase it. Gut healing is important for most children with chronic conditions.

The Gut Rx: Putting Out the Fire in the Gut: A Brief Overview

With 70–80 percent of the immune system and trillions of bacteria residing in the gut, putting out the fire in the gut will give your child's body a fighting chance to heal. Everyone is different, but starting with the key basics and then adjusting as you need to is the best way to go. You will need to first stop putting gasoline on the fire by avoiding all the foods that are likely contributing to your child's imbalances. You'll then take steps to restore a healthy balance of bacteria, replenish nutrients, repair the lining of the gut, and generally rebalance his system.

The Kids' Gut Rx
5 Steps to Put Out the Fire

1. Remove Gasoline
Fake Foods / Processed Foods
- Gluten / Grains
- Dairy
- Processed Foods
- Sugar
- Food Sensitivities
- Infections

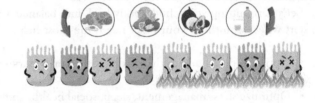

2. Replace
Pure Foods
- Nutrients
- Acid
- Enzymes

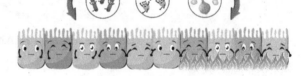

3. Repopulate
- Probiotics
- Prebiotics

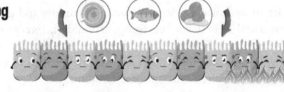

4. Repair Gut Lining
- Bone Broth
- Vitamin D
- Omega 3
- Supplements

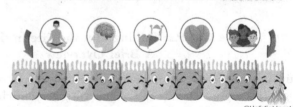

5. Rebalance
- Detoxification
- Stress Management
- Sleep
- Social Support
- Spiritual Health

@HolisticMomMD

Figure 5.2.

The idea of making major changes in your child's diet is very scary, but your child living a life sick all the time is far worse. Give it at least three to four weeks of gut healing by giving the body exactly what it needs to heal. I will briefly outline the steps here. If you would like more information, please take a look at my first book, *The Holistic Rx: Your Guide to Healing Chronic Inflammation and Disease.*

Step 1: Remove What Could Be Bothering Your Child

In order to put out the fire in the gut, we first need to remove *all* the possible offending triggers.

Food

Remember, I know some of these foods I've listed here can seem "healthy," but because we don't know what foods are contributing to problems and which ones aren't, it is best to take them all out. This will take some of the igniter fluid off the fire, allowing it to calm down and then see where you are. Taking them all out at once is a daunting task but will help to heal the child's gut more effectively. This is not forever; once your child feels better, you'll be ready to reintroduce each real food one at a time to see how she is affected. Do what is comfortable for you and your family. If it is too stressful to remove everything, start with eliminating gluten and dairy, as stress can lead to more problems.

With limited stress, start to eliminate the following as best as you can:

- Gluten/Grains
- Dairy
- Sugar
- All toxic foods—for example, nutrient-depleted foods and processed foods. Processed foods are full of poor-quality fats and oils (commercial liquid vegetable oils, hydrogenated oils, and trans fats) and GMOs.
- Specific food sensitivities
- Other fake foods

Most children will start to see improvement of symptoms when they remove these foods. If, after a couple of weeks, you're still not seeing any improvements, examine all the foundations of holistic parenting to see what other pieces are off balance.

If all of those check fine, work with a holistic functional medicine practitioner to locate your child's imbalances; he may even have further food sensitivities. Other problematic foods are beans/legumes (some people do okay
with lentils and navy beans), soy, eggs, nightshades, peanuts and nuts, and
caffeine, as these can lead to inflammation in some people (told you everyone
was different). Other sensitivities to consider are certain foods that may contain histamine, sulfates, salicylate, and oxalates. A practitioner will help you
navigate your child's healing journey. For those who have multiple food sensitivities or who are super frustrated with their condition, I have them follow
the Gut and Psychology Syndrome (GAPS) introduction diet without dairy.

Remove Infections

Some children/teens can have an overgrowth of microbes that are contributing to their symptoms, so removing these infections are important, as they can
increase intestinal inflammation. Have your functional medicine practitioner
look for pathogens like viruses, parasites, yeast, and even small intestinal bac-
terial/fungal overgrowth (SIBO/SIFO: good bacteria/fungus in the wrong
place).

Once you know what your child is dealing with, there are pharmaceutical or natural combinations—for example, berberine (active against *Candida
albicans* and *Staphylococcus aureus*), wormwood, caprylic acid, grapefruit seed
extract (antimicrobial and antifungal), garlic (active against bacteria, fungi,
viruses, and parasites), oregano oil, and peppermint oil.

Step 2: Replenish with Pure Food and the Ability to Digest

Next it's time to restore and replenish the vitamins, minerals, nutrients, and
essential ingredients for proper digestion and absorption that might have been
depleted by an impure diet or lifestyle and/or medications. To do this, incorporate healing real foods and replacing any deficiencies necessary for digestion.

Replenish with Healing Rainbow Food

The following need to be included into your child's diet (the more color, the
better):

- Vegetables
- Clean protein
- Healthy fat
- Bone broth

- Fermented foods (if tolerated)
- Herbs/spices
- Water

Bone broth and collagen are rich in bioavailable, easily absorbed minerals like calcium, magnesium, phosphorus, silicon, and sulfur as well as amino acids like L-glutamine (energy source for the intestinal cells), glucosamine, chondroitin, collagen gelatin, proline, and glycine. These nutrients are necessary to repair, seal, soothe, and restore gut mucosal lining and lower inflammation. Give your child at least one cup a day of bone broth.

Optimize the Ability to Digest

If your child is putting in the effort to eat healing rainbow foods, you also need to make sure she is actually digesting the foods she is eating. Digestive bitters, lemon water, and apple cider vinegar can help boost stomach acid, which is necessary for an optimal digestion. If your child needs more help with digesting, it is best to talk to a functional medicine doctor who can help you find out whether your child is even making enough stomach acid or whether she may need extra digestive support with digestive enzymes. The practitioner may check for optimal stomach acid with a baking soda test.

Step 3: Repopulate

Restoring the balance of good bacteria in the gut is absolutely crucial to overall health. Probiotics (helpful bacteria) and prebiotics packed with fiber and resistant starches will help cultivate your child's microbiome or inner garden.

Probiotics can be found in fermented foods such as unpasteurized natural sauerkraut, pickles, miso, and kimchi. They're also found in yogurt and kefir, but these are dairy products, so your child won't be eating them during this phase, as most don't tolerate them. Probiotics support the gut; improve nutrient absorption; reduce inflammation; nourish the cells in the colon and liver; create new compounds like B vitamins, vitamin K2, antioxidants, and enzymes; and lower the number of harmful pathogens like candida, fungi, and parasites. Food is the best way to get probiotics and, in some cases, the only way to get certain bugs like *Akkermansia*.

Prebiotics are "food" for probiotics. They optimize gut healing, decrease inflammation, and nourish and stimulate the growth of "good" bacteria while promoting the reduction in disease-causing bacteria. They work with the probiotics to optimize gut healing. Children should be eating their prebiotics, found in green leafy vegetables and other high-fiber foods, which are especially good at promoting growth of good bacteria; they also should eat asparagus, carrots, garlic, leeks, raw onions, radishes, avocados, broccoli, Brussels sprouts, cucumber, nuts/seeds, lentils, and tomatoes, as well as resistant starches like inulin and root vegetables. It is important to increase the biodiversity of the microbiome by exposing your family to the external world around them and the soil.

Step 4: Repair

Repairing the gut lining is important to ensure proper absorption of nutrients and gut function. Eat lots of food that will help repair the gut lining—for example, foods with zinc (lean beef and poultry, nuts such as cashews and almonds), vitamin A (carrots, dark leafy greens, winter squash, lettuce, dried apricots, cantaloupe, bell peppers, fish, liver, tropical fruits), vitamin C (bell peppers, dark leafy greens, kiwi, broccoli, berries, citrus fruits), vitamin D (sardines canned in oil, beef liver, egg yolks, or cod liver oil), omega-3, vitamin E, and selenium, which improves inflammation and heals the gut lining. As I've said before, I recommend that your child starts drinking bone broth. Find what best works for you; most children do well on a pure gut-healing diet with simply bone broth, fish oil, and probiotics. You can also include the following supplements (talk to your functional medicine practitioner about the correct supplement and dosage for your child):

Digestive enzymes: For children younger than five years old, you can add a pinch of digestive enzyme powder with each meal; for children older than five, you can add ½ teaspoon with each meal.

Glutamine powder: If your child is older than four years old, you can give 1.5 grams of glutamine powder twice daily with meals. Supplements should be added slowly and gradually, as some children with autism may regress with certain supplements like B12, GABA, or glutamate. Glutamine helps preserve the gut lining by lowering inflammation. L-glutamine can be found in bone broth and animal proteins, as well as raw spinach, red cabbage, and parsley.

Other supplements include Restore or ion biome, zinc carnosine (30 milligrams per day), colostrum powder, turmeric, slippery elm (200 milligrams per day), aloe vera (100 milligrams per day), licorice root, DGL (500 milligrams per day, specifically for leaky gut exacerbated by emotional stress), frankincense (an essential oil that helps heal leaky gut and lower inflammation), quercetin (500 milligrams three times per day with meals), chamomile, organic sulfur compounds, methylsulfonylmethane (MSM), boswellia powder, marshmallow root (100 milligrams per day), butyric acid or butyrate, and plantain.

Step 5: Rebalance by Living a Pure Life

Rebalancing by living a pure lifestyle—which includes detoxification, stress management, and optimizing sleep, social health, and spiritual health—can lower inflammation and aid in gut healing. Focus on activities that will add diversity of microbes from the soil to balance the microbiome and lower stress. Activities like gardening, spending time walking barefoot outside (which will help improve sleep, raise energy, and lower inflammation by stabilizing the internal bioelectrical environment), spending time in nature, and even getting a pet will diversify the microbiome.

Reintroducing Foods

Is your child really starting to miss certain real foods that were previously part of his diet? Are you at a point where his symptoms have improved or resolved enough that you want to start to reintroduce some pure food back into his diet? If symptoms haven't improved, I recommend that your child stay on the healing diet and consult with a holistic or functional health care practitioner. Healing takes time; it all depends on your child's condition and how long you have been dealing with the symptoms.

For those who are ready, start with the food that your child misses the most and have her eat that food in the purest form for a couple of days and notice how she feels. It's very important to reintroduce one food at a time and to pay careful attention to whether the symptoms return. That way, if she does have symptoms, you'll know exactly what food caused them, and she can choose to give up that food until further in her healing journey. If she has no reaction to the food, then she can move on to the next food. Sensitivities can take up to seventy-two hours to manifest—it is important to wait and see whether symptoms develop.

A relapse (meaning that your child's symptoms return) may happen because your child has eaten a food to which he's sensitive, or it may happen despite being on a good diet, as deficits in any of the other processes we talked about in part II may induce relapse. If your child relapses, it's okay. Take a deep breath, and think about all the positives that have come out of this healing journey. Slowly start to take a look at your child's life and see what could be out of balance. If his symptoms are not improving, then you may need to go back to the beginning of the Gut Rx above, start a stricter and more structured gut-healing approach (like the GAPS introduction diet without dairy), and see a functional medicine practitioner. A short-term gut-healing diet is better than a lifetime of pain and suffering!

LIVE IN A PURE ENVIRONMENT TO HEAL

Because our children literally are environmental sponges, cleaning up their environment is especially important. Identify what the toxic items in their environment can be, help them make sure their bodily fluids are moving, help them eat to detoxify, and swap out toxic cleaners for more natural products just like we discussed in chapter 3. Heavy metal detoxification is very important for improving autism, PANDAS (an acute-onset neuropsychiatric syndrome), or other chronic conditions. Optimizing gut health, limiting the daily toxin exposure, and even introducing integrative modalities (like homeopathy) will help protect against any adverse effects of vaccines.

Some children might need extra help to figure out what is leading to problems. One common and overlooked problem that bothers so many is mold.

Mold

If after a couple months your child still does not feel adequate, despite doing all the above, or perhaps if your child develops an autoimmunity, mold might be causing inflammation. Symptoms may include depression and other mood disorders, attention-deficit/hyperactivity disorder (ADHD), skin rashes, headaches, autoimmunity, sleep issues, fibromyalgia, or fatigue.

Mold can be found under floorboards, anywhere there's a crack in the wall or window frame, or in the carpet, making it even harder to detect. Mold is most common in damp and humid areas like the bathroom and basement, especially in older homes and in homes with basements, known leaks, crawl spaces, and flat roofs, as well as those built on a hillside. Some molds are easy to detect, like black mold, but others are not so easy to find. Mold can also be ingested, like on pistachios, cashews, peanuts, aged cheese, vinegars, pickled foods, dried fruit, and mushrooms.

Sometimes it is best to find a mold-free place to stay for a while and see whether your child feels better. If she does feel better away from home, and worse when your family returns home, your child could be reacting to mycotoxins. If this is the case, all the approaches in this book will be helpful. Testing is tricky, as the typical mold test only focuses on the air quality and the level of mold spores. Find a functional medicine physician who will be able to access this testing for your family in more detail.

OPTIMIZING STRESS MANAGEMENT, SLEEP, SOCIAL HEALTH, AND SPIRITUAL HEALTH

Managing Stress

Make sure you incorporate a stress management technique, an exercise routine, and time in nature to really optimize healing. Take a deep dive into your child's emotional health. See whether there is anything bothering her at school; talk to her friends to find out what could be leading to her stresses. Trauma can also lead to a lot of chronic conditions; investigate trauma and get her help to address this underlying issue. Your child is developing and learning, and this is the best time to instill lifelong coping mechanisms to increase resilience in life. When she is at an appropriate age, teach her prayer and abdominal breathing with mindful meditation.

Optimizing Sleep

Sleep is key to the healing process, so if your child is having problems with sleep, you need to figure out the underlying root cause of why he is not sleeping. Has this been a short- or long-term problem? Is there something in the bedroom or bed? Could it be a medication that can lead to sleep problems? Antidepressants, cold and flu medications that contain alcohol, pain relievers that contain caffeine (Midol, Excedrin), diuretics, corticosteroids, thyroid hormones, high blood pressure medications (beta blockers, calcium channel blockers), anticonvulsants, bronchodilators, decongestants, and stimulants can all lead to problems. Remember a sleep routine is critical for children.

Social Health

The people around your children can either make them or break them, so try to surround them with friends and family who will lift them up and not drag them down. Help them understand their "big" feelings, and help them find ways to cope (for example, cognitive behavioral therapy and nature).

Spiritual Health

This is probably the most important part of your child's healing journey. More often than not, a mother or patient will walk into my office for a follow-up visit and say, "Nothing is getting better!" Then, as I go through the child's initial list of symptoms, I realize that, indeed, most of the symptoms have improved!

If your child is constantly focusing on what is going wrong in his life, then it is very difficult for her to improve. This problem happens to parents, too, who then project it onto the child. Change the perspective, and that will bring healing. Immediately when your child wakes up in the morning, have her say ten things she is grateful for every day. We need to shift our negative world to a world where we are thankful.

Find an Integrative, Holistic, Functional Medicine Physician

Find a practitioner through a referral from a friend, family member, or your conventional doctor. It is key to always check a potential practitioner's education and credentials. To get more information about the practitioner and inquire whether he has expertise with kids, set up a pre-appointment phone call or make an appointment for a consultation.

FIX YOUR CHILD'S DEFICIENCIES

Living a healthy life and boosting immunity always begins with diet, and this step can't be replaced. Supplements can give your child the extra push in the right direction toward healing; they will support the immune system, allowing it to be healthy and balanced.

Nutritional deficiencies can interfere with your child getting better, so supplementing can give her the extra boost she needs to expedite healing. With our toxic conventional and commercial farming practices, the standard American diet is full of processed foods and low on microbial diversity; additionally, increased stress and toxins can decrease nutrient absorption and increase inflammation.

Medications can also lead to deficiencies; examples include the following:

- Proton pump inhibitors and H2 receptor antagonists cause depletions of beneficial flora; calcium; digestive enzymes; folic acid; B12; vitamins C, D, E, and K; biotin; chromium; and zinc.
- Antidepressant medications like SSRIs diminish melatonin, iodine, selenium, and folate. Do not give your child St. John's wort, 5-HTP, or SAMe without talking to his health care provider first. Other antidepressants diminish B2 and CoQ10.
- Oral contraceptive pills diminish vitamins B2, B5, B6, B12, and C; folate; magnesium; tyrosine; and zinc. Do not drink grapefruit juice

while on an oral contraceptive, as it can increase estrogen levels up to 30 percent.

- Antibiotics deplete good bacteria; vitamins B1, B2, B6, B3, and B12; vitamin K (if the antibiotic is taken for more than ten days); calcium; magnesium; and potassium.
- Blood pressure–lowering medication diminishes calcium; vitamins B6, B1, and C; zinc; sodium; potassium; and magnesium.
- Thyroid replacements like Synthroid diminish calcium.

How to Choose a Supplement

Vitamins and supplements are generally safe when used as directed, but taking high amounts can be very toxic. Water-soluble supplements can be excreted out into the urine, but fat-soluble vitamins like A, K, E, and D can gradually accumulate and lead to overdoses. Consuming a high number of supplements can lead to serious side effects.

If you decide to supplement, remember that the supplement industry is largely unregulated, so be sure you're using products made with integrity—and always read labels. Especially when it comes to children and teens, you want to make sure that you discuss dosages and supplements with your holistic functional medicine practitioner. More is not better—do not exceed the recommended dosage.

You want to make sure the brand is known for quality; look for large reputable brands and FDA approval. Make sure it is third-party tested and follows good manufacturing practices. Check for the initials USP, GMP, or NSF, to make sure the product doesn't contain additives, synthetic ingredients, or colorings. Purchasing from supplement companies that use organic ingredients is an added bonus. Check the expiration date and make sure the product is fresh. Make sure it is specifically formulated for your child/teen. Your best insurance is to purchase supplements from natural health stores or through a health care provider properly educated in quality, professional supplements.

Let's start with the key four supplements that will help put your child back into balance, boost immunity, and lower inflammation. As always, before beginning any new supplement program, check with your child's health care practitioner.

Vitamin D

Vitamin D is an interesting vitamin or prohormone that is an essential precursor to hundreds of disease-preventing proteins and enzymes; it binds to many receptors, causing changes to cell function. We make D3 as the sunlight hits our skin. When this happens, the liver and kidneys transform the vitamin D into a more active form, allowing our cells to read DNA instructions more effectively, which is important for our genetic code. Vitamin D regulates vital components of hormones and neurotransmitters like serotonin, helps control cell growth, is a cancer fighter, is essential in mineral metabolism, is a major player in bone strength, and regulates absorption and transport of calcium, magnesium, and phosphorus for bone mineralization and growth. Vitamin D is a disease preventer; it is vital in decreasing inflammation and lowering insulin resistance.

A study of more than six thousand American children showed that seven in ten of them have low levels of vitamin D.[1] Deficiencies of vitamin D can lead to problems in children, starting prenatally. A study showed that mothers' vitamin D levels during pregnancy were associated with their children's IQ, suggesting that higher vitamin D levels in pregnancy may lead to greater childhood IQ scores.[2] The risk of ADHD was 34 percent higher in children whose mothers had a vitamin D deficiency during pregnancy than in those children whose mothers' vitamin D level was sufficient during the first and second trimesters. The result was adjusted for maternal age, socioeconomic status, and psychiatric history.[3] A University of Michigan team study determined that low levels of vitamin D in elementary school could be linked to children's aggressive behavior as well as anxious and depressive moods during adolescence. The research team recruited about 3,202 children between the ages of five and twelve, and they found that children with low vitamin D levels were twice as likely to develop externalizing behavior problems (e.g., rule breaking and aggression).[4]

Vitamin D has many benefits for children, as it supports the immune system, helps balance hormones, and stabilizes mood. It improves symptoms of autism[5] and mood disorders, optimizes brain development and bone health, and supports healthy sleep. Vitamin D supplements support immune function in those children with autoimmune diseases, and they also can decrease the risk of childhood respiratory infections. Most patients are deficient in vitamin D. We look for a range of about 50–80 milligrams per milliliter to optimize health. It is best to have your child's physician check his vitamin D 25-OH lab value. If you work closely with a professional, she can prescribe the appropriate dose to quickly increase your child's vitamin D level.

Always make sure you and your child take vitamin D3, as vitamin D2 isn't metabolized by the body. A child needs vitamin D from two months old onward. Start at the age of two months with 400 IU per day. Once it is optimized, continuing on a dosage about twenty times the child's weight in pounds daily (or 2,000–4,000 IU per day) is appropriate. A vitamin D overdose is rare but possible, as a high vitamin D level (greater than 150 milligrams per milliliter) leads to excessively high calcium in the bloodstream, kidney damage, and even psychosis. Remember to take vitamin D and other fat-soluble vitamins with meals containing fats. Be cautious with vitamin D if you have hyperparathyroidism, Hodgkin's or non-Hodgkin's lymphoma, granulomatous disease (like sarcoidosis and tuberculosis), kidney stones, kidney disease, or liver disease. Foods that are also rich in vitamin D include sea vegetables, fish (especially sardines, salmons, and mackerel), beef liver, some cheeses, mushrooms like portobellos, eggs, raw milk, and cod liver oil.

Cod liver oil provides docosahexaenoic acid (DHA), vitamins A and D3, and, to a lesser extent, vitamins K and E (which help in the absorption and utilization of minerals and nutrients and help fight inflammation) because it is fermented, which preserves the essential oils in the fish. Some children don't tolerate vitamin D supplementation and do better with cod liver oil. Since fermented cod liver oil has twice the vitamin A and D3 of regular cod liver oil, only half the amount is needed. Doses of cod liver oil depend on the weight of the child. For children who weigh 25 pounds, give ¼ teaspoon per day; at 25 pounds to 35 pounds, give ⅓ teaspoon per day; at 35 pounds to 45 pounds, give ½ teaspoon per day; and at 45 pounds to 55 pounds, give ⅔ teaspoon per day. For anyone weighing more than 55 pounds, give 1 teaspoon per day. If you're not using fermented, I recommend butter oil in conjunction with a high-vitamin cod liver oil.

Magnesium

Magnesium is an essential mineral especially for nerve cells, muscles, and bones and has a major role in immunity. About 75–80 percent of the U.S. population is deficient in magnesium because of our acidic diet and constant fluoride exposure.[6] Cells need magnesium to work, including more than three hundred enzymes and hundreds of body processes that use or synthesize ATP, DNA, and RNA, which are cofactors in methylation and detoxification. Magnesium is vital in muscular contractions; production of testosterone and progesterone; production and utilization of fat, protein, and carbohydrates; and metabolism of calcium, sodium, and potassium. It is also a constituent of bone and teeth. Deficiencies have been linked to behavior issues in adolescents,[7] ADHD, and autism spectrum disorders.[8] Even though magnesium glycinate, chelate, and maleate are the best absorbed, magnesium citrate is great for constipation and sleep issues. Take the magnesium and calcium at least two hours apart from a multivitamin/mineral supplement. The daily requirements for children are birth to six months, 30 milligrams per day; six months to one year, seventy-five milligrams per day; one to three years, eighty milligrams per day; four to eight years, 130 milligrams per day; nine to thirteen, 240 milligrams per day; boys aged fourteen to eighteen, 410 milligrams per day; and girls aged fourteen to eighteen, 360 milligrams per day. Sources of magnesium are green leaves (e.g., frozen spinach or Swiss chard), avocados, dark chocolate, artichoke hearts, almonds, cashews, pumpkin and squash seeds, salmon, halibut, and meat.

Fish Oil

Fish oils are rich in essential fatty acids, like omega-3 and omega-6 fatty acids, which are needed for our cell membranes to work; fatty acids can't be produced by our body, so we need to consume them. These play a key role in growth and development, and they are associated with numerous health benefits.[9] Their use has been beneficial for a wide array of medical conditions. Sixty percent of a child's brain weight is made up of fat, and 25 percent of that fat is docosahexaenoic acid (DHA). A child's little body needs DHA to make myelin, and eicosapentaenoic acid (EPA), which is deficient in most of us, is very helpful in lowering inflammation.

Omega-3s are predominantly anti-inflammatory, as they reduce the expression of inflammatory genes and molecules in the body. Essential fatty acids (specifically omega-3s) help improve your child's immune system, heart health, and blood chemistry; promote brain health; improve symptoms of ADHD;[10] reduce asthma;[11] and lower triglycerides and increase HDL ("good") cholesterol.[12] Fatty acids also improve insulin sensitivity; protect against depression, digestive disorders, and arthritis; improve sleep;[13] improve skin, nail, and hair strength; increase nutrient absorption; improve fertility; and prevent and heal chronic disease by lowering inflammation.[14] An eight-week study of thirty-three boys linked doses between 400 milligrams and 1,200 milligrams of DHA daily to an increase in activation of the prefrontal cortex.[15]

Omega-3 foods are cold-water fatty fish like sardines, herring, wild-caught salmon, lake trout, mackerel, shellfish, clams, oysters, mussels, pasture-raised chickens, grass-fed meat (grass-fed beef has fewer omega-6s compared with soybean- or corn-fed cattle), antelope, shrimp, squid, eggs, walnuts, and flax and chia seeds. DHA is found in algae. If you are a vegetarian, eating a seaweed salad or a seaweed supplement with DHA is an effective way to benefit from omega-3s.

Always be sure to get fish oil that's clear of heavy metals, PCBs, pesticides, and other toxins, because if the fish was contaminated, then the fish oil is contaminated. Omega-3 causes platelet inhibition, so common side effects can be belching, halitosis, heartburn, nausea, loose stools, rash, increased bleeding, and bruising (mostly seen with 3 grams or more a day).

Remember, everyone is different, and you know your child better than anyone else. Find a practitioner who will work with you to explore what works for your child and what doesn't.

Probiotics

Probiotics are key to overall mental and physical health, as we discussed in detail above. They can be given to babies born via C-section and/or babies who have had a history of yeast, antibiotics, or steroids during pregnancy, labor, or while nursing. Probiotics can also be considered if there is a family history of increased intestinal permeability issues, like autoimmunity or metabolic syndrome, or if the child has had a lot of stressors or has a poor diet; otherwise, babies normally get enough probiotics from breast milk.

Probiotics can be given to a baby as early as a few years old. They can come in liquid or powdered forms and can be directly put in the child's mouth or in the formula milk. Dosage depends on age:

- Infant up to twelve months: 1–2 billion bacterial cells per day
- One to two years of age: 2–4 billion per day
- Two to four years of age: 4–8 billion per day
- Four to twelve years of age: 8–12 billion per day
- Twelve to sixteen years of age: 12–15 billion per day

Look for a mixture with at least ten strains, like lactobacilli (especially rhamnosus GG [shown to decrease eczema, allergies, and asthma], acidophilus, reuteri, plantarum, and brevis), bifidobacteria (infantis [strain most commonly found in infants], bifidum, longem, and lactis), and soil-based organisms, such as endospore probiotics like *Bacillus subtilis* and *Bacillus coagulans*. You can even change them every three to six months, but remember that the probiotic foods are key to optimizing gut health. If a child is dealing with small intestinal bacterial overgrowth, spore-forming probiotics are best. *Saccharomyces boulardii* is a good yeast that fights the bad yeast, so it can be used in situations of fungal overgrowth in a child. Look for a shelf-stable product that contains soil-based organisms that ensure the probiotic actually makes it into the gut to colonize. Avoid gummies. Probiotics are taken typically first thing in the morning before breakfast.

Remember, healing is a journey, not a destination. Focus on all the symptoms that are improving. Believe me, if you focus on that one symptom that isn't improving, your child will never get better. Any improvement is better than no improvement. Patience is key—it doesn't happen overnight, and everyone is different. I have seen seventy-year-olds improve in a week and autistic kids start speaking the day after they started this diet, but then I have also seen people with autoimmune disease take four or more years to heal (myself included), so it can take time. It may initially be a struggle, but you can educate your child, empower him, love him, give him hope, and put him back into balance. Never give up; there is so much hope. You and your child deserve a life filled with health and happiness!

· 6 ·

Testing and Integrative Modalities
for Healing

Children hate needles—actually, so do adults—but testing can help parents determine what their children's specific needs are and what the potential systemic causes may be for their chronic health conditions. Every child is different, so we need to look for your child's personal puzzle pieces that could be off balance. In one child, it might be gut issues, other mitochondrial issues, heavy metal issues, methylation issues, B vitamin issues, toxins, other nutrient deficiencies, or chronic infections. Lab tests will help guide the practitioner on which road to take to optimize your child's health.

LAB TESTS

Once you have found a health care practitioner who is willing to listen and spend the time to investigate your child's issues, work with the practitioner to get an initial set of lab tests. This will help you address your child's individual deficiencies and issues. The following tests are ones I always start with for all my patients. Your child's primary care doctor should feel comfortable ordering these tests; however, the doctor might give you a hard time, as it is not "standard of care" to check a child's blood work, so find one who can help you. If coded appropriately, most insurance plans cover them.

Now remember, there is a difference between optimal and normal. Optimal is what the body functions best at, and normal is anywhere within that large range that doesn't classify as low or high. I have provided the target/optimal ranges that I use and the interventions I typically recommend for my patients. You will see the ranges are similar to adults. Every individual is different, so always discuss results with your child's functional medicine practitioner,

149

as your child's personal physician may work with slightly different targets/ optimal ranges and interventions. Your child is unique and may require refinement of these recommendations based on his personal health circumstances.

The baseline labs I get on my pediatric patients are CBC, CMP, fasting insulin, fasting lipids, ferritin, homocysteine, hsCRP, vitamin D, HbA1c, TSH and thyroid antibodies, ANA, B12, and magnesium. See table 6.1 for interpretations of these tests.

Table 6.1. Labs and Interpretation

Labs	Optimal Fasting Levels	Interpretation/ Suggested Intervention
Complete Blood Count (CBC)	Normal values for the target range	If the hemoglobin levels become low, anemia and other abnormalities will need to be ruled out. Gut healing needs to be stressed.
Comprehensive Metabolic Profile (CMP)	Normal values for the target range: Fasting glucose: less than 90 mg/dL Calcium: less than 10 mg/dL	If fasting glucose is elevated, insulin resistance management is stressed, with lower refined carbohydrate intake. If calcium is higher than 10 mg/dL, carefully dose vitamin D to prevent parathyroid issues. If liver tests are elevated, look for other causes and improve your child's insulin resistance, if applicable.
Thyroid Stimulating Hormone (TSH)	Ideally less than 2.5 mIU/mL	If abnormal, work with a physician to find the underlying root cause and proper treatment options.
Free T4; Free T3; Reverse T3; TPO Antibody; Antithyroglobulin Antibody	Free T4 > 1.1 ng/dL Free T3 >3.2 pg/mL Reverse T3 <10:1 ratio RT3 to FT3 TPO antibody <9 IU/ mL or negative ATA <4 IU/mL or negative	If elevated, address autoimmunity and root causes. If reverse T3 is elevated, it can be due to excessive exercise, starvation diets, stress, or heavy metals.
Magnesium	More than 2 mg/dL	There isn't a great test to check the exact levels in the blood. But we can get a sense that your child is deficient. If it is less, you might need to supplement.
25-Hydroxy Vitamin D (vitamin D25-OH)	50–80 ng/mL	Adjust vitamin D dose up or down according to level. There are multiple ways to dose vitamin D; work with your child's doctor to determine how much supplemental vitamin D your child will need. Too much can be toxic, as it is stored in the liver; continue to monitor every few months.

Labs	Optimal Fasting Levels	Interpretation/ Suggested Intervention
Folate and Vitamin B12	In the top quartile of the reference (range for that lab) B12 >500 pg/mL	Interpret with homocysteine; if it is low, you will need to work with your child's doctor to supplement.
Homocysteine	4–8 mcmol/L	If elevated, add B complex with B12, folate, and B6. See a functional medicine practitioner for guidance. If low, add more protein to your child's diet.
Highly Sensitive C-Reactive Protein (hsCRP)	Less than 1.0 mg/L = low risk (ideal); 1–3 mg/L = intermediate risk; greater than 3 mg/L = high risk	If high, follow the foundations of holistic parenting and the HolisticMom, MD's Rx and see your child's practitioner for further guidance. Following a gut healing protocol will help improve the inflammation. Stress can also lead to elevated hsCRP, so it is important to incorporate a relaxation technique into your child's daily routine.
Fasting Lipids	Triglyceride/HDL cholesterol ratio less than 3	A ratio greater than 3 indicates probable insulin resistance. Decrease processed carbohydrate intake. This may indicate need for more fish oil.
HDL Cholesterol (good cholesterol)	HDL cholesterol greater than, 60 mg/dL	If HDL is less than 60, decrease carbohydrates, increase vegetables and berries and other low glycemic foods, increase fish oil, and increase exercise.
Fasting Insulin	Less than 10 mIU/L	If higher, concentrate lowering insulin resistance by following a low glycemic diet and intermittent fasting.
HbA1c	Less than 5.4 percent	If higher, concentrate on lowering insulin resistance.
Antinuclear Antibodies	Negative	For all autoimmunity, gut healing and looking for root causes are very important. If positive, discuss with your child's doctor.

Note: IU = international unit; mIU/mL = microIU/milliliter; mIU/L = microIU/liter; mg/dL = milligram/deciliter; ng/dL = nanogram/deciliter; pg/mL = picogram/milliliter; mcmol/L = micromole/liter; mg/L = milligram/liter.

LET'S TAKE IT A STEP FURTHER

Sometimes it is very overwhelming, and you need help. A functional medicine or holistic practitioner, nutritionist, or health coach will help you figure out the right food/lifestyle plan for you and your child. It is important to work with your child's doctor to assess food allergies/sensitivities and supplements/medications to support organ function, any persistent infections, individual gut imbalances (with a GI test), toxic load/liver detoxification/heavy metal poisoning, mold exposure, hormone regulation, and sometimes your child's specific genetic profile, to tailor the specific plan that will work best for your child.

Let's discuss some of these tests.

Gut Testing and Food Sensitivities

To help guide treatment, there are a number of testing methods for gut issues; some of these tests have been around for decades, and others are very new. I always start out with the cheapest option—listening to your child's body or taking a thorough history. A diagnostic stool evaluation is a noninvasive test to evaluate the gut microbiome to look for candida or yeast, any imbalances of good and bad bacteria, and parasites. The test will also evaluate immune markers—for example, secretory IgA (an antibody that is the first line of defense in our gut against infection); if your child's level is low, she is unable to produce this antibody, which signifies that she has an immune dysfunction. A lactose breath test or hydrogen or methane breath test can check for SIBO (small intestinal bacterial overgrowth); the leaky gut and organic acids test reveals vitamin and mineral deficiencies, as well as some sense of bacterial balance and presence of yeast. IgG and IgE tests can check for food sensitivities. Once you find out what your child is sensitive to, you can try to avoid that for a certain amount of time; also add in a gut-healing diet, so you can continue the healing process.

Nutritional Evaluation

Is your child getting enough nutrients? These tests can help determine whether he is getting enough of the nutrients he needs for optimal detoxification, mitochondrial function, and overall body function. Nutrients and mitochondrial function tests are critical to know how our children's brains and bodies function. For example, organic acid testing can look at mitochondrial function and the way your child processes energy. Nutritional evaluations can look at the nutrient levels for overall health, as well as mitochondrial and detoxification function. Other nutrient levels can be deficient, like omega-3, zinc, magnesium, B vitamins, vitamin A, vitamin D, and so many more.

Vitamin values in the following list are the minimum a child should take. Depending on the level of deficiency, the doctor will prescribe the dosage needed to correct it, so always consult with your practitioner before giving children supplements. It is best to get these nutrients through foods.

Calcium: Calcium is important for bones. Children aged four to eight years need 1,000 milligrams per day; children aged nine to thirteen need 1,300 milligrams per day. Accompany calcium with vitamin K and vitamin D.

Iron: Iron is important for blood cell, brain, and nerve formation. Children aged four to eight need 10 milligrams per day; children aged nine to thirteen only need 8 milligrams per day. Sources include chicken liver, shellfish, red meat, spinach, cashews, lentils, and beans, combined with vitamin C foods.

Zinc: Zinc is important for the immune system. Children aged four to eight need 5 milligrams per day; children aged nine to thirteen need 8 milligrams per day. Sources of zinc are oysters, crab, and red meat.

Vitamin A: Vitamin A is important for the eyes, bones, skin, and immune and neurological function. Recommended Dietary Allowance (RDA) levels of vitamin A are as follows: birth to six months, 400 micrograms per day; seven to twelve months, 500 micrograms per day; one to three years, 300 micrograms per day; four to eight years, 400 micrograms per day; nine to thirteen years, 600 micrograms per day; fourteen to eighteen years, 900 micrograms per day. Tolerable Upper Intake Levels (UL) for vitamin A have been established, and it is the highest level of intake that is likely to have no risk of harmful effect. Children aged birth to three need 600 micrograms per day (2,000 units); four to eight need 900 micrograms per day (3,000 units); nine to thirteen need 1,700 micrograms per day (5,667 units); and fourteen to eighteen receive 2,800 micrograms per day (9,333 units). Sources include butternut squash, kale, carrots, sweet potatoes, broccoli, spinach, and beef liver.

Vitamin B12: Vitamin B12 is important for the nervous system, growth, mood, heart health, hair, and skin. Children aged four to eight need 1.2 micrograms per day; children aged nine to thirteen need 1.8 micrograms per day. Sources of B12 include cage-free eggs, grass-fed meat, wild-caught fish, organ meats, and shellfish.

Vitamin C: Vitamin C supports collagen formation, heart health, skin, and immune function. Children aged four to eight need 25 milligrams per day; children aged nine to thirteen need 45 milligrams per day. Sources include fruits and vegetables (for example, kiwi, oranges, bell peppers, broccoli, papaya, pineapple, kale, broccoli sprouts, cauliflower, mango, and spinach).

Environmental Toxins

Environmental toxic tests can determine your child's overall toxic load. Is your child being exposed to something in his environment that is putting him out of balance? There are so many tests to see what exact toxin your child may be exposed to. For those with high toxic load, it may be beneficial to add supplements to optimize healing. As discussed previously, probiotics and digestive enzymes (specifically with lipase) optimize gut healing and improve digestion of fats. Glutathione, or N-acetyl cysteine—along with vitamin C and a liver support blend with alpha lipoic acid and milk thistle—can be taken on an empty stomach. If you do suspect mold, clean up the air with an air filter that will filter ultra-tiny particles. Avoid peanuts, raisins, dried fruit, nuts, coffee, and alcohol and focus on a low mold diet. But also carefully clean out the home with tea tree oil, distilled white vinegar, and grapefruit extract, including air ducts. Increase the detox practices (e.g., infrared saunas, IV detoxification, and neti pot), and increase alkaline water, dry brushing, and even detox supplements (glutathione, milk thistle, calcium d-gluconate, alpha lipoic acid, glycine, glutamine, taurine, n-acetyl cysteine [NAC], and such). Hire a certified mold remediator. Sometimes detox binders may be needed. Be cautious with supplements grown on aspergillus, medicinal mushrooms, saccharomyces, and kombucha. If you feel your child has a high toxic load, it can be very difficult to do a detox program on your own, so find a professional.

Chronic Infections

Especially if your child still continues to experience symptoms, it is important to look into chronic infections. Certain microbes are associated with certain autoimmune conditions. A functional medicine practitioner can test your child and treat her (with pharmaceuticals, nutraceuticals, or both) for the type of microbe that could be associated with her condition. Common ones could be a chronic viral infection, which can hide dormant and can become activated and trigger an inflammatory response.

Viruses like herpes simplex (e.g., 1, 2, 6), Epstein-Barr virus, hepatitis, and certain bacterial infections can go along with autoimmune conditions, including yersinia enterocolitica, H. pylori, SIBO/SIFO, Chlamydia pneumoniae, bartonella, mycobacterium avium subspecies paratuberculosis (MAP), mycoplasma, streptococcus, and babesia and borrelia burgdorferi (Lyme), as well as fungal infections like candida and parasitic infections like toxoplasmosis and blastocystitis hominis. If your child has been diagnosed with a bacterial infection, the practitioner may need a combination treatment that includes antibiotics, probiotics, and/or antimicrobial herbs like monolaurin (acid derived from coconut oil), humic acid, L-lysine, olive leaf extract, biocidin, oil of oregano, garlic, colloidal silver, and other microbial herbs. Healing foods and supplements for Lyme include thyme, lemon balm, zinc, licorice root, L-lysine, lomatium root, reishi mushroom, silver hydrosol, astaxanthin, and ascent iodine.

Genetic Testing

A professional can also test your child's genes to identify what genes are not working well. This test will help guide the practitioner to a specific nutritional plan and targeted nutrients your child might need. A professional can test for genetic mutations/variations or other errors in liver detoxification that can also slow recovery, like single nucleotide polymorphisms (SNPs), for example, MTHFR (no, I didn't just swear), GSTMI, and COMT SNP gene mutations. Children can also have genetic variations in B vitamin genes, so they may need higher doses and special forms of these nutrients.

Simple targeted interventions, depending on labs, can create a leap of healing. That is just the beginning. You can consult my first book, *The Holistic Rx: Your Guide to Healing Chronic Inflammation and Disease*, where I have listed in-depth healing and integrative modalities like supplements, homeopathy, acupressure, and even aromatherapy for more than eighty conditions for all ages. You can take that list of integrative modalities that you may be interested in to your child's doctor to find the best approach for her.

ADDITIONAL INTEGRATIVE MODALITIES

We as parents don't have the magic wand, and we can't control everything; however, we can do our best and provide our children with the tools to guide them on their own health journey. Along with the foundations of holistic parenting, integrative modalities are great tools to expedite healing, if used under the guidance of a practitioner. If your child has an acute or chronic issue, work with your doctor to address the issues medically and holistically, using modalities that I will discuss here to adjunct your conventional care. Your child might need antibiotics or other medications, and that is okay. In some cases, you need to put out the fire before you control the blaze. There is so much more you can do to adjunct healing by investigating and addressing your child's underlying root causes and improving his current symptoms with conventional and integrative modalities like supplements, homeopathy, acupressure, aromatherapy, and body work. There are so many other integrative modalities (and practitioners that you can see) that you can incorporate into your child's care, so the options are endless.

Supplements

Most kids do well with the bare minimum supplementation, as they should be getting most of their nutrients from their diet. There has been an increase of the rate of dietary supplement exposure from 2000 through 2012, where researchers found 275,000 accidental dietary supplement exposures, with about thirty-four deaths as a result of supplement overdose in the thirteen years reviewed.[1] The supplements more likely to be overdosed are fat-burning supplements, botanicals, hormonal supplements, and vitamin C. Vitamin C helps boost the immune system, acts as a natural antihistamine to help tame inflammation and swollen membranes, and increase glutathione. Children aged between one and three years old should only consume 400 milligrams of vitamin C, and those between four and eight years old should consume no more than 650 milligrams per day.

Botanical medicines should not be given to infants and toddlers—for example, aloe vera (none before age ten), buckthorn bark, cajeput oil, camphor, eucalyptus, fennel oil, horseradish, mint and peppermint oils (external application), nasturtium, rhubarb root, senna, and watercress. What follows are recommended doses for different acute and chronic conditions.

Acute Conditions

In conjunction with your conventional medical approach to treating the acute condition, you can also adjunct healing with the following:

Cold/flu: Vitamin D3 (5,000 IU per day, children 1,000 IU per day), fish oil, vitamin C (1 gram per day), echinacea, zinc, garlic, olive leaf extract, and other antiviral herbs like grapefruit extract and elderberry extract (10 milliliters daily). Cordyceps and mushroom extracts have provided immune-supporting properties, and oregano oil has antiviral, antibacterial, and anti-inflammatory properties.

Ear infections: Garlic oil has antimicrobial, antiviral, and antifungal properties;[2] putting three to four drops in the painful ear three to four times a day can help improve your child's pain. Additionally, you can try probiotics, zinc (>two years old: 10 milligrams twice a day), vitamin C (six to twelve years old: 500 milligrams twice daily), and vitamin D3 (ages two to twelve: 400 IU–2,000 IU, or more depending on the level of deficiency).

UTIs:[3] Probiotics, cranberry products, D-mannose, vitamin E,[4] and zinc.[5]

Chronic Conditions/Symptoms

Colic: Probiotics, fennel tea (¼ teaspoon three times daily) or chamomile tea (¼ cup three times daily).

Failure to thrive: Glutamine (250 milligrams/kilogram) and probiotics.

Picky eating: If you eliminate dairy, replace with calcium (900–1,000 milligrams, split into two doses) and add a new food every two weeks and 15 milligrams of zinc if your child is more than three years old; multivitamin, vitamin C (100 milligrams), vitamin D, vitamin A (2,500 IU or less), zinc, selenium, chromium, vitamin D (800–1,000 IU per day).

Dyspraxia: Fish oil, vitamin D complex, phosphatidylcholine.

Autism: 95 percent of autistic children have gut issues and inflammation, so working on gut health and detoxification is important. Start with high-potency probiotics, digestive enzymes, a multivitamin, and methylation support. Others you can add are fish oil (1,000–3,000 milligrams of EPA and DHA combined), high-potency probiotics, cod liver oil with vitamin D (2,000–5,000 IU daily with meals), B complex with B12 (1,000 micrograms daily) and B6 (0.6 milligrams per kilogram), multivitamin with zinc (10–20 milligrams daily), selenium (50–100 micrograms, depending on weight, daily), calcium and magnesium (6 milligrams per kilogram), vitamin E (100–400 IU per day) with essential amino acid combination, and vitamin C (400–1,000 milligrams per day).

Supplements for detoxification: High doses of methyfolate, vitamin C, vitamin A (5,000 IU per day minimum), NAC (600 milligrams daily), selenium (100 micrograms daily), glutathione (transdermally 100–200 milligrams twice daily), melatonin (1 milligram per day), and supporting methylation like methyl B12 injections (check with your child's integrative practitioner before giving B12), raise glutathione (IV, transdermal, and nebulized), folic acid, TMG (trimethylglycine; start with 250 milligrams twice daily; side effects are hyperactivity and more emotional behaviors) or DMG (dimethylglycine), NAC (can be taken orally, but in some kids it can lead to yeast overgrowth, so it should be given transdermally at 100–200 milligrams twice daily or higher to 2,000 milligrams per day).

PANDAS: Lower inflammation with vitamin D, omega 3 fatty acids, probiotics, curcumin, quercetin, NAC, fish oil, and SPMs (specialized pro-resolving mediators). Nutrients to lower abnormal blood brain barrier penetration include B vitamins, magnesium, melatonin, and a combination of antioxidant anti-inflammatory phytonutrients like resveratrol, pterostilbene, curcumin, and sulfurophane. Antimicrobial supplements include berberine, olive leaf, propolis, biocidin, garlic, grapefruit seed extract, oil of oregano, and colloidal silver. Others are zinc, selenium, trace minerals, and iron if needed.

Juvenile rheumatoid arthritis: 5 MTHF (200–400 micrograms daily), vitamin C (500–1,000 milligrams daily), calcium (1,000 milligrams daily), vitamin D (1,000–4,000 IU daily), CoQ10 (10–250 milligrams daily), vitamin E (200–400 IU daily), fish oil (2–4 grams of EPA daily), zinc (10–20 milligrams daily), selenium (20–200 micrograms daily), castor oil applied topically to the joints daily.

Attention-deficit/hyperactivity disorder (ADHD): Fish oil (1,000 milligrams per day of EPA/DHA); B complex (50 milligrams daily); multimineral supplement: 500 milligrams calcium, 100–300 milligrams magnesium (especially if your child has tics, is overfocused, and has sleep/anxiety issues), and/or 5–20 milligrams zinc twice daily (especially if your child has learning or memory issues); probiotic; powder inositol (2–6 grams twice daily) if your child is anxious, has sleep issues, or is overfocused; GABA (250 milligrams twice daily); L-theanine (100–300 milligrams twice daily for anxiety); 5HTP.

Anxiety: Vitamin C (1,000 milligrams in the morning); inositol (3–5 grams twice or three times daily); L-theanine; kava (if comfortable with risk); herbals like California poppy, lemon balm, and valerian.

- OCD: inositol, L-theanine, and/or herbals to reduce ambient anxiety; consider NAC.
- PTSD: inositol, L-theanine, and/or herbals.

Anemia: Iron (50–100 milligrams of well-absorbed iron like ferrous fumarate, glycerate, or citrate; take with vitamin C to help with absorption); B12 (1,000–2,000 micrograms daily in the methylcobalamin form sublingual); and folic acid (800–1,200 micrograms daily sublingual) if your child's doctor has diagnosed a deficiency. Green superfood powder: Spirulina (2,000 milligrams daily or one heaping teaspoon daily). Others include alfalfa, dandelion, burdock, yellowdock (one capsule or twenty drops of tincture).

Cancer: Though it is best for your child to get most of her nutrition from foods, there are some situations where you can add a dietary supplement. Several supplements have been shown to reduce the risk of developing cancer. Probiotics can optimize the immune system. Vitamin D has been shown to have a preventive effect on recurrence of malignancies and can support healthy bones. Vitamin C has antioxidant activity. Calcium/magnesium can support bone health. Studies suggest that patients with breast, prostate, and non-small lung cell cancer may derive biochemical and clinical benefits from omega-3.

Mushroom supplements are beneficial. Turmeric has antitumor activity. Others are green tea (EGCG, epigallocatechin gallate), L-glutamine (great for healing myositis and mucositis), and NAC.

Type 1 diabetes: Magnesium (100–400 milligrams daily), vitamin E (100–400 mg IU daily), alpha lipoic acid (100 milligrams daily), vitamin B3 (2–30 milligrams daily), chromium (50–200 micrograms daily), vitamin C (250–1,000 micrograms daily), fish oil (500–2,000 milligrams EPA/DHA per day), vitamin D (600–4,000 IU per day), milk thistle (80 percent silymarin [200 milligrams daily]).

Type 2 diabetes: Alpha lipoic acid (100 milligrams daily), chromium (50–200 micrograms daily), magnesium (100–200 milligrams daily), vitamin D (400–4,000 IU daily), zinc (5–20 milligrams daily), cassia cinnamon (1–2 grams three times daily), gymnasia (100 milligrams twice daily), milk thistle (80 percent silymarin [200 milligrams daily]), panax (ginseng root extract 15 percent ginsenosides [200 milligrams daily]).

Obesity: Fish oil (1–2 grams daily), pycnogenol (50–150 milligrams daily), psyllium (6 grams daily), vitamin B3 (10–20 milligrams daily), green tea (1–3 cups daily), plant sterols (1.5–2.3 grams daily).

Constipation: Magnesium (100–250 milligrams daily), probiotics, castor oil rubbed clockwise on the abdomen, zinc (20–40 milligrams daily), fish oil.

Crohn's disease: Fish oil (EPA/DHA 3 grams daily), probiotics, vitamin D (1,000–5,000 IU daily), NAC (3–6 grams daily), glutamine (5,000 milligrams daily), bromelain (250–1,000 milligrams daily), butyrate (4 grams daily), fiber, L-carnitine (500–2,000 milligrams daily), turmeric standardized extract (400–600 milligrams daily).

Ulcerative colitis: Probiotics, fish oil (3 grams EPA/DHA daily), vitamin D (1,000–4,000 IU daily), bromelain (250–1,000 milligrams daily), butyrate (500–1,000 milligrams daily), vitamin C (500–2,000 milligrams daily), curcumin (500–1,000 milligrams daily).

Excessive menstrual bleeding: Vitamin C (500–1,000 milligrams three times per day), fish oil, chasteberry extract, bioflavonoids (1,000 milligrams per day). Others include chlorophyll (25 milligrams per day), iron (30 milligrams twice a day with meals), chasteberry.

Premenstrual syndrome: Calcium (800–2,000 milligrams daily), vitamin B1 (100 milligrams daily), vitamin B6 (20–40 milligrams daily), fish oil (EPA/DHA 2–4 grams daily), magnesium (100–200 milligrams daily), vitamin D (1,000–4,000 IU per day), fennel extract liquid (thirty drops two times daily), ginkgo biloba leaf extract (50:1 ratio, 24 percent ginkgo heterosides, 6 percent terpene, lactone, 80 milligrams daily), saffron (60 milligrams daily), valerian root (0.8 percent), valerenic acid (250 milligrams daily), chasteberry (5 percent), vitexin (20–40 milligrams daily).

Tooth decay: Fermented cod liver oil (total of ½–1½ teaspoons per day), magnesium, gelatin, vitamin C, vitamin D, vitamin K2, vitamin A, B vitamins (B6, B9, B12), CoQ10, omega-3, oral probiotics, zinc, calcium.

Acne: Vitamin A (1,000–5,000 IU daily), probiotics, cod liver oil, collagen, L-glutamine, zinc (10 milligrams daily).

Eczema: Fish oil (EPA/DHA 1,000–4,000 milligrams daily), probiotics, vitamin D (1,000–4,000 IU per day), zinc (10–20 milligrams daily).

Allergic rhinitis: Bromelain (80–320 milligrams daily), probiotics (2–10 billion CFU daily), mixed carotenoids (1,000–5,000 IU daily), quercetin (200–400 milligrams divided into two to three doses daily), mixed tocopherols (100–400 IU daily), vitamin C (500–1,000 milligrams daily), stinging nettle leaf (100–500 milligrams daily).

Allergies: Bromelain (200–500 milligrams daily), flavonoids (200–400 milligrams divided into two to three daily doses), quercetin (250–500 milligrams divided into two to three doses daily), vitamin C (500–1,000 milligrams daily), stinging nettle leaf (250–500 milligrams daily), turmeric (100 milligrams daily).

Sinusitis: Bromelain (80–320 milligrams daily), multivitamin one per day, fish oil (1 gram of EPA/DHA per day), NAC (100–600 milligrams by mouth daily), nasal lavage (you can add five drops of goldenseal and five drops of NAC to the salt solution for an added benefit).

Homeopathy

Developed in the late 1700s, homeopathy is a medical system based on the belief that the body can cure itself. It uses tiny amounts of nature substances from plants and minerals and is an excellent and effective choice for children. Use the same types and dosages similar to adults. There are constitutional remedies and acute remedies; please see *The Holistic Rx: Your Guide to Healing Chronic Inflammation and Disease* for more information, as I have gone through all the chronic conditions and different remedies in a great amount of detail.

Acupressure

Acupressure works by placing pressure on specific points that lie along the meridians, or channels, in your body. The adult points can also be used for children and can be administered while massaging, bathing, dressing, or nursing. Infants respond promptly to acupressure, so only apply light pressure in a small circular motion for ten to thirty seconds at a time in ten- to fifteen-minute sessions; stretching isn't required for infants.

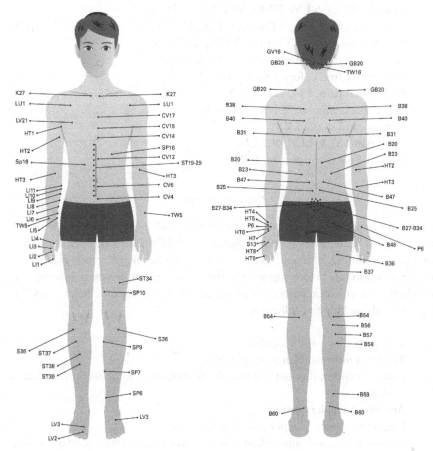

Figure 6.1.   Acupressure

Acupressure Points

Colic points: L12, B47, K3, HP3, LV3
Teeth pain: TW5, LU9, LI4, LI11, ST3, SI18
Sleep: GB20, SP4, SP6, H5, HP4
Pain: LI4, LV3
Digestion and nausea: P6, ST36
Anxiety: GV20
Ear pain: TW21, SI19, and GB2; TB17, K3, LI4 help ease pain
Cold: LI 4, GB20, LU7, ST 36, LU7, DU17
Inflammation and joint pain: The Yang Lin Qian point
ADHD: CV12, LI11, P6, H7, LU1, SP6
Anxiety: HP7, HP6, TW5, H7, H5, LU1

Obesity: ST25, ST36, ST40, SP6, B20, B21, CV12
Improved circulation: ST36, LI4, B40, H7, P6, SP6, K3, GV24.5, GB21
Constipation: LV3, LI4, LI11, ST36, CV12
Abdominal pain, constipation, and gas: CV6
Indigestion (use before a meal): CV12
Abdominal pain: LI4, LI11, LV3
Lower back pain: B25, B31, and B40
Tension and stress: LV3
Sinus pain: ST3, LI20, B2, LI4
Relief of nasal congestion: GB20

Aromatherapy

Essential oils are very beneficial for children and are very potent, so you only need a small amount to achieve efficacy. A child's skin is thinner, so dilute in a carrier oil (e.g., coconut oil, almond oil, jojoba oil, olive oil, grape seed oil, or avocado oil) before applying to the child. Aromatherapy is amazing for children, and you don't need to worry about skin reactions. Some uses for essential oils include the following:

Teething: clove and grapefruit oils
Temper tantrums: ylang-ylang, rose
Colic: lavender, Roman chamomile, fennel, marjoram, bergamot, ylang-ylang
Anxiety: lavender, vetiver
Immune support: Peppermint, frankincense
Antimicrobial and antioxidant effects: clove oil, tea tree oil, oregano oil, myrrh oil, frankincense, thieves' oil
Calming effects: ylang-ylang, neroli, orange, lavender, rose and sandalwood, chamomile, vetiver
Anti-inflammatory and analgesic effects: ginger, juniper, vetiver, ylang-ylang, turmeric, frankincense, myrrh, orange essential oils
Focus: vetiver, cedarwood, cardamom, peppermint basil, thyme
Fatigue: rose, jasmine, geranium
Pain: black pepper, rosemary, ginger
Digestive issues: peppermint oil, ginger, carrot seed, orange, fennel, spearmint, chamomile
Balance blood sugar: coriander, cinnamon
Balance female hormones: geranium, rose oils
Reduce stress: geranium, rose oil, lavender, bergamot, jasmine

Age-appropriate essential oils:

> Three days to three months: Roman chamomile, lavender, and mandarin
> Three months to five years: Roman chamomile, lavender, mandarin, plus
> bergamot, cedarwood, Eucalyptus smithii, frankincense, geranium, ginger, lemon, sweet marjoram, sweet orange, rose, rosemary, sandalwood, tea tree, thyme linalool, ylang-ylang
> Five years to puberty: all oils that are good for adults are considered safe for children, but use in smaller amounts

Body Work

Massage and chiropractic/osteopathic manipulations are very beneficial for children and are great ways to show affection and love. Touch stimulates the body to help release hormones that help the child develop appropriately; it's a great way to bond, and it improves overall circulation and healing. Hydrotherapy is very healing for a child.

Other Integrative Modalities

You can also try acupuncture, hypnosis, neurofeedback, biofeedback, energy work (reiki and craniosacral therapy), cognitive behavioral therapy, dialectical behavioral therapy, emotional freedom technique, exposure therapy, pulsed electromagnetic field therapy, or bioregulation therapy.

A WORD ABOUT FEVERS

A fever is so scary, but before you run immediately to the medicine cabinet, stop and ask yourself the question, "Why does my child have a fever?" Let's start with the basics. A fever is usually caused by infections from pathogens like bacteria or viruses. Noninfectious causes of fevers include an underlying inflammatory response or neoplastic condition.

Your child's body gets hot as it tries to fight infections; it is trying to create an inhospitable environment for bad bugs. Remember, the American Academy of Pediatrics said that fevers below 104 degrees Fahrenheit are not damaging, and the fever may help to allow a child's body to overcome the infection more quickly.[6] Also, fever reducers come with their own set of problems; for example, acetaminophen overdosage can be a major cause of acute liver failure in children.[7] The fever itself isn't dangerous. Fever reducers should be reserved for distressed children; the aim is to improve the child's well-being rather than to achieve normothermia because fever reducers have not been shown to prevent recurrence of febrile seizures.[8] So just because they are available over the counter doesn't mean they are actually safe. The acetaminophen in Tylenol binds to a super antioxidant in the body called glutathione, and it can actually increase the risk of developing allergies, eczema, and asthma, especially when given in the early years of life.[9]

The best approach for dealing with a fever is to support the immune system and keep your child (and you) comfortable with plenty of rest and lukewarm baths. Remember, suppressing the fever actually increases the amount of the influenza flu virus a person sheds, prolongs the duration of the shedding (so people stay contagious for longer!), and increases the transmission rate, which leads to larger epidemics with greater morbidity and mortality! Always talk to your primary care physician and weigh the risks versus the benefits. In 2020, researchers at the Johns Hopkins Bloomberg School of Public Health found that exposure to acetaminophen in the womb may increase a child's risk for attention-deficit/hyperactivity disorder (ADHD) or autism spectrum disorder.[10]

Important note: Fevers in newborns and immunosuppressed kids (or a fever more than 104 degrees Fahrenheit or 40 degrees Celsius) can indicate a dangerous infection and severe illness. If your child (or you) appears severely ill with (or without) a high fever, reach out for medical care immediately.

Additional Integrative Modalities

Supplements

Vitamin D3: 5,000 IU per day; children: 1,000 IU per day.

Fish oil: 1–2 grams of EPA/DHA per day (fish oil can maintain wintertime immunity).

Vitamin C: Don't take more than the following amounts of vitamin C: young children aged one to three: 400 milligrams per day; children aged four to eight: 650 milligrams per day; children aged nine to thirteen: 1,200 milligrams per day; teens: 1,800 milligrams per day.

Echinacea: Check the package insert for recommended dosages.

Zinc: 50 milligrams daily dose for adults; children (birth to three years): 2 to 4 milligrams per day; children aged four to six years: 5 milligrams per day; children aged seven to ten years: 7 to 9 milligrams per day. It is important, however, to check the package insert for recommended dosages.

Other antivirals include the following: olive leaf extract (two 500 milligram capsules four times per day with meals); grapefruit extract and elderberry extract (10 milliliters daily); cordyceps and mushroom extracts, which have immune-supporting properties; and oregano oil, which has antiviral, antibacterial, and anti-inflammatory properties. It is important to check the package insert for recommended dosages.

Other supplements that can help immune function include the following: colloidal silver, serum bovine immunoglobulins (binds to gut endotoxins), lipopolysaccharides, specialized pro-resolving mediators (SPMs; immune modulators that help resolve inflammation), and melatonin (helps lower inflammation).

Homeopathy

There are so many homeopathic combinations that can help.

Cold Calm (for colds)
Occillococinum (for flus)
Sinusalia (for sinus issues)
Sabidil (for allergies)

Aromatherapy

Lavender reduces inflammation and helps to calm anxiety.
Peppermint and frankincense essential oils can be applied on the neck and the bottom of the feet to support the immune system.
Clove oil has amazing antimicrobial and antioxidant properties and can protect the body against infections and speed recovery from flu.

Acupressure

Massage DU14, LI 4, GB 20, LU 7, San Jiao 5, ST 36

Other

Chiropractic care for flu prevention can help boost the immune system.

There are so many tools a parent has to optimize a child's brain, body, and immune system. There's so much hope!

Conclusion

Love, Educate, Empower, Hope

When a child enters this world, that child is a blank canvas. Your love, your words, the food we feed this child, and their life experiences will all determine the masterpiece. If we don't help our children create this masterpiece, someone else will do it for them—preparing them for a changing world.

March 2020 changed our lives forever. In a blink of an eye, our hugs and social routines, our business travel, and our vacations were taken from us. Almost overnight, the world shut down; we became filled with fear of the unknown, fear of sickness, and fear of interaction. Digital meetings replaced social gatherings and conferences. Online classrooms replaced schools. Many people who had stable jobs suddenly found themselves jobless and no longer able to pay their bills. Some faced the reality of hunger and homelessness. We went from a world we felt we controlled to a world that was out of our control. So many of us became overwhelmed and filled with hopelessness. The world was turned upside down.

Life is unpredictable. Preparing our children for an unpredictable life and increasing their resilience to whatever life throws at them is necessary as their lives continue to change.

Role Modeling Self Care

Healthy brains and bodies start with you. Take care of yourself, as you can't give from an empty vessel. Fill your cup and give out what overflows into your saucer. When I take time out for me, I am a better mother, wife, sister, and daughter. Protecting your peace is critical for healthy children, so prioritize your own self-care, and ignore all the judgment and the pressures to be perfect. No one is perfect. You just need to be you and just show up for your kids with unconditional love.

167

My parenting rules are straightforward: educate and be a great role model. It is really that simple. Children don't follow what we say; they follow what we do.

MAKING IT A FAMILY AFFAIR

Before the pandemic, I was a busy physician, entrepreneur, international speaker, and author. In March 2020, homebound with my four boys aged four through twelve, I had to add several other titles to my CV: lunch lady, PE teacher, art teacher, music teacher, janitor, and, most important, principal.

What was I going to do? It was overwhelming, and I was on the verge of spiraling down into a dark, endless abyss. But the tools of holistic functional medicine and holistic parenting helped us hold on and, ultimately, step out of the world of hysteria and come back into a world of reason.

I was definitely not equipped or trained to manage the daily schedules of four children. So, I took matters in my own hands—I turned regular schooling into a full family affair, or "life schooling." I turned my personal and professional work into work we now can do together as a family. Holistic medicine went from "me" to "we."

My writing projects turned into *our* projects. My interviews turned into *our* interviews. My books turned into *our* books. My mission turned into *our* mission. By changing the *me* to *we*, we became a team, working together, and the kids rose up to the mission and continue to grow into leaders, one day, one meal, and one hug and kiss at a time.

OUR HEALING ROUTINES

> "You will never change your life, until you change something you do daily. The secret of your success is found in your daily routine."
>
> —John C. Maxwell

The healthy routine that we worked on together and continue to instill has saved my sanity and made us grow stronger as a family, despite a changing world.

I communicate with my children regularly about each part of my own daily routine, educating them why I am doing what I am doing. Through years of discussion, they know why gratitude, sunshine, nature, rainbow foods, meditation, and good sleep are important for optimal health.

With a grateful mind-set, we then instilled our "healing routine." We start the day with morning sunshine outdoors. We spend the early morning harvesting our garden, sampling the produce, and using the food we picked to create a delicious breakfast together.

The children know that each bite we take can either hurt us or help us. They know that we need to put nutrient-dense foods in our bodies—foods that will keep our gut bacteria happy and optimize our hormone levels. They know the effects of different types of foods, and they can recognize the difference between real foods and "fake" foods filled with chemicals.

For breakfast, lunch, snacks, and dinner, we concentrate on "eating the rainbow"; we eat lots of veggies, clean proteins, and healthy fats. We have a list that helps them to focus on foods they can eat, not foods they can't eat. Develop a healing routine that is right for your family.

HOLISTIC PARENTING CREATES MINDFUL, RESILIENT CHILDREN

Mindful children are resilient children. I teach my boys to pay attention to what's happening in their bodies, their minds, and their souls. They are aware of their passions, desires, and emotions. They are aware of what is going on internally and externally. They are able to grow with life's challenges; they are resilient.

Growing up, I thought being constipated, tired, and having chronic rashes were part of "my normal" until holistic integrated medicine taught me otherwise. I had to learn to be mindful. I wanted my children to have that right from the start, and it is really working.

The boys now have learned to adjust their lifestyle to help bring their bodies back into balance when they feel their bodies teetering in the wrong direction—on their own. That's the power of knowledge! The boys know that their bodies "talk" to them via their out-of-the-norm symptoms. The children are very aware of their bodies and surroundings, and if anything is off balance, they have learned to correct it, without me in the picture!

Through education, role modeling, and conversing about our bodies, environment, and decisions, the boys have learned that every bite and every action can have an influence on their internal and external world. They're learning the power of their own choices.

FROM FEAR TO HOPE

With limited control over what was going on in the outside world, I took control of what I could—the things that go on in my house. In a world filled with negativity, I wanted the children to wake up to a world of positivity, hopes, and dreams; I wanted them to feel confident that they are able to accomplish anything to which they put their minds and their efforts. I want them to rise daily to a world filled with possibilities.

With so much change, fear, and unknown, we have doubled down on gratitude practices, laughter, games, and fun. My job is to help them plant the seeds. Gratitude watered those seeds. It fills their lives with hope and allows them to convert problems to solutions. Our job is to empower our children with the ability to be resilient, so that they take charge of their brains, bodies, and behavior before someone else does.

Children are not just our future; they are our future leaders. Children are braver, stronger, and smarter than most of us realize. We, as parents, are teachers, guides, leaders, protectors, providers, and educators. Children know the direction, and they are intuitively able to guide others. I want to nurture that innate leadership. If I can do it, you can, too! With unconditional love, all is possible. I am here for you! Together we can build a healthier, balanced future!

When we empower children, they can empower others. Each child can be a drop in the ocean to create a ripple effect that can change the world, inside and out. You've got this!

Gratefully
Dr. Madiha

Appendix

The Holistic Rx Resource Guide
for Healthy Brain and Body

WELL-CHILD VISITS,
AGE TWO WEEKS TO THREE YEARS

Two-Week Visit
Your Baby's Development at Two Weeks

- Your baby is adjusting to the world.
- She is beginning to trust.
- He is learning to communicate.

Parents' Responsibilities

Comfort and Love Your Baby and Develop a Relationship

- Holding and rocking your baby stimulates her sensation of touch.
- Quickly responding to your baby's crying teaches her she can trust you and that she is a good communicator. Trust is an important foundation for future relationships.
- Babies are able to calm down more quickly when they become upset if they are consistently held and cuddled.
- Consistent sensitive and responsive caregiving helps babies develop secure emotional bonds. This lasts into the toddler years.
- Skin-on-skin contact has so many benefits for you and your baby.

Protect Your Baby's Brain

- Support the head until your infant's neck is strong enough to hold up her head. Her neck muscles will strengthen over the next six weeks. You can help this process by trying to have her move her head as you move an object. If she is focused on you or a toy, then move it (or you) from side to side for her to follow with her eyes (and eventually her head).
- Don't shake your baby! Shaking causes her brain to move around and smash into her hard skull, causing bruising and bleeding of her brain. It can be frustrating when a baby will not stop crying or fussing. Take a break by placing your baby in the crib or bassinet, have your partner take over, or ask a friend to help out. *Don't shake your baby!*

Develop Your Baby's Brain

- Gentle touch, holding, and eye contact are important for your baby's weight gain.
- Your voice will reinforce his bond with you, and your touch will strengthen the connections in his brain. This will provide a good framework for his future brain development.
- Sing and talk to your baby during routine activities like feeding him, changing him, or giving him a bath. He will love your voice, even if you are not a good singer.
- Read books to your baby.

Keep Your Baby Safe

- Put him on his back to sleep, and don't have loose blankets or stuffed animals in the crib or bassinet. This will help prevent Sudden Infant Death Syndrome (SIDS).
- Place him in a rear-facing car seat in the back seat of your car.
- Have a working smoke detector and/or carbon monoxide monitor on each floor of your house.
- Don't smoke around your baby; if you must smoke, do it outside. Smoking increases the risk of SIDS.
- Offer your baby a pacifier when he goes to sleep. This may reduce the risk of SIDS.

Adjusting to Parenthood

- Learning to be a parent is a slow process made up of physical and emotional demands.
- Be flexible. The best-made plans may need to be changed. Find a routine that is comfortable for you and your family members.
- Communicate. Take time to talk with your spouse or other support person about day-to-day life. If you are part of a couple, go out as a couple and keep your romance alive.
- Take care of yourself. Meeting your own personal needs helps you meet the needs of other family members.
- Make rest and sleep a priority.
- Get away by yourself for some personal time. Always protect your peace.
- Don't be "house proud." Let housework slide and enjoy your baby.
- Use your resources and ask family and friends for help.
- Share your feelings with other new parents.
- Take advantage of community services, such as family centers, play groups, babysitting co-ops, and other programs like Mother's Day Out.

Keeping Inflammation at Bay

Digestive Health and Detoxification

Pay attention to subtle signs that your child's health may be becoming imbalanced. If your child is having any symptoms of colic, gas, spitting up, or indigestion; abdominal pain, constipation, or other digestive issues; congestion, rash or hives, cough, or difficulty breathing; chronic ear infections; cradle cap; projectile vomiting; fits/tics; sinus issues; or adenoids, these may be risk factors for developing bigger health problems down the road like autism, autoimmune disease, or mood disorders. If you notice these symptoms, remove one or two of the problematic foods at a time, starting from the food that your child or you eat the most, following the Gut Rx. Breastfeeding mothers can follow the same protocol, eliminating foods and watching for symptoms in your baby; formula-fed babies may need to change their formula. If your child needs formula, it isn't the end of the world. Some women just can't make as much milk as others, and it is okay. Choose organic formulas when possible.

Clean up your child's surroundings. Pesticides and other environmental toxins can lead to neurodevelopmental damage while disrupting the endocrine system. Optimizing gut health and limiting the daily toxin exposure will help protect against any adverse effects of vaccines. Homeopathics can also be used to prevent or limit vaccine side effects.

The Four S's: Stress Management, Sleep, Social Health, and Spiritual Health

Managing stress is essential in any healing and disease-prevention program, as our thoughts, feelings, and emotions directly affect our children's physical health. Parenting can directly affect the child's brain chemicals. Developing bonds of love, respect, and honor, as well as being involved in a child's life can help activate a sensory nerve in the child's brain that releases oxytocin and natural opioids, which decrease stress response systems and provide the child with feelings of well-being and help the brain develop.

Two-Month Visit

Your Baby's Development at Two Months

- Your baby now recognizes you and has a special smile just for you.

Parents' Responsibilities

Protect Your Baby

- Use a rear-facing only car seat.
- Always put your baby on her back when sleeping.
- Keep a hand on your baby when dressing or changing her, or when she is on a sofa or bed.
- Never leave your child alone in bathwater.

Develop Your Baby's Brain

- Stimulate her vision. The vision center of your newborn's brain is the most active part. She especially is intrigued by human faces and can see thing clearly about a foot away. During feedings, she may look intently at your face. At other times when she is alert, show her photos of family members and other babies. She will also be drawn to contrasts between light and dark. Your baby may prefer to look at things from the sides of her eyes (peripheral vision); after three months, babies develop better central vision.
- Encourage language skills. Even at such a young age, you baby's language is quite developed. He can distinguish several hundred different spoken words. If you talk to him often, he may be able to speak up to three hundred more words by the age of two years compared to children whose parents do not actively converse with them. Use many words with your baby, and repeat them in later conversations. Tell

him what you are buying in the store, or what color clothes you are putting on him.
- Give your baby something to reach for and hold onto—for example, a finger or toy. Allow your baby to touch objects with different textures and shapes.

Increase Your Baby's Sense of Security

- Develop a bedtime, feeding, and playtime routine.
- Continue to respond quickly to his crying with a soothing voice and loving touch.
- Help your baby calm herself by guiding her fingers to her mouth or giving her a blanket or soft object that is special to her.

Strengthen Your Baby's Neck Muscles

- Engage in "tummy time" with your baby. Get on the floor with your baby and play with her. This will encourage her to use her neck muscles. It will also help prevent her from getting a misshapen head from only lying on her back.

Take Care of Yourself: Protect Your Peace

- Babies whose mothers reported high stress cried and fussed more than babies whose mothers reported little stress.
- Beat stress by setting priorities, practicing gratitude, treating yourself right, engaging in aerobic exercise for twenty minutes or more daily, relaxing for twenty minutes each day, changing your routine, letting someone else do the job, and laughing (it will help put your problems in perspective).

Don't Feel Guilty

- Guilt may be defeating. The only positive benefit of guilt is considering your past mistakes and resolving to make better decisions in the future.
- Common mistakes parents make from guilt include overprotecting the child, giving unnecessary gifts, not setting limits or giving into demands, or ignoring misbehavior.
- Going back to work can be stressful; start to store an ounce at a time of breast milk.

- It is okay if you can't breastfeed; do what is best for you and your child. Choose organic formula if needed. Let go of the guilt. You are amazing!

Keep Inflammation at Bay

Digestive Health and Detoxification

Look for soft signs of chronic inflammation, and if present, start a gut-healing diet immediately. Clean up your child's surroundings. Feed your baby on demand. Give your baby vitamin D drops (400 IU) per day. Continue to take your prenatal vitamin.

The Four S's: Stress Management, Sleep, Social Health, and Spiritual Health

Managing stress is essential in any healing and disease-prevention program, as our thoughts, feelings, and emotions directly affect our children's physical health. Continue to prioritize your sleep and optimize your social and spiritual health. Focus on all the things that are going right in your life.

Four-Month Visit

Your Baby's Development at Four Months

- Your baby's vision is nearly as good as an adult's vision now.
- Your baby's brain is more like an adult's brain now.
- She may be sleeping through the night.
- She may reach for objects and even grasp them.
- She continues to communicate with you by cooing, babbling, or gurgling.
- Your baby does a good job of supporting her head.
- Your baby may be able to roll over now.
- Your baby is learning to use all of his senses at once, which is called sensory integration.

Parents' Responsibilities

Stimulate Conversations

- When your baby babbles at you, talk back to him with real words. You will notice he will pause in his conversation, waiting for you to join in; when you pause, he will start babbling to you. He is learning how to carry on a conversation.

- Read to your baby.

Encourage Hand-Eye Coordination

- Hold an interesting toy above your infant, and let her reach for it. She will likely reach for it with both hands, and she may even bring it to her for a closer peek. She may try to put it in her mouth, so make sure that the toy is large enough so she cannot put the whole thing in her mouth.

Help Integrate Your Baby's Senses

- Feeding time is actually a great way for your baby to integrate all her senses. She smells her organic formula or breast milk, feels your caring touch, tastes her food, hears your soothing voice, and sees you while you feed her.
- Calm your baby with your loving touch when she's fussy.
- Offer colorful toys to hold.

Advance Your Baby's Diet

- Between now and the next visit, you may want to introduce solid foods to your baby's diet. Start with broth and follow the Healing Infant Feeding Guide (to come).

Teach Manners

- The way you play with your baby now provides the foundations for good manners and social skills.
- Talking with your fussy baby while you are getting ready to breastfeed or preparing a bottle can teach him to wait; it also teaches him words.
- Back-and-forth games are the first instruction in taking turns. When he reaches for a toy, make sure the toy is within his reach so he can grab it.

Encourage Predictability

- Your baby loves predictability and likes to anticipate what will happen next.

- Peek-a-boo give her a chance to think about your return after you have "disappeared."
- Continue to develop your routine. Bedtime routines help her know what to expect leading up to bedtime. A bath, a book, and a soft lullaby will provide uninterrupted time that is fully devoted to your baby. It will let her know that you love her, even though she must go to bed.

Keep Inflammation at Bay

Digestive Health and Detoxification

Look for soft signs of chronic inflammation, and if present, start a gut-healing diet immediately. Clean up your child's surroundings. Continue vitamin D and probiotics. Clean baby's gums and teeth with a soft cloth or toothbrush with a no-fluoride toothpaste.

The Four S's: Stress Management, Sleep, Social Health, and Spiritual Health

Managing stress is essential in any healing and disease-prevention program, as our thoughts, feelings, and emotions directly affect our children's physical health. Continue to prioritize your sleep and optimize your social and spiritual health. Focus on all the things that are going right in your life by singing the "gratitude song." Don't use digital media to calm your baby.

Six-Month Visit

Your Baby's Development at Six Months

- Your baby can roll over and scoot.
- She will soon be able to sit up by herself.
- He has good reaching and grasping ability.
- She will bring her feet to her mouth.
- He will turn to a voice when he is called.
- She recognizes strangers.
- He is learning to eat solid foods.
- She may get her first tooth.

Parents' Responsibilities

Keep Your Baby Safe

- Work on childproofing your home. Get on your hands and knees and remove anything that potentially could be dangerous (small or sharp objects, chemicals, electrical cords, medications, ant traps, toiletries, and such). Cover electric outlets and put safety locks on cabinet doors.
- Do not use a baby walker. These are dangerous. Stationary exercise stations are okay; however, they can put added stress on your baby's growing spine.
- Adjust mattress heights on your crib so that your baby will not fall out when he learns to pull up.

Develop Your Baby's Eating Skills

- Your baby needs to practice how to swallow food and thrust her tongue. She will be messy at first, but giving her solids from a spoon and not from a bottle will help her acquire this new skill.
- Offer your baby sips from a cup.
- Once her first tooth comes in, you should use a small, soft toothbrush to brush it.

Advance Your Baby's Diet

- If you have not started already, begin adding solids, starting with broth and advancing as tolerated. Follow the Healing Infant Feeding Guide to optimize gut health and keep inflammation at bay.
- Offer your baby solid foods two to three times per day; let her decide how much to eat.
- Add iron-dense foods to her diet like pureed red meat, liver, and spinach.
- When using baby food from a jar, place a small amount of food into a bowl and feed from a bowl; put the rest of the jar in the refrigerator. Feeding your baby from a jar places bacterium into the jar each time the spoon is dipped into the jar.
- Don't give any food that could make your baby choke. Avoid anything the size and consistency of a peanut (popcorn, raisins, whole grapes, carrot sticks, and so on).

- Feeding time will be messy, so don't scold her for her efforts to learn to eat. She is also practicing hand-eye coordination and developing her sense of touch.

Use Everyday Moments for Learning

- Bath time is not only for cleaning but also for learning. Your baby will want to imitate you. Show him how he can fill a container with water and then empty it, or make his rubber ducky squeak and splash. In the process of having fun, he is discovering simple math and science concepts like floating and sinking, full and empty, and liquids and solids. He also realizes that you are a good teacher. You can also name his body parts.
- Talk to your baby.

Make Your Baby Feel Comfortable around Strangers

- In the next several months, your baby may begin to be fearful of new people or family members not often seen. To help with this fear, you can introduce him from the safety of your arms. It may also help if the new person has one of your baby's favorite things, such as a toy or book.

Keep Inflammation at Bay

Digestive Health and Detoxification

Look for soft signs of chronic inflammation, and if present, start a gut-healing diet immediately. Clean up your child's surroundings. Keep feeding your baby nutrient-dense foods. You may need to offer your baby the specific food ten to fifteen times before she likes it. Continue to practice good dental hygiene.

The Four S's: Stress Management, Sleep, Social Health, and Spiritual Health

Managing stress is essential for disease prevention, as our thoughts, feelings, and emotions directly affect our children's physical health. Continue to prioritize your sleep and optimize social and spiritual health. Focus on all the things that are going right in your life by singing the "gratitude song."

Nine-Month Visit

Your Baby's Development at Nine Months

- Your child is able to now sit alone.
- Your baby is learning to crawl.
- She will be able to pull to standing and even cruise around furniture while holding on.
- He can wave bye-bye.
- She can repeat sounds.
- He may develop separation anxiety.
- She is able to hold things between her thumb and forefinger.

Parents' Responsibilities

Keep Your Baby Safe

- Your baby should be in a rear-facing car seat until she is two years old or reaches the highest weight or height allowed by your car seat manufacturer.
- Continue to childproof your home. Make sure small objects are not available for your baby to place in his mouth and choke.

Build Your Baby's Brain

- Communicate with your baby. Have conversations with her, and sing and read to her daily.
- Do not allow screen time.
- Love and cuddle your baby.
- Give your baby toy blocks, balls, and puzzles.
- Let your baby explore the outside and inside environment. Take your baby out in nature.

Advance Your Baby's Diet

- Let your baby feed himself some foods, such as soft, mashed foods.
- Focus on lots of veggies, clean protein, healthy fats, and bone broth.
- Encourage your baby to drink from a cup, with the goal of weaning off the bottle by the age of fifteen months.

Encourage Good Behavior

- Distraction works well at this age as a tool for stopping unwanted activities. If your baby is playing with the cord to the light, move him from that area and offer a favorite toy. Instead of saying "no" to one thing, you can usually say "yes" to something else.
- Continue to be consistent with discipline.
- Don't use "no" often; use "no" only when he is going to get hurt or hurt others.
- Start to ask your baby to help you. She can hold a fork for you or get you something. Start to involve your baby in your daily routine.

Help Establish Object Permanence

- Peek-a-boo and disappearing games are fun because your baby believes you or the toy has actually disappeared. However, when you or the toy "reappears," your baby is learning that objects are still present even when he can't see them. These games will help him know that you will always return, and they are even good practice for good-byes.

Anticipate Separation Anxiety

- Separation anxiety will likely begin to surface around ten months and continue for half a year. When you are out of sight, your baby will become greatly distressed until she is able to see you again.
- The best preparation for separation anxiety is a healthy relationship with your baby. You may also practice "leaving" for a short time. When she crawls or scoots into another room, wait a few minutes and then follow her. When you leave a room, tell her that you are going and you will be back. When she begins to fuss, try to soothe her with your voice instead of running right back into the room.
- Remember that she will stop crying within a few minutes of your leaving, and she will also be glad to see you when you return.
- Don't sneak out; this will only make your baby worry that you will disappear at any time without warning.

Practice Language Skills

- Your baby has a good understanding of words and can even follow simple directions. Continue to speak in simple sentences and give words to her actions.

- Offer your baby choices and encourage him to point, reach, or vocalize to show you what he wants. Being able to tell you what he wants is much better than him being fussy.

Don't Cry It Out; Love It Out

- Go to your baby at night and reassure her that you are still there, but don't pick her up. Soothe her and let her know you are there for her.
- Tell her you love her, and hold her hand and comfort her. Make sure she has something that gives her comfort, like a blanket or favorite stuffed toy. This will help her soothe herself. You can play her favorite music in the background.

Keep Inflammation at Bay

Digestive Health and Detoxification

Look for soft signs of chronic inflammation, and, if present, start a gut-healing diet immediately. Clean up your child's surroundings. Start to talk to your child about how his decisions can affect him. Start talking about good food and bad fake food.

The Four S's: Stress Management, Sleep, Social Health, and Spiritual Health

Managing stress is essential in any healing and disease-prevention program, as our thoughts, feelings, and emotions directly affect our children's physical health. Spend a lot of time in nature. Continue to prioritize sleep and optimize social and spiritual health. Focus on all the things that are going right in your life by singing the "gratitude song." Continue to develop a routine that works for you and your family.

Twelve-Month Visit

Your Baby's Development at Twelve Months

- Your baby will start taking his first steps alone.
- She is becoming more independent.
- He is cruising while holding onto furniture quite well.
- She can hold a cup and even drink from it.
- He can feed himself with his fingers.
- She can say a few words and babbles a lot.

Parents' Responsibilities

Explore with Your Child

- Follow your child's lead as she explores the world. On walks, describe things to her and ask her questions.
- Play both outdoors and indoors.
- Give your baby a new toy to play with, such as musical instruments like drums.
- Engage in make-believe games with your child to stimulate her imagination.

Stimulate Your Toddler's Motor Skills

- Provide toys that can be pushed and pulled. Offer a ball to toss or a rattle to shake.
- Make "obstacle courses" with pillows to climb over and boxes to climb through.
- Place favorite toys around the room and ask your baby to bring them to you.
- Set up a container of objects to dump out and place back.
- Let him do things over and over.

Support Your Child's Responsibilities

- Let your child "help" you in setting the table or making dinner.
- Encourage him to help in getting himself dressed.
- Give him a spoon to try feeding himself.
- Involve your child in your daily routine and allow him to help you around the house.

Advance Your Toddler's Diet

- Begin the transition from formula to raw A2 milk if tolerated. If signs of inflammation develop, change to a clean seed, nut, or coconut milk.
- Continue to focus on veggies, clean protein, and healthy fats.
- Feed your child at the table with the family and involve her with meals. Encourage your child to feed herself.
- Continue to brush your child's teeth. Use a pea-sized amount of natural toothpaste.

Keep Your Toddler Safe

- Monitor your toddler closely, especially around animals, water, machines, cars, and streets.
- Do not let your child play with plastic bags or small objects that could cause choking.
- Choose shoes that are flexible and not too tight. Shoes should not be rigid.

Encourage Language Development

- Avoid TV/screen time.
- Continue to read with your toddler and play games with him.
- Narrate what you and your child are doing, using phrases such as "peeling an orange" or "steaming carrots on the stove for your snack."
- Use the "real" word in a sentence after your child uses part of the word. When he says "wawa," you say, "You want water?"
- Label his feelings for him and provide a reason for them, such as "You're happy because I gave you a new toy."

Develop Healthy Behaviors

- Distraction remains a good tool for getting you toddler to swap an inappropriate activity for one that is acceptable.
- Do not allow hitting or biting from your toddler.
- Encourage taking turns and sharing by saying, "Now it's my turn."
- Continue to talk to your child about how the decisions she makes affect her.
- Continue to read to your child.
- Take your child to a holistic dentist.
- Develop a healing routine together.

Make Everyday Moments Teachable and Help Your Child Become a Good Problem Solver

- If your child is struggling, use that moment as a teachable moment and help her problem solve.
- Encourage creative play, read a book together, and such.

Keep Inflammation at Bay

Digestive Health and Detoxification

Look for soft signs of chronic inflammation, and if present, start a gut-healing diet immediately. Clean up your child's surroundings.

The Four S's: Stress Management, Sleep, Social Health, and Spiritual Health

Managing stress is essential in any healing and disease-prevention program, as our thoughts, feelings, and emotions directly affect our children's physical health. Continue to prioritize sleep and optimize social and spiritual health. Focus on all the things that are going right in your life by singing the "gratitude song." Appreciate your child when he does what you ask him to do. If he tries to help you but messes it up, don't get upset; instead, acknowledge the effort.

Fifteen-Month Visit

Your Child's Development at Fifteen Months

- Your child will begin to name objects.
- She understands words/phrases.
- He can play hide and seek.
- She will try to throw and catch a ball.
- He has good climbing abilities.
- She has temper tantrums.

Parents' Responsibilities

Keep Your Toddler Safe

- Lower the crib mattress to the lowest setting.
- Continue to use the car seat for every car ride.
- Your toddler is becoming a great climber. Make sure that dressers, changing tables, and bookshelves are stable and cannot be pulled down by a climbing child. A good idea is to buy inexpensive shelf brackets to bolt furniture to the walls.

Encourage Healthy Eating Habits

- Eat together as a family. Continue to focus on veggies, clean protein, and healthy fats.
- Allow your child to continue using a spoon and a cup. Cut things into bite-sized portions. Of course, he will be messy, so be prepared with a bib, high-chair tray, and even floor covering.
- Do not put your child to bed with a bottle. This practice can cause damage to teeth and gums and creates an unwanted bedtime routine.

Develop Healthy Behaviors

- Continue following your daily routine that your toddler is used to.
- Keep bedtime a consistent time; put your toddler down for a daily nap.
- Show more enthusiasm for good behaviors rather than negative responses for bad behaviors. This is called "positive reinforcement" and tends to work better than punishment at this age. Remember, most times, instead of saying "no," you can offer a "yes" alternative.
- Temper tantrums will become more common; a tantrum is a way for your toddler to express frustration. The best way to deal with these temper tantrums is to ignore them. Determine if the tantrum is from the upstairs brain versus the downstairs brain. Use connection.
- Set limits and discipline mindfully.
- Most children are not ready for toilet training at this age.
- Increase the responsibilities and chores you give your child.

Develop Your Child's Brain

- Limit TV/screen time to only one hour per day.
- Encourage games and make-believe games.
- Continue to read with your toddler.
- Repetitive tasks or games help strengthen the connections in your child's brain. He may enjoy throwing a ball repeatedly, but he may do it a little differently every time. He may bounce it off the floor or off the couch, for example. By doing repetition, and changing it slightly, he is experimenting with his world and becoming prepared for different situations.

Encourage Language Skills

- Label emotions for your child.
- Label objects and events for your child. Point to things while shopping or driving and tell him what they are.
- Narrate activities for your child. For example, say out loud the steps in making dinner, setting the table, or changing a diaper.

Nurture Your Child's Positive Self-image

- Make sure you let your child know how proud you are of her.
- Tell her that you realize she is working hard and learning new things; tell her that you are proud of her efforts.
- Give your child choices.
- Limit saying "no."

Keep Inflammation at Bay

Digestive Health and Detoxification

Talk to your child about real food and fake food. Look for soft signs of chronic inflammation, and if present, start a gut-healing diet immediately. Clean up your child's surroundings. Optimizing gut health and limiting the daily toxin exposure will help protect against any adverse effects of vaccines. Supplement with probiotics, vitamin D, fish oil, and multivitamins, if indicated.

The Four S's: Stress Management, Sleep, Social Health,
and Spiritual Health

Managing stress is essential in any healing and disease-prevention program, as our thoughts, feelings, and emotions directly affect our children's physical health. Continue to prioritize sleep and optimize social and spiritual health. Focus on all the things that are going right in your life. Continue to sing the "gratitude" song. Continue to develop your healing routine.

Eighteen-Month Visit

Your Child's Development at Eighteen Months

- Your child is saying many words.
- She can sing, jump, and dance.
- He can undress himself and help put on some clothes.

Parents' Responsibilities

Encourage Appropriate Eating Options

- Focus on lots of veggies, clean protein, healthy fats, and bone broth.
- Limit high sugar and inflammatory snacks like pop, candy, chips, and such.
- Wean your child from the bottle.
- Continue to brush your toddler's teeth.

Keep Your Child Safe

- Keep the poison control center phone number near your telephone and program it into your smartphone (800-222-1222).
- Childproof your home. Get on your hands and knees to examine safety from your toddler's perspective.
- Do not smoke in the house or in the car. Children exposed to smoke at a young age are more likely to develop asthma.
- Avoid foods that are choking hazards, including gum, hard candy, nuts, popcorn, raisins, large raw vegetables, and large pieces of meat or hot dogs.

Assist with Emotional Maturation

- Label the emotion your child is experiencing, as well as those of people around him. This will help your child know what his is feeling, as well as help him learn to read social cues of others.
- Labeling emotions also helps your toddler know that you understand his feelings.
- Regulating behavior is an emerging skill for your toddler. He may be able to put off his wants for a few minutes, which is called delaying gratifications.

Develop Healthy Behaviors

- Children learn by repetition and practice. They need to practice acceptable behaviors, and they need repeated exposure to limits on their behavior.
- View discipline as a way of teaching your toddler about regulating his own behavior and about appropriate forms of behavior.
- Model behavior that is acceptable to accomplish what your toddler wishes.

- Decide what limits are important. Be consistent in enforcing them.
- Plan ahead with difficult situations.
- Don't get into the habit of bribing your children to get good behavior.
- Increase the responsibilities and chores you give your child.

Stimulate Your Child's Brain

- Encourage play with other toddlers. Often the best way for your toddler to learn is to play with other children who are slightly more developmentally advanced. These interactions provide much learning.
- Have a bowl of sand available so your child can perform scientific experiments of scooping, pouring, filling, and emptying. A slotted spoon will provide an interesting problem for your child to solve, as she tries to keep the sand in the spoon or fill another container before it falls out. The texture of the sand helps develop her sense of touch.
- Finger painting is a great exercise to improve fine motor control. Thicker-paged books may be a great starting point. With practice, he will be able to turn regular pages. Don't worry if he rips a page; just tape it up and use it as a learning experience.
- Remember to give your child independent playtime.

Keep Inflammation at Bay

Digestive Health and Detoxification

Continue to teach your child about real food and fake food. Go through the colors of the rainbow of food. Look for soft signs of chronic inflammation, and if present, start a gut-healing diet immediately. Clean up your child's surroundings. Supplement with probiotics, vitamin D, fish oil, and multivitamins, if indicated.

The Four S's: Stress Management, Sleep, Social Health, and Spiritual Health

Managing stress is essential in any healing and disease-prevention program, as our thoughts, feelings, and emotions directly affect our children's physical health. Continue to prioritize sleep and optimize social and spiritual health. Focus on all the things that are going right in your life. Continue to sing the "gratitude" song. Continue to develop your healing routine.

Two-Year Visit

Your Child's Development at Two Years

- Your child can run, climb, and go up and down stairs.
- Your child can make sentences.

Parents' Responsibilities

Support Your Child's Exploration of the World

- Continue to maintain a safe environment for playing.
- Expect your child to be curious about body parts; use the correct terms.

Model Healthy Habits

- It is hard to be a good role model for your children all the time; however, it is probably the most important job of your life.
- Continue to talk about the association between your child's choices and how he feels.
- Talk about good food versus fake food.
- Begin morning gratitude and meditations or prayers.
- Brush your teeth with your child. It is another moment to spend together and shows him that tooth brushing is important for adults, too.
- Read books with him, and let him read the newspaper or magazines with you. You are showing him that adults read, too.
- Your toddler should only watch a maximum of one hour of TV per day. However, the less TV you watch, the more you are able to devote to your child and the better role model you are.
- Model sharing to your toddler. Most toddlers are not good at sharing with other children. Your toddler is most likely focused on himself, even while playing. It is hard for him to share his feelings and anticipate feelings of others. Help your child label his emotions.
- Increase the responsibilities and chores you give your child.
- Prioritize your self-care and self-compassion.
- Take time to exercise, detoxify, and spend time in nature.

Promote Your Child's Development

- Begin toilet training when your child is ready, and when you are ready. You may know that she is ready when she notices that she is wet, tells you when she is peeing and/or pooping, can take off her pants by herself, or is concerned about being dirty. Praise her when she pees on the potty, but do not scold her when she has an accident or goes in her diaper or pull ups. Sometimes children are initially interested but then lose interest for a while. She will return to the job of potty training when she is ready.

- Provide plenty of opportunities for your toddler to practice fine motor skills. Examples include using utensils to eat, putting on shoes, washing his hands, letting him zip or button, painting with brushes, drawing with crayons, playing with play-dough, building with blocks, putting puzzles together, playing musical instruments, stringing beads, and playing dress up.
- Encourage activities that use gross motor skills. Make safe spaces for dancing, running, jumping, hopping, and such.
- Read to your child every day.
- Name your child's emotions.
- Engage in make-believe games with your imaginative toddler. He may begin to imitate adult activities like house or serving dinner. You can jump right in and play the role he assigns to you. Be sure to ask open-ended questions such as "What are you cooking?" This allows him a chance to again be imaginative with his answer.
- Turn your child's words and phrases into sentences.

Be Clear with Rules and Be Consistent

Start to establish household rules, for example, what to do when you wake up (brush your teeth and make your bed) and what to do after you are done eating. Create a bedtime routine together.

Keep Inflammation at Bay

Digestive Health and Detoxification

Talk about the importance of nourishing your body with the foods you eat. Look for soft signs of chronic inflammation, and if present, start a gut-healing diet immediately. Clean up your child's surroundings. Supplement with probiotics, vitamin D, fish oil, and multivitamins, if indicated. Start talking about the importance of detoxification.

The Four S's: Stress Management, Sleep, Social Health, and Spiritual Health

Managing stress is essential in any healing and disease-prevention program, as our thoughts, feelings, and emotions directly affect our children's physical health. Continue to prioritize sleep and optimize social and spiritual health. Focus on all the things that are going right in your life. Continue to sing the "gratitude" song. Continue to develop your healing routine together.

Three-Year Visit

Your Child's Development at Three Years

- Your child can name friends.
- Your child can speak three-to-four-word sentences clearly.
- Your child can speak two to three sentences at a time.
- She climbs and runs well.
- He dresses and undresses without help.
- She takes turns when playing with others.
- Your child shows a wide range of feelings.

Parents' Responsibilities

Build Self-confidence

- Build self-esteem. Appreciate, give lots of hugs, and let your child know she is loved and fun to be with.
- Help your child make sense of the world. Help him understand and cope with rules; help him through complex situations and to think through challenges.
- Share your toddler's excitement about her accomplishments. Take time to watch and delight in your child's accomplishments.
- Join in your child's pretend play. Use play to help her work through difficult feelings and experiences.
- Help your child be a good problem solver. Empathize with her frustrations. Ask if she has ideas and offer suggestions.
- Let your child know it's smart to ask for help.

Help with Self-control

- Set and enforce clear and consistent limits. Use words and gestures to communicate your message and teach alternatives. Redirect your child's attention and meet goals in an acceptable way. Avoid negotiating.

- Give your child the skills she needs to manage her emotions. Point out consequences of your child's behavior. Give her a chance to figure things out before stepping in; give her appropriate opportunities to make choices.
- Help your child learn to cope with his strong emotions. Empathize with your child and plan ahead.
- Look for clues to understand the meaning behind your child's behavior, and help her understand her feelings and behavior.
- Respond to tantrums in a way that helps self-control. Stay calm and take a break from the cause. Reconnect after the tantrum and praise her when she does well calming herself down.
- Give your child choices. Don't offer choices as a threat.
- Explore alternatives to time-outs; time-outs only serve to punish and isolate the child. Time-outs do not help children learn from the experience, and they do not teach correct behavior.
- Model self-calming.
- Give your child credit when he shows self-control.
- Continue educating about the association between how your child feels and his lifestyle.
- Talk to your child about the importance of taking care of her body.
- Teach your child about mindful awareness and self-regulation.
- Tell stories, play, and read books to help sculpt the behavior you want.
- Continue to build on the chores and responsibilities you give your child.
- Involve them in your day.

Help Thinking Skills Develop

- Pay attention to what your child is trying to help you with, and work with his ideas to build something great.
- Spend lots of time pretending with your child.
- Build your child's logical thinking skills. Don't ask questions right away; ask what he thinks first.
- Figure out what objects do and how things go together. Notice patterns and connect ideas.
- Sort and categorize as you go through your day together.
- Think and talk about feelings.

Improve Language Skills

- Talk together.
- Ask open-ended questions that don't have a yes/no answer.
- Notice the number, color, size, and shape of things around you.
- Make up rhymes, recite child-friendly poems, and sing songs with your child.
- Help your child build and grow her sentences and tell stories.
- Ask to help out with "big kid" tasks.
- Celebrate her attempts.

Keep Inflammation at Bay

Digestive Health and Detoxification

Talk about her favorite real foods, and why fake foods are not good for her. Have her choose all the rainbow foods she loves and make a plate for herself. Look for soft signs of chronic inflammation, and if present, start a gut-healing diet immediately. Clean up your child's surroundings. Supplement with probiotics, vitamin D, fish oil, and multivitamins, if indicated.

The Four S's: Stress Management, Sleep, Social Health, and Spiritual Health

Managing stress is essential in any healing and disease-prevention program, as our thoughts, feelings, and emotions directly affect our children's physical health. Continue to prioritize sleep, optimize social and spiritual health. Focus on all the things that are going right in your life. Continue to sing the "gratitude" song. Continue to create your healing routine.

THE HEALING INFANT FEEDING GUIDE

It's a confusing world out there, especially when it comes to feeing your infant. When to start? What to start? What to do with picky eaters? How much to feed? The questions are endless!

Let me make it simple: To keep inflammation and subsequent chronic conditions at bay, we need to feed our children the most nutrient-dense foods that will optimize their gut health and keep glucose, insulin, and hormones balanced.

Keep the following in mind:

- Stick with veggies, clean protein, and healthy fats at each meal as you continue to introduce more and more solids.
- Fat is critical for babies. Fat is necessary for your baby's vital functions and composes about 60 percent of your baby's rapidly growing brain.
- Contemporary first baby foods (rice cereal, etc.) don't contain enough of the specific nutrients that babies absolutely require, are rough on the babies' developing digestive system, and don't provide adequate energy. Most babies are functionally grain intolerant and are not ready for grains because a complete set of carbohydrate enzymes won't be present until about three years of age.
- If you want to try grains, try hypoallergenic ones like quinoa and brown rice.
- Always avoid inflammatory foods as outlined.

HEALING FOOD INTRODUCTION TIMELINE

To optimize health and happiness and keep inflammation at bay—especially if you have a family history of chronic disease or food sensitivities—follow the healing food introduction timeline detailed in table A.1. This guide will give you an idea of how to introduce foods; however, each child is different, so adjust as needed.

When to start: Start the very first foods at four months for babies fed commercial formula. Start at six months when breastfeeding. But each child is different, so look for signs that your baby is ready to start foods—for example, your baby can sit up well without support, is ready and willing to chew, is developing a pincer grasp, is eager to participate in mealtime, and may try to grab food and put it in his mouth. Wait three to five days before introducing another food.

At each stage, continue to offer foods from the previous stage. Avoid all the inflammatory foods as long as possible. Watch for food sensitivities/allergies and stop those foods. You may introduce the offending food again once the gut is healed, depending on the severity of the sensitivity/allergy.

Your baby is worth it! A healthy start gives your baby a jump start to a healthy and happy life. Do what you can—just take it meal by meal and day by day. This is an exciting time for your baby to experience a whole new world!

Table A.1.   Food Introduction Timeline

Age	Food
Zero to four/six months	Start with breast milk or organic formula. Nursing moms should eat an anti-inflammatory diet full of veggies, clean protein, and healthy fat. They should supplement with vitamin D, fish oil, probiotics, and magnesium, if indicated.
Week 1 (begin at four months for formula-fed babies; six months for breastfed babies)	Start with homemade meat stock with the fat and freshly pressed vegetable juice mixed with warm water between meals (start with carrot juice, then add cabbage, celery, and lettuce).
Week 2	Continue with previous foods. Add probiotic gradually, homemade sauerkraut juice, and soups with pureed non-starchy vegetables. If handmade raw organic yogurt is well tolerated, you can gradually increase the daily amount; introduce sour cream, fermented with yogurt culture.
Week 3	Continue with previous foods. Add pureed boiled meats (starting with chicken); introduce ripe avocado, starting with a teaspoon added to the vegetable puree, gradually increasing the amount.
Weeks 4 and 5	Continue with previous foods. Add egg yolks to vegetable puree (do a sensitivity test first); add cooked apples; increase amount of butter, coconut oil, and/or ghee. Add grated frozen liver (start liver early if there is an iron deficiency or a formula issue, if the mother is a vegetarian, and/or if the baby is failing to thrive).
Weeks 6 and 7	Carry on with previous foods. Gradually increase egg yolks to two a day, adding to your baby's soup or cups of meat stock. Increase the meat intake, particularly gelatinous meats around the joints and bones (well cooked in water).
Weeks 8 and 9	Continue with previous foods. Add pancakes made with nut butter and eggs. Increase the amount of freshly pressed juices. Try to add some fresh apple to the juice mixture. Add raw vegetables starting with lettuce and peeled cucumbers (blended in a food processor and added to soup or vegetable puree). After these two vegetables are well tolerated, gradually add other vegetables, finely blended. Examples include cooked sweet potato and carrots cooked in soup with marrow, ghee, and other organ meats.
Week 10 and onward	Carry on with previous foods. Add scrambled egg with raw butter or animal fat, with avocados and raw or cooked vegetables. Try some ripe raw apples (without the skin) and ripe banana (with all fruit given between meals). Continue marrow, as well as other lacto-fermented veggies and tropical fruit.
Ten months of age	Carry on with previous foods. You can add filtered water, beets, well-steamed leafy greens, more herbs, and coconut water.

(continued)

Table A.1. *(continued)*

Age	Food
Eleven months of age	Carry on with previous foods. Add wild-caught fish and its stocks.
Twelve to fifteen months of age	Carry on with previous foods. Add honey, tomato, citrus fruits, whole eggs, peppers, sweeteners like maple syrup, soaked nuts, raw dairy milk (if tolerated), spices like paprika and cinnamon, whole stevia plant, radishes, uncooked berries, cranberries, and beets.
Fifteen to eighteen months of age	Continue previous foods. Add kombucha, carob, and sprouted seeds.
Eighteen to twenty-one months of age	Continue previous foods. Add raw greens (all except kale and collard greens are still cooked).
Twenty-one to twenty-four months of age	Continue with previous foods. You can add properly prepared legumes and shellfish.
Two years +	Continue veggies, clean protein, healthy fat, bone broth, and adequate hydration.

HOLISTIC KIDS' RESOURCES

Books

Basic Children's Health and Parenting

A Compromised Generation: The Epidemic of Chronic Illness in America's Children by Beth Lambert
The Dirt Cure by Dr. Maya Shetreat
Family Health Revolution by Carla Atherton
The Rule of Five: A Parent's Guide to Raising Healthy Kids in an Unhealthy World by Dr. Ana Maria Temple
The Science of Parenting by Margot Sunderland
The Wellness Mama 5-Step Lifestyle Detox: The Essential DIY Guide to a Healthier, Cleaner, All-Natural Life by Katie Wells

Pregnancy

Green Mama: Giving Your Child a Healthy Start and a Greener Future by Manda Aufochs Gillespie

Nutrition

The Pegan Diet: 21 Practical Principles for Reclaiming Your Health in a Nutritionally Confusing World by Dr. Mark Hyman

Super Nutrition for Babies: The Right Way to Feed Your Baby for Optimal Health by Kelly Genzlinger and Dr. Katherine Erlich

Integrative, Functional, and Holistic Therapies

The Autism Revolution: Whole Body Strategies for Making Life All It Can Be by Dr. Martha Herbert and Karen Weintraub

Brain Inflamed: Uncovering the Hidden Causes of Anxiety, Depression, and Other Mood Disorders in Adolescents and Teens by Dr. Kenneth Bock

Brain under Attack: A Resource for Parents and Caregivers of Children with PANS, PANDAS and Autoimmune Encephalitis by Beth Lambert and Maria Rickert Hong

Cure Tooth Decay by Ramiel Nagel

The Family's Guide to Aromatherapy: A Safe Approach to Essential Oils for a Holistic Home by Erika Galentin

Gut and Psychology Syndrome by Dr. Natasha Campbell

Heal Your Child from the Inside Out: The 5-Element Way to Nurturing Healthy, Happy Kids by Robin Ray Green

Healing ADHD: The Breakthrough Program That Allows You to See and Heal the 7 Types of ADD by Dr. Danial G. Amen

Healing the New Childhood Epidemics: Autism, ADHD, Asthma and Allergies: The Groundbreaking Program for the 4-A Disorders by Dr. Kenneth Bock and Cameron Stauth

Healing without Hurting: Treating ADHD, Apraxia and Autism Spectrum Disorders Naturally and Effectively without Harmful Medications by Jennifer Giustra-Kosek

Healthy Kids, Happy Moms: 7 Steps to Heal and Prevent Common Childhood Illness by Dr. Sheila Kilbane

The Holistic Rx: Your Guide to Healing Chronic Inflammation and Disease by Dr. Madiha Saeed

It's Gonna Be Ok: Proven Ways to Improve Your Child's Mental Health, by Dr. Roseann Capanna-Hodge

Life Will Get Better: Simple Solutions for Parents of Children with Attention, Anxiety, Mood and Behavioral Challenges by Dr. Nicole Beurkens

Nourishing Hope for Autism: Nutrition and Diet Guide for Healing Children by Julie Matthews

Outsmarting Autism, Updated and Expanded: Build Healthy Foundations for Communication, Socialization, and Behavior at All Ages by Patricia S. Lemer

Teletherapy Toolkit: Therapist Handbook for Treating Children and Teens by Dr. Roseann Capanna-Hodge

Treatment Alternatives for Children by Dr. Lawrence Rosen and Jeff Cohen

Children's Books

Adam's Healing Adventure Series by Dr. Madiha Saeed
A Healthy New Me & ADHD Free by Jennifer Giustra-Kosek
The Incredible Microbiome by Sean Davies and Tori Davies

Cookbooks

Against All Grain: Delectable Paleo Recipes to Eat Well and Feel Great by Danielle Walker
Junior Chef: 100 Super Delicious Recipes for Kids by Kids by Will Bartlett, Katie Dessinger, Paul Kimball, Abigail Langford, and Anthony Spears
The Paleo Kids Cookbook: Transition Your Family to Delicious Grain- and Gluten-Free Food for a Lifetime of Healthy Eating by Jennifer Robins
The Wellness Mama Cookbook by Katie Wells

Holistic Websites for Children's Health

Documenting Hope: https://www.documentinghope.com
Dr. Ana Maria Temple: https://www.dranamaria.com
Dr. Nicole Beurkens, Holistic Child Psychologist: https://www.drbeurkens.com
Dr. Sheila Kilbaine: http://www.sheilakilbane.com
Happy Kids, Healthy Kids by Dr. Elisa Song: https://healthykidshappykids.com
HolisticMom, MD: https://holisticmommd.com
Integrative Pediatrics by Dr. Joel Warsh: https://integrativepediatrics.com
Katie Kimball and Kitchen Stewardship: https://www.kitchenstewardship.com
KnoWEwell: https://www.knowewell.com
The Stern Method by Ryan and Teddy Sternagel: https://thesternmethod.com
Wholistic Kids and Families by Dr Pejman Katiraei: https://wholistickids.com
Ziva Meditation: https://zivameditation.com

NUTRIENTS AND FOOD

Table A.2 gives a list of foods that are great sources of the vitamins and minerals our kids' bodies and brains need.

KID-FRIENDLY HEALING RECIPES

Breakfast

Cassava Flour Waffles

Ingredients
   ¾ cup cassava flour
   1 tablespoon honey
   ½ teaspoon baking soda
   ¼ teaspoon salt
   3 eggs

Table A.2. Power Foods

Vitamin A	Fish, shellfish, carrots, winter squash, lettuce, dried apricots, bell peppers, tropical fruit, cantaloupe, liver
Vitamin B1	Trout, sunflower seeds, acorn squash, peas
Vitamin B2	Mushrooms, spinach, almonds, lean meats
Vitamin B3	Yellowfin tuna, lean meats, peanuts, mushrooms, sunflower seeds, peas, avocado
Vitamin B6	Root vegetables, red meat, leafy greens
Vitamin B9	Avocados, beets, green vegetables
Vitamin B12	Red meat, shellfish and fish
Vitamin C	Berries, green leafy vegetables, yellow bell peppers, kale, broccoli, kiwi, citrus fruits, guava
Vitamin D	Sea vegetables, fish (salmon, sardines, mackerel), beef liver, mushrooms, eggs, raw milk, cod liver oil
Vitamin E	Avocados, leafy greens, fish
Vitamin K2	Fermented vegetables, liver, fish
Calcium	Green leafy vegetables, okra, broccoli, bok choy, flaxseeds, sesame seeds, almonds, spinach, walnuts, sardines, Brazil nuts, salmon, kale
Iron	Liver, red meat, squash, pumpkin seeds, nuts, lentils, shellfish, dark leafy greens
Magnesium	Avocados, green vegetables, dark chocolate, artichoke hearts, almonds, cashews, pumpkin, squash, meat, fish
Selenium	Fish, poultry, red meat
Zinc	Oysters, poultry, red meat
Copper	Mushrooms, organ meats, shellfish
Iodine	Fish, shellfish, sea vegetables
DHA/EPA	Fish, shellfish, sea vegetables
Glutamine	Fish, poultry, red meat; insoluble fiber is abundant in celery, cruciferous vegetables, leafy greens
Folic acid	Black beans, lentils, spinach, asparagus, sunflower seeds, romaine lettuce, broccoli, turnip greens, mango, peanuts

    ¼ cup water
    ¼ cup avocado oil

Directions
    1. Mix all ingredients into a batter.
    2. Ladle batter into a ceramic waffle iron.
    3. Remove from waffle iron when cooked.

Blueberry Muffins

Ingredients
    3 cups almond flour
    ½ cup honey

1 teaspoon baking soda
1 teaspoon salt
6 eggs
½ cup avocado oil
Blueberries

Directions

1. Preheat oven to 350 degrees Fahrenheit. Stir together the ingredients.
2. Pour batter into paper-lined muffin pan cups. Bake for 15 minutes or until golden.

Anti-inflammatory Omelet

Ingredients

6 eggs
1 tablespoon avocado, ghee, or coconut oil
½ teaspoon curry powder
Salt, to taste
1 tablespoon cilantro, chopped
5–6 cherry tomatoes, diced
1 cup chopped spinach
¼ teaspoon black pepper
¼ teaspoon paprika

Directions

1. In a bowl, beat the eggs with a fork.
2. Add in all the other ingredients.
3. Add avocado, ghee, or coconut oil to a ceramic nontoxic pan over medium-low heat.
4. Add the eggs to the skillet and cook without stirring until the edges begin to set. With a silicon spatula, push the edges toward the center of the pan and tilt the pan so the uncooked eggs move to the edge.
5. Repeat until the eggs are almost set, so it will be easier to flip the omelet. Once flipped, let each side cook until done.

Green "Hulk" Smoothie

Ingredients

Frozen power greens
Frozen blueberries
Frozen strawberries
Frozen cauliflower, riced
Water or nondairy milk

½ avocado
Banana
1 zucchini
1 scoop collagen
Spirulina
1 scoop amla

Directions
1. Add ¼ cup of each ingredient. Mix in a blender.
2. Add stevia if needed to add sweetness. I also add supplements into the smoothie, like glutathione, glutamine, and zinc.
3. Additional note: Other add-ins my kids love are passion fruit, turmeric, ginger, jack fruit, acerola, aronia berries, figs, kiwi, dates, pomegranate, dandelion greens, microgreens, and dragon fruit. So experiment and have fun!

Halwa Poori: Traditional Pakistani Breakfast

Traditionally, halwa is made from semolina and sugar, and poori is a fried bread. We will make the halwa from nuts and honey. Halwa poori can be served with chick pea curry, fermented vegetables, and so much more! Yum!

Halwa

Ingredients
¼ cup ghee
Cardamom (a few seeds)
1 cup almond flour
1 cup walnuts (pulsed in food processor to a granular flour)
Honey, to taste
½ cup water
Raisins
Coconut flakes

Directions
1. Heat ghee in skillet.
2. Add cardamom seeds.
3. Add almond flour and walnut flour. Sauté until golden brown.
4. Add in water and honey to taste.
5. Cover on low heat, stirring regularly.
6. Add in raisins and coconut flakes, as desired.

Poori

Ingredients
> 2 cups arrowroot flour
> ½ cup almond flour
> 2 eggs
> 1 cup nondairy milk/water
> ½ teaspoon garlic
> ¼ teaspoon black pepper
> 1 teaspoon salt
> Cumin

Directions
> 1. Mix all ingredients together in a bowl.
> 2. Add oil to a ceramic skillet over medium-low heat.
> 3. Ladle the batter onto the skillet to make a very thin crepe.
> 4. Turn over to cook both sides evenly.

This recipe is a great naan, tortilla, poori, or pita and can be a great substitute in any of your favorite dishes!

French Toast

Ingredients
> 5 slices of Base Culture Bread
> ¼ cup of coconut milk
> 1 egg
> 1 tablespoon coconut sugar
> Pinch of salt
> 1 tablespoon avocado oil or butter

Directions
> 1. Mix together coconut milk, egg, coconut sugar, and salt.
> 2. In a hot skillet, melt avocado oil or butter.
> 3. Dip the bread in the egg coconut milk mixture.
> 4. Fry slices until golden brown, and then flip to cook both sides.

Serve with fresh berries and organic maple syrup.

Lunch

Chicken Bites

Ingredients
> 1 pound chicken cut into bite-sized pieces
> ½ teaspoon garlic

½ teaspoon salt
¼ teaspoon black pepper
1 tablespoon lemon juice
¼ teaspoon paprika
2 tablespoons chickpea flour

Directions

1. Mix all ingredients together, and, with 1 tablespoon of oil, cook each side for 2–3 minutes over medium heat.

Pasta

Ingredients

1 onion, chopped
1 tablespoon avocado oil
1 pound ground grass-fed beef or organic turkey
1 teaspoon salt
½ teaspoon black pepper
1 tablespoon Italian seasoning
1 teaspoon garlic
1 3-ounce packet broccoli sprouts
1 cup riced cauliflower
1 jar pasta sauce
1 box lentil pasta

Directions

1. In a large saucepan, sauté chopped onions in a little bit of avocado oil until translucent.
2. Combine ground beef and spices together. Add beef and spices to the saucepan and add vegetables. Cook until ground beef is no longer pink and the vegetables are tender.
3. Add in pasta sauce and cook until thickened.
4. Boil and cook lentil pasta according to instructions on the box.
5. When pasta is cooked, drain pasta and add to sauce.

Blackened Fish Tacos

Ingredients

6 pieces wild-caught haddock
1 tablespoon smoked paprika
1 teaspoon onion powder
1 teaspoon garlic powder
1 teaspoon salt

1 teaspoon taco seasoning
Cassava flour taco shells
Cabbage, sliced
Salsa, to taste

Directions
1. Dip each side of the fish into the spices.
2. In a cast iron skillet, with a tablespoon of oil, cook fish until tender.
3. Combine fish into cassava flour tortilla shell; add salsa and cabbage to taco.

Chicken Burritos

Ingredients
1 pound chicken, diced
1 bell pepper, diced
½ onion, diced
1 teaspoon garlic powder
1 teaspoon salt
1 teaspoon taco seasoning
Cassava flour burrito tortillas
1 can refried organic beans
Cabbage, sliced
Salsa, to taste
Almond milk cream cheese (optional)

Directions
1. Dice chicken and cook in a medium skillet with vegetables and spices.
2. Once cooked, move to a plate.
3. Warm tortilla in an oiled skillet just until it is soft and pliable.
4. Transfer the warmed tortilla to a plate. In the center of the tortilla, add cabbage slices topped with chicken mixture. Add refried beans, salsa, and almond milk cream cheese.
5. Fold both sides in and then fold the top in, burrito-style.
6. Heat oil in a ceramic skillet over medium-high heat. Cook the burrito 2 minutes each side to make the tortilla crispy.
7. Serve with veggies, avocado, and even enchilada sauce.

Salmon/Sardine Salad

Ingredients
2 cans wild-caught salmon or sardines

⅓ cup avocado mayo
1 medium celery stalk, finely chopped
½ teaspoon salt
½ teaspoon black pepper
Chopped onions and fresh herbs like dill (optional)

Directions

1. In a small bowl, combine all ingredients and mix well.
2. Serve with veggies, almond flour or seed crackers, sweet potato chips, or on top of a bed of lettuce for wraps.

Yellow Soup

Ingredients

2 tablespoons avocado oil
1 large onion, diced
3 cups chicken bone broth
1 can butternut squash
1 can pumpkin
1 cup frozen cauliflower rice
1 cup frozen carrots
1 tablespoon rosemary
1 teaspoon garlic
½ teaspoon salt
Optional spices: ¼ teaspoon sage and ginger

Directions

1. Heat the oil in a large pot over medium heat.
2. Add in the onions and sauté until soft.
3. Add in bone broth, veggies, and spices. Bring to a boil.
4. Cover and simmer until veggies are tender.
5. Let cool slightly; then pour the soup into a blender, and blend until smooth. You may need to do this in smaller batches.

Unwrapped Egg Roll

Ingredients

2 tablespoons of avocado oil
¼ of onion, sliced
Whole rotisserie chicken, shredded
1 12-ounce bag of coleslaw
3 tablespoons coconut aminos

2 tablespoons sesame oil
1 teaspoon garlic
Salt, to taste
½ cup peanut butter ·
Konjiac noodles (optional)
Sesame seeds for garnish

Directions
1. In a skillet, add oil and sliced onions and sauté until softened.
2. Add in chicken, coleslaw mix, coconut aminos, sesame oil, and spices.
3. Once the cabbage has wilted down and cooked, add in peanut butter.
4. Mix in noodles if desired.
5. Serve hot, topped with sesame seeds.

Dinner

Quick Rainbow Broccoli Salad

Ingredients
1 10-ounce bag broccoli florets
1 12-ounce bag coleslaw mix
½ cup avocado mayonnaise
1 tablespoon honey
¼ cup halved grapes
¼ cup goji berries

Directions
1. Mix all ingredients together.

Coconut Shrimp Curry

Ingredients
2 tablespoons avocado oil
1 large onion, diced
1 cup chicken bone broth
2 cans coconut milk
2 pounds wild-caught shrimp
½ cup of mushrooms, sliced
½ cup of carrots, sliced
½ cup of any other veggies
1 teaspoon curry powder
1 teaspoon turmeric
½ teaspoon paprika
½ teaspoon salt

Directions
1. Heat the oil in a large pot over medium heat.
2. Add in the onions and sauté until soft.
3. Add in bone broth, coconut milk, shrimp, veggies, and spices. Bring to a boil.
4. Cover and simmer until veggies are tender and soup thickens.

Chicken Wings

Ingredients
4 pounds chicken wings, cut into flats and drumettes
½ teaspoon salt
2 teaspoons garlic powder
Pinch of cracked pepper

Directions
1. Toss chicken wings in spices and air fry until done.
2. Serve with favorite sauce and salad.

Rainbow Pasta Salad

Ingredients
1 box lentil pasta
1 can black olives
½ yellow bell pepper, chopped
1 red bell pepper, chopped
2 cups cherry tomatoes
1 green bell pepper, chopped
1 cup spinach, chopped
1 can heart of palms, chopped
2 tablespoons of olive oil
Squeeze of lemon, as desired
2 teaspoons Italian seasoning

Directions
1. In a large pot of salted boiling water, cook pasta according to box directions. Once the pasta is done, drain and rinse under cold water.
2. Add in veggies, spices, oil, and lemons.

Fish Fingers

Ingredients
Avocado oil

    6 pieces haddock or cod
    1 cup chickpea flour
    ¼ cup water
    1 teaspoon salt
    1 teaspoon garlic
    ½ teaspoon paprika

Directions
    1. Heat ½ inch of avocado oil in a skillet over medium heat.
    2. Slice up fish into strips.
    3. Combine chickpea flour, water, and spices until it makes a thick paste.
    4. Dip fish into the chickpea flour mixture.
    5. Place battered fish into hot oil and cook both sides until crispy.

Note: One can also make a batter with one egg and ¼ cup of cassava flour, with a little bit of water to create a paste; then dip the fish into the batter and fry similar to the above.

Green Beans

Ingredients
    2 tablespoons avocado oil
    ½ diced onion
    1 12-ounce bag green beans
    1 4-ounce container of shiitake mushrooms
    2 tablespoons coconut aminos
    1 teaspoon garlic
    1 teaspoon salt

Directions
    1. In a skillet, heat the oil.
    2. Add onions and cook until soft.
    3. Add in vegetables, coconut aminos, and spices.
    4. Serve as a side dish.

Lasagna

Ingredients
    1 pound ground beef
    ½ onion, diced
    4 ounces mushrooms, diced
    1 12-ounce bag frozen cauliflower, riced
    3 ounces broccoli sprouts

2 cloves garlic
1 jar tomato sauce
1 teaspoon Italian seasoning
1½ teaspoons basil
Salt
Almond-flour lasagna sheets
¼ cup black olives, sliced
2 large tomatoes, sliced

Cheese layer
16 ounces almond milk ricotta
½ cup parsley, chopped
1 egg

Directions
1. Brown beef, onion, diced mushrooms, riced cauliflower, broccoli sprouts, and garlic over medium-high heat until no pink remains.
2. Stir in pasta sauce and spices. Let sauce simmer.
3. Mix together ricotta, parsley, and egg.
4. Add one cup of meat sauce to a 9 x 13 pan. Top with a lasagna noodle.
5. Layer with ⅓ cheese mixture and 1 cup meat sauce.
6. Repeat and top the final noodle layer with sauce.
7. Slice up olives and tomatoes to garnish on top.
8. Cover with parchment paper and foil and bake for 45 minutes.
9. Rest 15 minutes before cutting.

Calamari

Ingredients
2 10-ounce packs calamari
½ cup tapioca flour
1 egg
½ teaspoon garlic
½ teaspoon paprika
¼ teaspoon pepper
1 cup avocado oil for frying

Sauce
½ cup avocado mayo
1 tablespoon sriracha

Directions
1. Pat calamari dry.

2. Add tapioca flour, egg, and spices.
3. Fry one by one in the hot oil until golden brown.
4. Remove from oil and place on paper towels to drain oil.
5. Combine avocado mayo and sriracha for dipping sauce.
6. Serve hot.

Dessert

Banana Bread

Ingredients
    3 cups almond flour
    ½ cup honey
    1 teaspoon baking soda
    1 teaspoon salt
    6 eggs
    ½ cup avocado oil
    5 bananas
    ½ cup walnuts, chopped

Directions
1. Preheat oven to 350 degrees Fahrenheit.
2. In a large mixing bowl, combine all the ingredients except walnuts and blend until smooth.
3. On a unbleached parchment–lined cookie sheet, pour out batter and top with chopped walnuts.
4. Bake for 15 minutes.
5. Remove and let cool before cutting to serve.

Pineapple Upside-Down Cake

Ingredients
    3 cups almond flour
    ½ cup oil
    ½ cup honey
    6 eggs
    1 teaspoon baking soda
    1 teaspoon salt
    1 15-ounce can pineapple (drained), reserving juice
    ½ cup reserved juice from canned pineapple (100%)
    Sliced red fruit to place within the pineapple circles

Directions
1. Preheat oven to 350 degrees Fahrenheit.
2. In a large mixing bowl, combine all ingredients except pineapple circles and blend until smooth.
3. On an unbleached parchment–lined cookie sheet, place pineapple circles as desired on the cookie sheet, with either cherries, raspberries, or strawberries placed in the middle of the pineapple circles.
4. Pour the almond flour mixture over the pineapple circles.
5. Bake for 15 minutes.
6. Remove from oven, flip, and let cool before cutting to serve.

Chocolate Chip Peanut Butter Cookies

Ingredients
   3 cups almond flour
   ½ cup peanut butter or another nut butter
   ½ cup honey
   3 eggs
   1 teaspoon baking soda
   1 teaspoon salt
   No-sugar chocolate chips

Directions
1. Preheat oven to 350 degrees Fahrenheit.
2. In a large mixing bowl, combine all the ingredients and blend until smooth.
3. On an unbleached parchment–lined cookie sheet, roll out cookies.
4. Bake for 15 minutes.

Tigernut Flour Chocolate Chip Cookies

Ingredients
   2 cups Tigernut flour
   ⅔ cup honey
   ⅓ cup avocado oil
   1 tablespoon gelatin
   1 teaspoon baking soda
   ½ teaspoon salt
   No-sugar chocolate chips

Directions

1. Preheat oven to 350 degrees Fahrenheit.
2. In a large mixing bowl, combine all the ingredients and blend until smooth.
3. On an unbleached parchment–lined cookie sheet, roll out cookies.
4. Bake for 15 minutes.

Chocolate-Covered Strawberries

Ingredients
   Strawberries
   No-sugar chocolate chips

Directions

1. Melt chocolate chips in a glass bowl over a pan with boiling water.
2. Dip strawberries into the melted chocolate and lay on parchment paper.
3. Add toppings like coconut or crushed nuts as needed.
4. Refrigerate until solid.

Dairy-Free Custard

Ingredients
   2 cans coconut milk
   12 egg yolks
   1.5 scoops gelatin
   ¼ cup honey
   Pinch of salt

Directions

1. In a glass or stainless steel bowl, mix together egg yolks, coconut milk, and honey.
2. Using the double boiler method, cook the egg in the coconut honey mixture, whisking together to combine (don't stop whisking).
3. When the mixture is hot, whisk in the gelatin.
4. When the custard starts to thicken, take off the heat.
5. Place a strainer over a clean bowl and pour custard into the strainer to remove lumps.
6. For fruit tart, add custard to paleo pie crust (my favorite crust is Dr. Izabella Wentz's cassava flour pie crust from *Hashimoto's Food Pharmacology*). For trifle, layer on top of fruit, alternating with almond flour cake.
7. Refrigerate for at least 2 hours before serving.

Notes

INTRODUCTION: FROM MEDICAL DOCTOR TO HOLISTICMOM, MD

1. World Health Organization, "Obesity and Overweight," accessed February 24, 2021, https://www.who.int/news-room/fact-sheets/detail/obesity-and-overweight.
2. Joshua Aspril and Johns Hopkins Bloomberg School of Public Health, "U.S. Autism Rates up 10 Percent in New CDC Report," Johns Hopkins Bloomberg School of Public Health, March 26, 2020, https://www.jhsph.edu/news/news-releases/2020/us-autism-rates-up-10-percent-in-new-cdc-report.html.
3. Karen Weintraub, "The Prevalence Puzzle: Autism Counts," *Nature* 479, no. 7371 (2011): 22–24, https://doi.org/10.1038/479022a.
4. Amy Morin, "The Truth about Troubled Teens," *Verywell Mind*, March 26, 2020, https://www.verywellmind.com/what-is-happening-to-our-children-2606269.
5. Gillian Ray, "Mental and Behavioral Health in Children: A Crisis Made Worse by the Pandemic," Children's Hospital Association, February 24, 2021, https://www.childrenshospitals.org/Newsroom/Press-Releases/2021/Mental-and-Behavioral-Health-Crisis-in-Children.

CHAPTER 1: TODAY'S DILEMMA: IS OUR CHANGING WORLD THREATENING OUR FUTURE?

1. Centers for Disease Control and Prevention, "Heart Disease Facts," September 8, 2020, https://www.cdc.gov/heartdisease/facts.htm.
2. World Health Organization, "Suicide: One Person Dies Every 40 Seconds," accessed February 24, 2021, https://www.who.int/news/item/09-09-2019-suicide-one-person-dies-every-40-seconds.

3. Centers for Disease Control and Prevention, "About the Center," January 19, 2021, https://www.cdc.gov/chronicdisease/center/index.htm.

4. Rob Stein, "Sperm Counts Plummet in Western Men, Study Finds," NPR, July 31, 2017, https://www.npr.org/2017/07/31/539517210/sperm-counts-plummet-in-western-men-study-finds.

5. J. Van Cleave, S. L. Gortmaker, and J. M. Perrin, "Dynamics of Obesity and Chronic Health Conditions among Children and Youth," *Journal of the American Medical Association* 303, no. 7 (2011): 623–30, https://doi.org/10.1001/jama.2010.104.

6. Harvard School of Public Health, "More Than Half of U.S. Children Will Have Obesity as Adults If Current Trends Continue," June 22, 2018, https://www.hsph.harvard.edu/news/press-releases/childhood-obesity-risk-as-adults/.

7. Van Cleave, Gortmaker, and Perrin, "Dynamics of Obesity and Chronic Health Conditions among Children and Youth."

8. Sid Kirchheimer, "Year 2000 Babies High Risk for Diabetes," WebMD, October 7, 2003, https://www.webmd.com/diabetes/news/20031007/year-2000-babies-high-risk-for-diabetes.

9. Fateme Shafiei, Asma Salari-Moghaddam, Bagher Larijani, and Ahmad Esmaillzadeh, "Adherence to the Mediterranean Diet and Risk of Depression: A Systematic Review and Updated Meta-Analysis of Observational Studies," *Nutrition Reviews* 77, no. 4 (2019): 230–39, https://doi.org/10.1093/nutrit/nuy070.

10. Greta A. Bushnell, Stephen Crystal, and Mark Olfson, "Trends in Antipsychotic Medication Use in Young Privately Insured Children," *Journal of the American Academy of Child & Adolescent Psychiatry*, October 19, 2020, https://doi.org/10.1016/j.jaac.2020.09.023.

11. R. C. Sun and D. T. L. Shek, "Student Classroom Misbehavior: an Exploratory Study Based on Teachers' Perceptions," *Scientific World Journal* (2012), https://doi.org/10.1100/2012/208907; Tori Rodriguez, "Impact of the COVID-19 Pandemic on Adolescent Mental Health," *Psychiatry Advisor*, April 30, 2021, https://www.psychiatryadvisor.com/home/topics/child-adolescent-psychiatry/adolescent-mental-health-issues-are-further-exacerbated-by-the-covid-19-pandemic/.

12. Sally C. Curtin and Melonie Heron, "Death Rates Due to Suicide and Homicide among Persons Aged 10–24: United States, 2000–2017," NCHS Data Brief, October 2019, https://www.cdc.gov/nchs/data/databriefs/db352-h.pdf.

13. S. H. Lee, G. Paz-Filho, C. Mastronardi, J. Licinio, and M-L Wong, "Is Increased Antidepressant Exposure a Contributory Factor to the Obesity Pandemic?" *Translational Psychiatry* 6, no. 3 (2016), https://doi.org/10.1038/tp.2016.25.

14. Danielle C. DeVille, "Suicidal Ideation, Suicide Attempts, and Self-Injury in Children Aged 9 to 10 Years," *JAMA Network Open*, February 7, 2020, https://doi.org/10.1001/jamanetworkopen.2019.20956.

15. K. Weintraub, "The Prevalence Puzzle: Autism Counts," *Nature* 479, no. 7371 (2011): 22–24, https://pubmed.ncbi.nlm.nih.gov/22051656/.

16. Arndt Manzel, Dominik N. Muller, David A. Hafler, Susan E. Erdman, Ralf A. Linker, and Markus Kleinewietfeld, "Role of 'Western Diet' in Inflammatory Autoimmune Diseases," *Current Allergy and Asthma Report* 14, no. 1 (January 2014), http://www.www.doi.org/10.1007/s11882-013-0404-6.

17. Centers for Disease Control and Prevention, "FastStats—Asthma," January 25, 2021, https://www.cdc.gov/nchs/fastats/asthma.htm.

18. Scholastic, "Classroom Behavior Problems Increasing, Teachers Say," accessed May 17, 2021, https://www.scholastic.com/teachers/articles/teaching-content/class room-behavior-problems-increasing-teachers-say/; Amy Morin, "The Truth about Troubled Teens," *Verywell Mind*, March 26, 2020, https://www.verywellmind.com /what-is-happening-to-our-children-2606269; United States Department of Justice, "102. Juvenile Crime Facts," January 22, 2020, https://www.justice.gov/archives/jm /criminal-resource-manual-102-juvenile-crime-facts.

19. Nora D. Volkow, "Prevalence of Substance Use among Young People in the US," *JAMA Pediatrics*, March 29, 2021, https://doi.org/10.1001/jamapediatrics .2020.6981.

20. Food and Agriculture Organization, "Fertilizer Use to Surpass 200 Million Tonnes in 2018," February 16, 2015, http://www.fao.org/news/story/en/item /277488/icode/.

21. Food and Agriculture Organization, "Fertilizer Use to Surpass 200 Million Tonnes in 2018"; Susan Cosier, "The World Needs Topsoil to Grow 95% of Its Food—but It's Rapidly Disappearing," *Guardian*, May 30, 2019, https://www.the guardian.com/us-news/2019/may/30/topsoil-farming-agriculture-food-toxic-amer ica; United Nations, "24 Billion Tons of Fertile Land Lost Every Year, Warns UN Chief on World Day to Combat Desertification," UN News, June 16, 2019, https:// news.un.org/en/story/2019/06/1040561.

22. Daniel Stolte, "One-Third of Plant and Animal Species Could Be Gone in 50 Years," University of Arizona News, February 12, 2020, https://news.arizona.edu /story/onethird-plant-and-animal-species-could-be-gone-50-years.

23. Food and Agriculture Organization, "What Is Happening to Agrobiodiversity?" accessed February 24, 2021, http://www.fao.org/3/y5609e/y5609e02.htm.

24. Jenny Howard, "Dead Zones, Facts and Information," *National Geographic Environment*, July 31, 2019, https://www.nationalgeographic.com/environment /article/dead-zones.

25. Kelsie Sandoval, "Kids in the U.S. Are Eating More Fast Food, the CDC Reports," NBCNews.com, August 14, 2020, https://www.nbcnews.com/health/kids -health/kids-u-s-are-eating-more-fast-food-cdc-reports-n1236756.

26. M-F O'Connor and M. R. Irwin, "What Is Inflammation? And Why Does It Matter for Child Development?" Center on the Developing Child at Harvard University, November 13, 2020, https://developingchild.harvard.edu/resources/what-is -inflammation-and-why-does-it-matter-for-child-development/.

27. O'Connor and Irwin, "What Is Inflammation?"

28. T. M. Wright and C. A. Feghali, "Cytokines in Acute and Chronic Inflammation," *Frontiers in Bioscience: A Journal and Virtual Library* 2 (January 1997): 12–26, https://doi.org/10.2741/a171.

29. Neeti D. Mehta, Ebrahim Haroon, Xiaodan Xu, Bobbi J. Woolwine, Zhihao Li, and Jennifer C. Felger, "Inflammation Negatively Correlates with Amygdala-Ventromedial Prefrontal Functional Connectivity in Association with Anxiety in

Patients with Depression: Preliminary Results," *Brain, Behavior, and Immunity*, October 2018, https://doi.org/10.1016/j.bbi.2018.07.026.

30. Tristen K. Inagaki, Keely A. Muscatell, Michael R. Irwin, Steve W. Cole, and Naomi I. Eisenberger, "Inflammation Selectively Enhances Amygdala Activity to Socially Threatening Images," *NeuroImage* 59, no. 4 (2012): 3222–26, https://doi .org/10.1016/j.neuroimage.2011.10.090.

31. Pauline Anderson, "Inflammatory Dietary Pattern Linked to Brain Aging," *Medscape*, July 19, 2017, https://www.medscape.com/viewarticle/883038.

32. Ekin Secinti, Ellen J. Thompson, Marcus Richards, and Darya Gaysina, "Research Review: Childhood Chronic Physical Illness and Adult Emotional Health—A Systematic Review and Meta-Analysis," *Journal of Child Psychology and Psychiatry* 58, no. 7 (2017): 753–69, https://doi.org/10.1111/jcpp.12727.

33. Allison A. Appleton, Stephen L. Buka, Marie C. McCormick, et al., "Emotional Functioning at Age 7 Years Is Associated with C-Reactive Protein in Middle Adulthood," *Psychosomatic Medicine* 73, no. 4 (2011): 295–303, https://doi.org/10.1097/psy .0b013e31821534f6; University of Birmingham, "Childhood Cognitive Problems Could Lead to Mental Health Issues in Later Life," *ScienceDaily*, accessed April 7, 2021, https://www.sciencedaily.com/releases/2021/04/210407110411.htm.

34. Marica Leone, Ralph Kuja-Halkola, Amy Leva, Brian M. D'Onofrio, Henrick Larsson, Paul Lichtenstein, and Sarah E. Bergen, "Association of Youth Depression with Subsequent Somatic Diseases and Premature Death," *JAMA Psychiatry*, December 9, 2020, https://doi.org/10.1001/jamapsychiatry.2020.3786.

35. R. Dantzer, Jason C. O'Connor, M. A. Lawson, and K. W. Kelley, "Inflammation-Associated Depression: From Serotonin to Kynurenine," *Psychoneuroendocrinology* 36, no. 3 (2011): 426–36, https://doi.org/10.1016/j.psyneuen.2010.09.012.

36. S. I. Hanswijk, M. Spoelder, L. Shan, et al., "Gestational Factors throughout Fetal Neurodevelopment: The Serotonin Link," *International Journal of Molecular Sciences* 21, no. 16 (2020): 5850, https://doi.org/10.3390/ijms21165850.

37. M. D. Rudolph, A. M. Graham, E. Feczko, O. Miranda-Dominguez, J. M. Rasmussen, R. Nardos, S. Entringer, P. D. Wadhwa, C. Buss, and D. A. Fair, "Maternal IL-6 during Pregnancy Can Be Estimated from Newborn Brain Connectivity and Predicts Future Working Memory in Offspring," *Nature Neuroscience* 21, no. 5 (2018): 765–72, https://doi.org/10.1038/s41593-018-0128-y.

38. A. M. Graham, J. M. Rasmussen, M. D. Rudolph, C. M. Heim, J. H. Gilmore, M. Styner, S. G. Potkin, S. Entringer, P. D. Wadhwa, C. Buss, and D. A. Fair, "Maternal Systemic Interleukin-6 during Pregnancy Is Associated with Newborn Amygdala Phenotypes and Subsequent Behavior at 2 Years of Age," *Biological Psychiatry* 83, no. 2 (2018): 109–19, https://doi.org/10.1016/j.biopsych.2017.05.027.

39. J. Posner, J. Cha, A. K. Roy, B. S. Peterson, R. Bansal, H. C. Gustafsson, E. Raffanello, J. Gingrich, and C. Monk, "Alterations in Amygdala–Prefrontal Circuits in Infants Exposed to Prenatal Maternal Depression," *Translational Psychiatry* 6, no. 11 (November 2016): e935, https://doi.org/10.1038/tp.2016.146.

40. Massachusetts General Hospital, "Childhood Psychiatric Symptom Risk Strongly Linked to Adverse Exposures during Gestation," *ScienceDaily*, accessed April 28, 2021, https://www.sciencedaily.com/releases/2021/04/210428140901.htm.

41. University College London, "New Mothers Twice as Likely to Have Post-natal Depression in Lockdown, Study Finds," *ScienceDaily*, accessed May 11, 2021, https://www.sciencedaily.com/releases/2021/05/210511123619.htm.

42. M. Gevezova, V. Sarafian, G. Anderson, and M. Maes, "Inflammation and Mitochondrial Dysfunction in Autism Spectrum Disorder," *CNS & Neurological Disorders—Drug Targets* 19, no. 5 (2020): 320–33, https://doi.org/10.2174/1871527319666200 628015039.

43. K. F. E. Van de Loo, J. A. E. Custers, S. Koene, et al., "Psychological Functioning in Children Suspected for Mitochondrial Disease: The Need for Care," *Orphanet Journal of Rare Diseases* 15, no. 76 (2020), https://doi.org/10.1186/s13023-020 -1342-8.

44. MedlinePlus, "What Is Noncoding DNA?" accessed February 24, 2021, https://ghr.nlm.nih.gov/primer/basics/noncodingdna.

45. S. Strang, C. Hoeber, O. Uhl, B. Koletzko, T. F. Münte, H. Lehnert, R. J. Dolan, S. M. Schmid, and S. Q. Park, "Impact of Nutrition on Social Decision Making," *Proceedings of the National Academy of Sciences of the United States of America* 114, no. 25 (June 20, 2017): 6510–14, https://doi.org/10.1073/pnas.1620245114.

46. C. S. Mott Children's Hospital, "Mott Poll Report: Healthy Eating for Children: Parents Not Following the Recipe," National Poll on Children's Health, February 20, 2017, https://mottpoll.org/reports-surveys/healthy-eating-children-parents -not-following-recipe.

47. Centers for Disease Control and Prevention, "Children Eating More Fruit, but Fruit and Vegetable Intake Still Too Low," press release, August 5, 2014, https://www .cdc.gov/media/releases/2014/p0805-fruits-vegetables.html.

48. "Worldwide Trends in Body-Mass Index, Underweight, Overweight, and Obesity from 1975 to 2016: A Pooled Analysis of 2416 Population-Based Measurement Studies in 128.9 Million Children, Adolescents, and Adults," *Lancet*, December 16, 2017, https://www.thelancet.com/journals/lancet/article/PIIS0140 -6736(17)32129-3/fulltext.

49. N. M. Giollabhui et al., "Executive Dysfunction in Depression in Adolescence: The Role of Inflammation and Higher Body Mass," *Psychological Medicine* (March 2019): 1–9, https://www.cambridge.org/core/journals/psychological-medicine/article /abs/executive-dysfunction-in-depression-in-adolescence-the-role-of-inflammation -and-higher-body-mass/70A07BF9EE0E8E204792E4C36230E1C5.

50. "Poor Diets May Lower Children's IQ," *Guardian*, February 7, 2011, https:// www.theguardian.com/science/2011/feb/07/diet-children-iq.

51. P. M. Rodier, "Developing Brain as a Target of Toxicity," *Environmental Health Perspectives* 103, suppl. 6 (September 1995): 73–76, https://doi.org/10.1289/ehp .95103s673; B. P. Lanphear, "The Impact of Toxins on the Developing Brain," *Annual Review of Public Health* 36 (March 2015): 211–30, https://doi.org/10.1146 /annurev-publhealth-031912-114413.

52. B. P. Lanphear, C. V. Vorhees, and D.C. Bellinger, "Protecting Children from Environmental Toxins," *PLoS Medicine* 2, no. 3 (2005): e61, https://doi.org/10.1371 /journal.pmed.0020061; J. Liu and G. Lewis, "Environmental Toxicity and Poor Cognitive Outcomes in Children and Adults," *Journal of Environmental Health* 76, no.

6 (January–February 2014): 130–38, https://www.ncbi.nlm.nih.gov/pmc/articles /PMC4247328/.

53. Benoit Denizet-Lewis, "Why Are More American Teenagers Than Ever Suffering from Severe Anxiety?" *New York Times Magazine*, October 11, 2017, https:// www.nytimes.com/2017/10/11/magazine/why-are-more-american-teenagers-than -ever-suffering-from-severe-anxiety.html.

54. Daniel Arkin, "Covid Stress Taking a Toll on Children's Mental Health, CDC Finds," NBCNews.com, November 12, 2020, https://www.nbcnews.com/health /kids-health/covid-stress-taking-toll-children-s-mental-health-cdc-finds-n1247540.

55. S. Suffren, V. La Buissonnière-Ariza, A. Tucholka, M. Nassim, J. R. Séguin, M. Boivin, M. Kaur Singh, L. C. Foland-Ross, F. Lepore, I. H. Gotlib, R. E. Tremblay, and F. S. Maheu, "Prefrontal Cortex and Amygdala Anatomy in Youth with Persistent Levels of Harsh Parenting Practices and Subclinical Anxiety Symptoms over Time during Childhood," *Development and Psychopathology*, March 22, 2021, https:// doi.org/10.1017/S0954579420001716.

56. Corinne David-Ferdon, Jeffery E. Hall, Khiya J. Marshall, Linda L. Dahlberg, and Alana M. Vivolo-Kantor, "A Comprehensive Technical Package for the Prevention of Youth Violence and Associated Risk Behaviors," National Center for Injury Prevention and Control, Division of Violence Prevention, Centers for Disease Control and Prevention, 2016, https://www.cdc.gov/violenceprevention/pdf/yv -technicalpackage.pdf.

57. "Preventing Bullying | Violence Prevention | Injury Center | CDC," Centers for Disease Control and Prevention, October 21, 2020, https://www.cdc.gov/violence prevention/youthviolence/bullyingresearch/fastfact.html.

58. A. Nagano-Saito et al., "Stress-Induced Dopamine Release in Human Medial Prefrontal Cortex—[18]F-Fallypride/PET Study in Healthy Volunteers," *Synapse* 67, no. 12 (December 2013): 821–30, https://doi.org/10.1002/syn.21700.

59. Erin Digitale, "Stanford Study Finds Stronger One-Way Fear Signals in Brains of Anxious Kids," Stanford Medicine News Center, April 21, 2020, https://med .stanford.edu/news/all-news/2020/04/stanford-study-finds-stronger-one-way-fear -signals-in-brains-of-.html.

60. A. F. T. Arnsten, "Stress Signalling Pathways That Impair Prefrontal Cortex Structure and Function," *Nature Reviews Neuroscience* 10, no. 6 (June 2009): 410–22, https://doi.org/10.1038/nrn2648.

61. Centers for Disease Control and Prevention, "Do Your Children Get Enough Sleep?" March 2, 2020, https://www.cdc.gov/chronicdisease/resources/infographic /children-sleep.htm.

62. Michael J. Breus, "Lack of Sleep Disrupts Our Genes," *Psychology Today*, March 21, 2013, https://www.psychologytoday.com/us/blog/sleep-newzzz/201303/lack -sleep-disrupts-our-genes.

63. S. M. Flood and K. R. Genadek, "Time for Each Other: Work and Family Constraints among Couples," *Journal of Marriage and Family* 78, no. 1 (2016): 142–64, https://doi.org/10.1111/jomf.12255.

64. S. F. Waters, E. A. Virmani, R. A. Thompson, S. Meyer, H. A. Raikes, and R. Jochem, "Emotion Regulation and Attachment: Unpacking Two Constructs and

Their Association," *Journal of Psychopathology and Behavioral Assessment* 32 (2010): 37–47, https://doi.org/10.1007/s10862-009-9163-z; Y. Dvir, J. D. Ford, M. Hill, and J. A. Frazier, "Childhood Maltreatment, Emotional Dysregulation, and Psychiatric Comorbidities," *Harvard Review of Psychiatry* 22, no. 3 (2014): 149–61, https://doi.org /10.1097/HRP.0000000000000014.

65. Ericsson, "Ericsson Mobility Report: 70 Percent of World's Population Using Smartphones by 2020," press release, June 3, 2015, https://www.ericsson.com/en /press-releases/2015/6/ericsson-mobility-report-70-percent-of-worlds-population -using-smartphones-by-2020.

66. M. G. Hunt et al., "No More FOMO: Limiting Social Media Decreases Lone-liness and Depression," *Journal of Social and Clinical Psychology* 37, no. 10 (November 2018): 751–68, https://doi.org/10.1521/jscp.2018.37.10.751; B. A. Primack et al., "Social Media Use and Perceived Social Isolation among Young Adults in the U.S.," *American Journal of Preventive Medicine* 53, no. 1 (July 2017): 1–8, https://doi.org /10.1016/j.amepre.2017.01.010.

67. J. T .F. Lau et al., "Incidence and Predictive Factors of Internet Addiction among Chinese Secondary School Students in Hong Kong: A Longitudinal Study," *Social Psychiatry and Psychiatric Epidemiology* 52, no. 6 (June 2017): 657–67, https://doi .org/10.3390/ijerph17228547.

68. B. Popkin and C. Hawks, "The Sweetening of the Global Diet, Particularly Beverages: Patterns, Trends and Policy Responses for Diabetes Prevention," *Lancet Diabetes & Endocrinology* 4, no. 2 (February 2016): 174–86, https://doi.org/10.1016 /S2213-8587(15)00419-2.

69. J. Gramlich, "5 Facts about Crime in the U.S.," Pew Research Center, January 3, 2019, http://www.pewresearch.org/fact-tank/2019/01/03/5-facts-about-crime -in-the-u-s/.

70. A. Szabo, "Negative Psychological Effects of Watching the News in the Televi-sion: Relaxation or Another Intervention May Be Needed to Buffer Them!" *Interna-tional Journal of Behavioral Medicine* 14, no. 2 (2007): 57–62, https://doi.org/10.1007 /BF03004169.

71. J. A. Rosenkranz, E. R. Venheim, and M. Padival, "Chronic Stress Causes Amygdala Hyperexcitability in Rodents," *Biological Psychiatry* 67, no. 12 (June 2010): 1128–36.

72. K. I. Kolmychkova, A. V. Zhelankin, V. P. Karagodin, and A. N. Orekhov, "Mitochondria and Inflammation," *Patologicheskaia Fiziologiia I Eksperimental'naia Tera-piia* 60 no. 4 (2016): 114–21.

CHAPTER 2: THE SCIENCE OF HOLISTIC PARENTING

1. W. T. Greenough, J. E. Black, and C. S. Wallace, "Experience and Brain De-velopment," *Child Development* 58 (1987): 539–59, https://doi.org/10.2307/1130197.

2. D. T. Neal, W. Wood, and J. M. Quinn, "Habits—a Repeat Performance," *Current Directions in Psychological Science* 15, no. 4 (2006): 198–202, https://psycnet.apa .org/record/2006-12374-010.

3. S. Kuppens and E. Ceulemans, "Parenting Styles: A Closer Look at a Well-Known Concept," *Journal of Child and Family Studies* 28, no. 1 (2019): 168–81, https://doi.org/10.1007/s10826-018-1242-x.

4. J. P. Shonkoff and P. A. Fisher, "Rethinking Evidence-Based Practice and Two-Generation Programs to Create the Future of Early Childhood Policy," *Development and Psychopathology* 25 (2013): 1635–53, https://doi.org/10.1017/S0954579413000813.

5. The famous "triune brain theory" was originally developed by American neuroscientist Dr. Paul MacLean in the 1960s. See J. D. Newman and J. C. Harris's review of his works: "The Scientific Contributions of Paul D. MacLean (1913–2007)," *Journal of Nervous and Mental Disease* 197, no. 1 (January 2009): 3–5, https://doi.org/10.1097/NMD.0b013e31818ec5d9.

6. K. M. Hassevoort, N. A. Khan, C. H. Hillman, and N. J. Cohen, "Childhood Markers of Health Behavior Relate to Hippocampal Health, Memory, and Academic Performance," *Mind, Brain, and Education* 10 (2016): 162–70, https://doi.org/10.1111/mbe.12108.

7. Pia Rotshtein, Mark P. Richardson, Joel S. Winston, Stefan J. Kiebel, Patrik Vuilleumier, Martin Eimer, Jon Driver, and Raymond J. Dolan, "Amygdala Damage Affects Event-Related Potentials for Fearful Faces at Specific Time Windows," *Human Brain Mapping* 31, no. 7 (2009): 1089–1105, https://doi.org/10.1002/hbm.20921.

8. J. S. Feinstein et al., "The Human Amygdala and the Induction and Experience of Fear," *Current Biology* 21, no. 1 (2011): 34–38, https://doi.org/10.1016/j.cub.2010.11.042.

9. B. Kolb, "Brain and Behavioral Plasticity in the Developing Brain: Neuroscience and Public Policy," *Paediatrics & Child Health* 14, no. 10 (2009): 651–52, https://doi.org/10.1093/pch/14.10.651.

10. A. S. Hodel, "Rapid Infant Prefrontal Cortex Development and Sensitivity to Early Environmental Experience," *Developmental Review* 48 (2018): 113–44, https://doi.org/10.1016/j.dr.2018.02.003.

11. N. J. Kelley et al., "Stimulating Self-Regulation: A Review of Non-invasive Brain Stimulation Studies of Goal-Directed Behavior," *Frontiers in Behavioral Neuroscience* 12 (January 2019), https://doi.org/10.3389/fnbeh.2018.00337.

12. S. E. Cusick and M. K. Georgieff, "The Role of Nutrition in Brain Development: The Golden Opportunity of the 'First 1000 Days,'" *Journal of Pediatrics* 175 (2016): 16–21, https://doi.org/10.1016/j.jpeds.2016.05.013.

13. Centers for Disease Control and Prevention, "Early Brain Development and Health," accessed February 22, 2021, https://www.cdc.gov/ncbddd/childdevelopment/early-brain-development.html.

14. J. Jirout, J. LoCasale-Crouch, K. Turnbull, et al., "How Lifestyle Factors Affect Cognitive and Executive Function and the Ability to Learn in Children," *Nutrients* 11, no. 8 (2019): 1953, https://doi.org/10.3390/nu11081953.

15. K. Sukhpreet et al., "Bacteroides-Dominant Gut Microbiome of Late Infancy Is Associated with Enhanced Neurodevelopment," *Gut Microbes* 13, no. 1 (2021), https://doi.org/10.1080/19490976.2021.1930875.

16. D. Moreau, L. J. Kirk, and K. E. Waldie, "High-Intensity Training Enhances Executive Function in Children in a Randomized, Placebo-Controlled Trial," *Elife* 6 (August 2017), https://elifesciences.org/articles/25062.

CHAPTER 3: DIGESTIVE HEALTH AND DETOXIFICATION

1. Ruby J. Graham et al., "Estimates of the Heritability of Human Longevity Are Substantially Inflated Due to Assortative Mating," *Genetics* 2010, no. 3 (November 1, 2018): 1109–24, https://doi.org/10.1534/genetics.118.301613.

2. J. L. Harris, J. A. Bargh, and K. D. Brownell, "Priming Effects of Television Food Advertising on Eating Behavior," *Health Psychology* 28, no. 4 (July 2009): 404–13, https://doi.org/10.1037/a0014399; E. J. Boyland et al., "Food Choice and Overconsumption: Effect of Premium Sports Celebrity Endorser," *Journal of Pediatrics* 163, no. 2 (August 2013): 339–43.

3. J. A. Emond et al., "Exposure to Child-Directed TV Advertising and Preschoolers' Intake of Advertised Cereal," *American Journal of Preventive Medicine* 56, no. 2 (2019): e35–e43.

4. L. Schnabel, E. Kesse-Guyot, B. Allès, M. Touvier, B. Srour, S. Hercberg, C. Buscail, and C. Julia, "Association between Ultraprocessed Food Consumption and Risk of Mortality among Middle-Aged Adults in France," *JAMA Internal Medicine* 179, no. 4 (2019): 490–98, https://doi.org/10.1001/jamainternmed.2018.7289.

5. L. G. Baraldi, S. E. Martinez, D. S. Cannella, and C. A. Monteiro, "Consumption of Ultra-processed Foods and Associated Sociodemographic Factors in the USA between 2007 and 2012: Evidence from a Nationally Representative Cross-sectional Study," *BMJ Open* 8, no. 3 (2018): e020574.

6. B. Caballero, "The Global Epidemic of Obesity: An Overview," *Epidemiologic Reviews* 29 (2007): 1–5, https://doi.org/10.1093/epirev/mxm012.

7. W. P. T. James, "WHO Recognition of the Global Obesity Epidemic," *International Journal of Obesity*, December 2008, https://pubmed.ncbi.nlm.nih.gov/19136980/.

8. GBD 2017 Diet Collaborators, "Health Effects of Dietary Risks in 195 Countries, 1990–2017: A Systemic Analysis for Global Burden of Disease Study 2017," *Lancet* 393, no. 10184 (May 2019): 1958–72.

9. Christina Roberto and Mary Gorski, "Public Health Policies to Encourage Healthy Eating Habits: Recent Perspectives," *Journal of Healthcare Leadership* 7 (2015): 81–90, https://doi.org/10.2147/JHL.S69188.

10. J. B. Furness, W. A. Kunze, and N. Clerc, "Nutrient Tasting and Signaling Mechanisms in the Gut; Part II, The Intestine as a Sensory Organ: Neural, Endocrine, and Immune Responses," *American Journal of Physiology* 277, no. 5 (1999): G922–28, https://doi.org/10.1152/ajpgi.1999.277.5.G922.

11. "Your Changing Microbiome," Learn Genetics, accessed February 24, 2021, https://learn.genetics.utah.edu/content/microbiome/changing/.

12. "Human Microbiome Project Defines Normal Bacterial Makeup of the Body," National Institutes of Health, accessed February 24, 2021, https://www.nih.gov/news-events/news-releases/nih-human-microbiome-project-defines-normal-bacterial-makeup-body.

13. I. Yang, E. J. Corwin, P. A. Brennan, S. Jordan, J. R. Murphy, and A. Dunlop, "The Infant Microbiome: Implications for Infant Health and Neurocognitive Development," *Nursing Research* 65, no. 1 (2016): 76–88, https://doi.org/10.1097/NNR.0000000000000133.

14. T. Paus, M. Keshavan, and J. N. Giedd, "Why Do Many Psychiatric Disorders Emerge during Adolescence?" *Nature Reviews Neuroscience* 9 (2008): 947–57, https://doi.org/10.1038/nrn2513.

15. C. L. Johnson and J. Versalovic, "The Human Microbiome and Its Potential Importance to Pediatrics," *Pediatrics* 129, no. 5 (May 2012): 950–60, https://doi.org/10.1542/peds.2011-2736.

16. M. G. Dominguez-Bello, E. K. Costello, M. Contreras, M. Magris, G. Hidalgo, N. Fierer, et al., "Delivery Mode Shapes the Acquisition and Structure of the Initial Microbiota across Multiple Body Habitats in Newborns," *Proceedings of the National Academy of Sciences* 107 (2010): 11971–975, https://doi.org/10.1073/pnas.1002601107; J. E. Koenig, A. Spor, N. Scalfone, A. D. Fricker, J. Stombaugh, R. Knight, et al., "Succession of Microbial Consortia in the Developing Infant Gut Microbiome," *Proceedings of the National Academy of Sciences* 108, suppl. 1 (2011): 4578–85, https://doi.org/10.1073/pnas.1000081107; T. Yatsunenko, F. E. Rey, M. J. Manary, I. Trehan, M. G. Dominguez-Bello, M. Contreras, et al., "Human Gut Microbiome Viewed across Age and Geography," *Nature* 486 (2012): 222–27, https://doi.org/10.1038/nature11053.

17. Hedvig E. Jakobsson, Thomas R. Abrahamsson, Maria C. Jenmalm, Keith Harris, Christopher Quince, Cecilia Jernberg, Bengt Björkstén, Lars Engstrand, and Anders F. Andersson, "Decreased Gut Microbiota Diversity, Delayed Bacteroidetes Colonisation and Reduced Th1 Responses in Infants Delivered by Caesarean Section," *Gut* 63, no. 4 (2014): 559–66, https://doi.org/10.1136/gutjnl-2012-303249.

18. Jakobsson et al., "Decreased Gut Microbiota Diversity."

19. Yang et al., "The Infant Microbiome."

20. Work Group on Breastfeeding, "Breastfeeding and Use of Human Milk," *Pediatrics* 129, no. 3 (2012): e827–41; revised from *Pediatrics* 100, no. 6 (December 1997): 1035–39, https://doi.org/10.1542/peds.100.6.1035.

21. Mark A. Underwood, J. Bruce German, Carlito B. Lebrilla, and David A. Mills, "Bifidobacterium Longum Subspecies Infantis: Champion Colonizer of the Infant Gut," *Pediatric Research* 77 (2015): 229–35, https://doi.org/10.1038/pr.2014.156.

22. Daniel Garrido, David C. Dallas, and David A. Mills, "Consumption of Human Milk Glycoconjugates by Infant-Associated Bifidobacteria: Mechanisms and Implications," *Microbiology* 159, pt. 4 (2013): 649–64, https://doi.org/10.1099/mic.0.064113-0.

23. D. Barile and R. A. Rastall, "Human Milk and Related Oligosaccharides as Prebiotics," *Current Opinion in Biotechnology* 24, no. 2 (February 2013): 214–19, https://doi.org/10.1016/j.copbio.2013.01.008.

24. D. A. Lopez, J. J. Foxe, Y. Mao, W. K. Thompson, H. J. Martin, and E. G. Freedman, "Breastfeeding Duration Is Associated with Domain-Specific Improvements in Cognitive Performance in 9-10-Year-Old Children," *Frontiers in Public Health*, April 26, 2021, https://doi.org/10.3389/fpubh.2021.657422.

25. Courtney M. Gardner, Kate Hoffman, Heather M. Stapleton, and Claudia K. Gunsch, "Exposures to Semivolatile Organic Compounds in Indoor Environments and Associations with the Gut Microbiomes of Children," *Environmental Science & Technology Letters* 8, no. 1 (2020): 73–79, https://pubs.acs.org/doi/10.1021/acs.estlett.0c00776.

26. N. Michels, T. Van de Wiele, F. Fouhy, S. O'Mahony, G. Clarke, and J. Keane, "Gut Microbiome Patterns Depending on Children's Psychosocial Stress: Reports versus Biomarkers," *Brain, Behavior, and Immunity* 80 (August 2019): 751–62, https://doi.org/10.1016/j.bbi.2019.05.024.

27. J. E. Flannery, K. Stagaman, A. R. Burns, et al., "Gut Feelings Begin in Childhood: The Gut Metagenome Correlates with Early Environment, Caregiving, and Behavior," *mBio* 11, no. 1 (2020): e02780-19, https://doi.org/10.1128/mBio.02780-19.

28. J. P. Karl, A. M. Hatch, S. M. Arcidiacono, et al., "Effects of Psychological, Environmental and Physical Stressors on the Gut Microbiota," *Frontiers in Microbiology* 9 (2018): 2013, https://doi.org/10.3389/fmicb.2018.02013.

29. R. Diaz Heijtz, S. Wang, F. Anuar, Y. Qian, B. Björkholm, A. Samuelsson, M. L. Hibberd, H. Forssberg, and S. Pettersson, "Normal Gut Microbiota Modulates Brain Development and Behavior," *Proceedings of the National Academy of Sciences* 108, no. 7 (2011): 3047–52, https://doi.org/10.1073/pnas.1010529108; Yang et al., "The Infant Microbiome."

30. Yang et al., "The Infant Microbiome."

31. M. C. Arrieta, L. Bistritz, and J. B. Meddings, "Alterations in Intestinal Permeability," *Gut* 55, no. 10 (2006): 1512–20, https://doi.org/10.1136/gut.2005.085373.

32. Stephan C. Bischoff, Giovanni Barbara, Wim Buurman, Theo Ockhuizen, Jörg-Dieter Schulzke, Matteo Serino, Herbert Tilg, Alastair Watson, and Jerry M. Wells, "Intestinal Permeability—A New Target for Disease Prevention and Therapy," *BMC Gastroenterology* 14, no. 189 (2014), http://www.ncbi.nlm.nih.gov/pmc/articles/PMC4253991/.

33. Bischoff et al., "Intestinal Permeability."

34. S. Gaidos, "The Inconstant Gardener," *Science News*, November 15, 2013, https://www.sciencenews.org/article/inconstant-gardener?mode=.

35. Irene Knuesel, Laurie Chicha, Markus Britschgi, Scott A. Schobel, Michael Bodmer, Jessica A. Hellings, Stephen Toovey, and Eric P. Prinssen, "Maternal Immune Activation and Abnormal Brain Development across CNS Disorders," *Nature Reviews Neurology* 10 (2014): 643–60, https://doi.org/10.1038/nrneurol.2014.187; Lorelei Pratt, Li Ni, Nicholas M. Ponzio, and G. Miller Jonakait, "Maternal Inflammation Promotes Fetal Microglial Activation and Increased Cholinergic Expression in the Fetal Basal Forebrain: Role of Interleukin-6," *Pediatric Research* 74, no. 4 (2013): 393–401, https://doi.org/10.1038/pr.2013.126.

36. H. E. Vuong, J. M. Yano, T. C. Fung, and E. Y. Hsiao, "The Microbiome and Host Behavior," *Annual Review of Neuroscience* 25, no. 40 (July 2017): 21–49, https://doi.org/10.1146/annurev-neuro-072116-031347.

37. E. Jašarević, C. D. Howard, K. Morrison, A. Misic, T. Weinkopff, P. Scott, C. Hunter, D. Beiting, and T. L. Bale, "The Maternal Vaginal Microbiome Partially Mediates the Effects of Prenatal Stress on Offspring Gut and Hypothalamus," *Nature Neuroscience* 21, no. 8 (August 2018): 1061–71, https://doi.org/10.1038/s41593-018-0182-5.

38. Wang Li, Scot E. Dowd, Bobbie Scurlock, Veronica Acosta-Martinez, and Mark Lyte, "Memory and Learning Behavior in Mice Is Temporally Associated with Diet-Induced Alterations in Gut Bacteria," *Physiology & Behavior* 96, no. 4–5 (2009): 557–67, http://www.sciencedirect.com/science/article/pii/S003193840800382X.

39. C. L. Johnson and J. Versalovic, "The Human Microbiome and Its Potential Importance to Pediatrics," *Pediatrics* 129, no. 5 (2012): 950–60, https://doi.org/10.1542/peds.2011-2736.

40. Jeroen Visser, Jan Rozing, Anna Sapone, Karen Lammers, and Alessio Fasano, "Tight Junctions, Intestinal Permeability, and Autoimmunity," *Annals of the New York Academy of Sciences* 1165, no. 1 (May 2009): 195–205, https://doi.org/10.1111/j.1749-6632.2009.04037.x.

41. Nina Batchelor, Jennifer Kelly, Hyun Choi, and Brona Geary, "Towards Evidence-Based Emergency Medicine: Best BETs from the Manchester Royal Infirmary. BET 2: Probiotics and Crying Time in Babies with Infantile Colic," *Emergency Medicine Journal* 32, no. 7 (July 2015): 575–76, https://doi.org/10.1136/emermed-2015-204984.2.

42. J. Niu, L. Xu, Y. Qian, et al., "Evolution of the Gut Microbiome in Early Childhood: A Cross-sectional Study of Chinese Children," *Frontiers in Microbiology* 11 (2020): 439, https://doi.org/10.3389/fmicb.2020.00439.

43. Gregory Bouchaud, Pascal Gourbeyre, Tiphaine Bihouée, Philippe Aubert, David Lair, Marie-Aude Cheminant, Sandra Denery-Papini, Michel Neunlist, Antoine Magnan, and Marie Bodinier, "Consecutive Food and Respiratory Allergies Amplify Systemic and Gut but Not Lung Outcomes in Mice," *Journal of Agricultural and Food Chemistry* 63, no. 28 (July 2015): 6475–83, https://doi.org/10.1021/acs.jafe.5b02338.

44. A. W. Campbell, "Autoimmunity and the Gut" [Review article], *Autoimmune Diseases* (2014), https://doi.org/10.1155/2014/152428; Arrieta, Bistritz, and Meddings, "Alterations in Intestinal Permeability."

45. Greta Fowlie, Nicholas Cohen, and Xue Ming, "The Perturbance of Microbiome and Gut-Brain Axis in Autism Spectrum Disorders," *International Journal of Molecular Sciences* 19, no. 8 (2018): 2251, https://doi.org/10.3390/ijms19082251.

46. Gonca Özyurt, Yusuf Öztürk, Yeliz Çağan Appak, Fatma Demet Arslan, Maşallah Baran, İnanç Karakoyun, Ali Evren Tufan, and Aynur Akay Pekcanlar, "Increased Zonulin Is Associated with Hyperactivity and Social Dysfunctions in Children with Attention Deficit Hyperactivity Disorder," *Comprehensive Psychiatry* 87 (November 2018): 138–42, https://doi.org/10.1016/j.comppsych.2018.10.006.

47. A. T. Soliman, M. Yasin, and A. Kassem, "Leptin in Pediatrics: A Hormone from Adipocyte That Wheels Several Functions in Children," *Indian Journal of Endo-*

crinology and Metabolism 16, suppl. 3 (2012): S577–87, https://doi.org/10.4103/2230 -8210.105575.

48. M. T. Osborne et al., "Amygdalar Activity Predicts Future Incident Diabetes Independently of Adiposity," *Psychoneuroendocrinology* 100 (February 2019): 32–40, https://doi.org/10.1016/j.psyneuen.2018.09.024.

49. A. G. de Lange, A. C. S. Bråthen, D. A. Rohani, A. M. Fjell, and K. B. Wal-hovd, "The Temporal Dynamics of Brain Plasticity in Aging," *Cerebral Cortex* 28, no. 5 (May 2018): 1857–65, https://doi.org/10.1093/cercor/bhy003.

50. D. D. Clarke and L. Sokoloff, "Circulation and Energy Metabolism of the Brain," in *Basic Neurochemistry: Molecular, Cellular, and Medical Aspects*, eds. G. Siegel, B. Aranoff, and R. Albers (Philadelphia, PA: Lippincott-Raven, 1999).

51. L. B. Achanta, B. D. Rowlands, D. S. Thomas, G. D. Housley, and C. D. Rae, "Beta-Hydroxybutyrate Boosts Mitochondrial and Neuronal Metabolism but Is Not Preferred over Glucose under Activated Conditions," *Neurochemical Research* 42 (2017): 1710–23, https://doi.org/10.1007/s11064-017-2228-6.

52. F. Bellisle, "Effects of Diet on Behaviour and Cognition in Children," *British Journal of Nutrition* 92, suppl. 2 (2004): S227–32, https://doi.org/10.1079/BJN 20041171.

53. Y. Li, Q. Dai, J. C. Jackson, and J. Zhang, "Overweight Is Associated with De-creased Cognitive Functioning among School-Age Children and Adolescents," *Obesity* 16, no. 8 (2008): 1809–15, https://doi.org/10.1038/oby.2008.296.

54. N. Mac Giollabhui et al., "Executive Dysfunction in Depression in Adoles-cence: The Role of Inflammation and Higher Body Mass," *Psychological Medicine* (March 2019): 1–9, https://doi.org/10.1017/S0033291719000564.

55. J. M. Lee, D. Appugliese, N. Kaciroti, R. F. Corwyn, R. H. Bradley, and J. C. Lumeng, "Weight Status in Young Girls and the Onset of Puberty," *Pediatrics* 119, no. 3 (March 2007): e624–30, https://doi.org/10.1542/peds.2006-2188.

56. Bernard Gesch, "Adolescence: Does Good Nutrition = Good Behaviour?" *Nutrition and Health* 22, no. 1 (January 2013): 55–65, https://doi.org/10.1177 /0260106013519552.

57. S. Schoenthaler, S. Amos, and W. Doraz, "The Effect of Randomized Vitamin-Mineral Supplementation on Violent and Non-violent Antisocial Behavior among Incarcerated Juveniles," *Journal of Nutritional & Environmental Medicine* 7, no. 4 (1997), https://doi.org/10.1080/13590849762475.

58. L. L. Iannotti, M. Tielsch, M. M. Black, and R. E. Black, "Iron Supplementa-tion in Early Childhood: Health Benefits and Risks," *American Journal of Clinical Nutrition* 84 (2006): 1261–76, https://doi.org/10.1093/ajcn/84.6.1261.

59. A. M. Di Girolamo and M. Ramirez-Zea, "Role of Zinc in Maternal and Child Mental Health," *American Journal of Clinical Nutrition* 89 (2009): 940S–45S, https://doi .org/10.3945/ajcn.2008.26692C.

60. S. E. Saint, L. M. Renzi-Hammond, N. A. Khan, C. H. Hillman, J. E. Frick, and B. R. Hammond, "The Macular Carotenoids Are Associated with Cogni-tive Function in Preadolescent Children," *Nutrients* 10 (2018): 193, https://doi.org /10.3390/nu10020193.

61. J. C. Lieblein-Boff, E. J. Johnson, A. D. Kennedy, C. S. Lai, and M. J. Kuchan, "Exploratory Metabolomic Analyses Reveal Compounds Correlated with Lutein Concentration in Frontal Cortex, Hippocampus, and Occipital Cortex of Human Infant Brain," *PLoS ONE* 10 (2015): e0136904, https://doi.org/10.1371/journal.pone.0136904.

62. D. Benton, "The Impact of Diet on Anti-social, Violent and Criminal Behaviour," *Neuroscience and Biobehavioral Reviews* 31, no. 5 (2007): 752–74, https://doi.org/10.1016/j.neubiorev.2007.02.002.

63. H. Zahedi, H. R. Kelishadi, R. Heshmat, M. E. Motlagh, S. H. Ranjbar, G. Ardalan, M. Payab, M. Chinian, H. Asayesh, B. Larijani, and M. Qorbani, "Association between Junk Food Consumption and Mental Health in a National Sample of Iranian Children and Adolescents: The CASPIAN-IV Study," *Nutrition* 30, no. 11–12 (November–December 2014): 1391–97, https://doi.org/10.1016/j.nut.2014.04.014.

64. A. Borrmann and G. B. Mensink; KiGGS Study Group, "Obst- und Gemüsekonsum von Kindern und Jugendlichen in Deutschland, and Ergebnisse der KiGGS-Welle 1" [Fruit and vegetable consumption by children and adolescents in Germany: Results of KiGGS wave 1], *Bundesgesundheitsblatt Gesundheitsforschung Gesundheitsschutz* 58, no. 9 (September 2015): 1005–14, https://doi.org/10.1007/s00103-015-2208-4.

65. K. B. Pandey and S. I. Rizvi, "Plant Polyphenols as Dietary Antioxidants in Human Health and Disease," *Oxidative Medicine and Cellular Longevity* 2, no. 5 (November–December 2009): 270–78.

66. E. M. Holt, L. M. Steffen, A. Moran, S. Basu, J. Steinberger, J. A. Ross, C.-P. Hong, and A. R. Sinaiko, "Fruit and Vegetable Consumption and Its Relation to Markers of Inflammation and Oxidative Stress in Adolescents," *Journal of the American Dietetic Association* 109, no. 3 (2009): 414–21, https://doi.org/10.1016/j.jada.2008.11.036.

67. M. M. Kaczmarczyk, M. J. Miller, and G. G. Freund, "The Health Benefits of Dietary Fiber: Beyond the Usual Suspects of Type 2 Diabetes Mellitus, Cardiovascular Disease and Colon Cancer," *Metabolism* 61, no. 8 (August 2012): 1058–66, https://doi.org/10.1016/j.metabol.2012.01.017.

68. Pandey and Rizvi, "Plant Polyphenols as Dietary Antioxidants in Human Health and Disease."

69. Holt et al., "Fruit and Vegetable Consumption and Its Relation to Markers of Inflammation and Oxidative Stress in Adolescents."

70. M. Ahmad, M. N. Ansari, A. Alam, and T. H. Khan, "Oral Dose of Citrus Peel Extracts Promotes Wound Repair in Diabetic Rats," *Pakistan Journal of Biological Sciences* 16, no. 20 (2013): 1086–94, https://doi.org/10.3923/pjbs.2013.1086.1094.

71. Willy J. Malaisse, "Insulin Release: The Receptor Hypothesis," *Diabetologia* 57, no. 7 (July 2014): 1287–90, https://doi.org/10.1007/s00125-014-3221-0.

72. F. Bonatto, M. Polydoro, M. E. Andrades, M. L. Conte de Fronte Jr., F. Dal-Pizzol, L. N. Rotta, D. O. Souza, M. L. Perry, and J. C. F. Moreira, "Effects of Maternal Protein Malnutrition on Oxidative Markers in the Young Rat Cortex and Cerebellum," *Neuroscience Letters* 406 (2006): 281–84, https://doi.org/10.1016/j.neulet.2006.07.052.

73. S. E. Cusick and M. K. Georgieff, "The Role of Nutrition in Brain Development: The Golden Opportunity of the 'First 1000 Days,'" *Journal of Pediatrics* 175 (2016): 16–21, https://doi.org/10.1016/j.jpeds.2016.05.013.

74. S. Grantham-McGregor and H. Baker-Henningham, "Review of the Evidence Linking Protein and Energy to Mental Development," *Public Health Nutrition* 8 (2005): 1191–1201, https://doi.org/10.1079/PHN2005805.

75. D. Mozaffarian et al., "Plasma Phospholipids Long-Chain w-3 Fatty Acids and Total and Cause-Specific Mortality in Older Adults: A Cohort Study," *Annals of Internal Medicine* 158, no. 7 (2013): 515–25, https://doi.org/10.7326/0003-4819-158 -7-201304020-00003.

76. J. Sarris, D. Mischoulon, and I. Schweitzer, "Omega-3 for Bipolar Disorder: Meta-analyses of Use in Mania and Bipolar," *Journal of Clinical Psychiatry* 73, no. 1 (August 2011): 81–86, https://doi.org/10.4088/JCP.10r06710.

77. M. Huss, A. Volp, and M. Stauss-Grabbo, "Supplementation of Polyunsaturated Fatty Acids, Magnesium, and Zinc in Children Seeking Medical Advice for Attention-Deficit/Hyperactivity Problems, an Observational Cohort Study," *Lipids in Health and Disease* 9 (2010): 105, https://doi.org/10.1186/1476-511X-9-105.

78. T. Nagakura, S. Matsuda, K. Shichijyo, H. Sugimoto, and K. Hata, "Dietary Supplementation with Fish Oil Rich in Omega-3 Polyunsaturated Fatty Acids in Children with Bronchial Asthma," *European Respiratory Journal* 16, no. 5 (November 2000): 861–65.

79. R. Chowdhury, S. Warnakula, S. Kunutsor, et al., "Association of Dietary, Circulating, and Supplement Fatty Acids with Coronary Risk: A Systemic Review and Meta-analysis," *Annals of Internal Medicine* 160, no. 6 (March 2014): 398–406, https:// doi.org/10.7326/M13-1788.

80. Susan M. Silbernagel, David O. Carpenter, Steven G. Gilbert, Michael Gochfeld, Edward Groth, Jane M. Hightower, and Frederick M. Schiavone, "Recognizing and Preventing Overexposure to Methylmercury from Fish and Seafood Consumption: Information for Physicians," *Journal of Toxicology* (July 2011), https://doi .org/10.1155/2011/983072.

81. S. van Vliet, N. A. Burd, and L. J. C. van Loon, "The Skeletal Muscle Anabolic Response to Plant- versus Animal-Based Protein Consumption," *Journal of Nutrition* 145, no. 9 (September 2015): 1981–91, https://doi.org/10.3945/jn.114.204305.

82. D. F. Birt, T. Boylston, S. Hendrich, et al., "Resistant Starch: Promise for Improving Human Health," *Advances in Nutrition* 4, no. 6 (November 2013): 587–601, https://doi.org/10.3945/an.113.004325.

83. W. J. Craig, "Health Effects of Vegan Diets," *American Journal of Clinical Nutrition* 89, no. 5 (May 2009): 1627S–33S, https://doi.org/10.3945/ajcn.2009.26736N.

84. Ann Reed Mangels, "Bone Nutrients for Vegetarians," *American Journal of Clinical Nutrition* 100, suppl. 1 (July 2014): 469S–75S, https://doi.org/10.3945/ajcn.113 .071423.

85. C. L. Baym, N. A. Khan, J. M. Monti, L. B. Raine, E. S. Drollette, R. D. Moore, M. R. Scudder, A. F. Kramer, C. H. Hillman, and N. J. Cohen, "Dietary Lipids Are Differentially Associated with Hippocampal-Dependent Relational Memory in Prepubescent Children," *American Journal of Clinical Nutrition* 99, no. 5 (2014): 1026–

32, https://doi.org/10.3945/ajcn.113.079624; K. Handeland, J. Øyen, S. Skotheim, I. E. Graff, V. Baste, M. Kjellevold, L. Frøyland, Ø. Lie, L. Dahl, and K. M. Stormark, "Fatty Fish Intake and Attention Performance in 14–15-Year-Old Adolescents: FINS-TEENS—a Randomized Controlled Trial," *Nutrition Journal* 16 (2017), https://doi.org/10.1186/s12937-017-0287-9.

86. Artemis P. Simopoulos, "Omega-3 Fatty Acids in Inflammation and Autoimmune Diseases," *Journal of the American College of Nutrition* 21, no. 6 (December 2002): 495–505, https://doi.org/10.1080/07315724.2002.10719248.

87. Mauricio G. Martín, Frank Pfrieger, and Carlos G. Dotti, "Cholesterol in Brain Disease: Sometimes Determinant and Frequently Implicated," *EMBO Reports* 15, no. 10 (2014): 1036–52, https://doi.org/10.15252/embr.201439225; Hansen Wang, "Lipid Rafts: A Signaling Platform Linking Cholesterol Metabolism to Synaptic Deficits in Autism Spectrum Disorders," *Frontiers in Behavioral Neuroscience* 8 (March 2014), https://doi.org/10.3389/fnbeh.2014.00104; Mucahit Emet, Atakan Yucel, Halil Ozcan, Sultan Tuna Akgol Gur, Murat Saritemur, Nevzat Bulut, and Musa Gumusdere, "Female Attempted Suicide Patients with Low HDL Levels Are at Higher Risk of Suicide Re-attempt within the Subsequent Year: A Clinical Cohort Study," *Psychiatry Research* 225, no. 1–2 (2015): 202–7, https://doi.org/10.1016/j.psychres.2014.11.026; Maria da Graça Cantarelli, Ana Carolina Tramontina, Marina C. Leite, and Carlos-Alberto Gonçalves, "Potential Neurochemical Links between Cholesterol and Suicidal Behavior," *Psychiatry Research* 220, no. 3 (2014): 745–51, https://doi.org/10.1016/j.psychres.2014.10.017.

88. M. Pesonen, A. Ranki, M. A. Siimes, and M. J. T. Kallio, "Serum Cholesterol Level in Infancy Is Inversely Associated with Subsequent Allergy in Children and Adolescents: A 20-Year Follow-Up Study," *Clinical & Experimental Allergy* 38, no. 1 (January 2008): 178–84, https://doi.org/10.1111/j.1365-2222.2007.02875.x.

89. Joseph R. Hibbeln, Levi R. G. Nieminen, and William E. M. Lands, "Increasing Homicide Rates and Linoleic Acid Consumption among Five Western Countries, 1961–2000," *Lipids* 39, no. 12 (2004): 1207–13, https://doi.org/10.1007/s11745-004-1349-5.

90. Gian Luigi Russo, "Dietary N−6 and N−3 Polyunsaturated Fatty Acids: From Biochemistry to Clinical Implications in Cardiovascular Prevention," *Biochemical Pharmacology* 77, no. 6 (March 2009): 937–46, https://doi.org/10.1016/j.bcp.2008.10.020; Jay Whelan, "The Health Implications of Changing Linoleic Acid Intakes," *Prostaglandins Leukotrienes & Essential Fatty Acids* 79, no. 3–5 (September–November 2008): 165–67, https://doi.org/10.1016/j.plefa.2008.09.013.

91. Paolo Bergamo, Gianna Palmieri, Ennio Cocca, Ida Ferrandino, Marta Gogliettino, Antonio Monaco, Francesco Maurano, and Mauro Rossi, "Adaptive Response Activated by Dietary Cis9, Trans11 Conjugated Linoleic Acid Prevents Distinct Signs of Gliadin-Induced Enteropathy in Mice," *European Journal of Nutrition* 55, no. 2 (March 2016): 729–40, https://doi.org/10.1007/s00394-015-0893-2.

92. G. Grosso, J. Yang, S. Marventano, A. Micek, F. Galvano, and S. N. Kales, "Nut Consumption on All-Cause, Cardiovascular, and Cancer Mortality Risk: A Systematic Review and Meta-analysis of Epidemiologic Studies," *American Journal*

of Clinical Nutrition 101, no. 4 (February 2015): 783–93, https://doi.org/10.3945/ajcn.114.099515.

93. B. Gopinath, V. M. Flood, G. Burlutsky, et al., "Consumption of Nuts and Risk of Total and Cause-Specific Mortality over 15 Years," *Nutrition, Metabolism and Cardiovascular Diseases* 25, no. 12 (December 2015): 1125–31, https://doi.org/10.1016/j.numecd.2015.09.006.

94. A. Dulloo, G. M. Fathi, N. Mensi, et al., "Twenty-Four-Hour Energy Expenditure and Urinary Catecholamines of Human Consuming Low-to-Moderate Amounts of Medium-Chain Triglycerides: A Dose-Response Study in a Human Respiratory Chamber," *European Journal Clinical Nutrition* 50, no. 3 (March 1996): 152–58.

95. Staffan Lindeberg, Eliasson Mats, Lindahl Bernt, and Ahrén Bo, "Low Serum Insulin in Traditional Pacific Islanders—the Kitava Study," *Metabolism* 48, no. 10 (October 1999): 1216–19, https://doi.org/10.1016/s0026-0495(99)90258-5.

96. Brenda Diaz, Lizeth Fuentes-Mera, Armando Tovar, Teresa Montiel, Lourdes Massieu, Herminia Guadalupe Martínez-Rodríguez, and Alberto Camacho, "Saturated Lipids Decrease Mitofusin 2 Leading to Endoplasmic Reticulum Stress Activation and Insulin Resistance in Hypothalamic Cells," *Brain Research* 1627 (November 2015): 80–89, https://doi.org/10.1016/j.brainres.2015.09.014; Mark M. Yore, Ismail Syed, Pedro M. Moraes-Vieira, Tejia Zhang, Mark A. Herman, Edwin A. Homan, Rajesh T. Patel, et al., "Discovery of a Class of Endogenous Mammalian Lipids with Anti-diabetic and Anti-inflammatory Effects," *Cell* 159, no. 2 (2014): 318–32, https://doi.org/10.1016/j.cell.2014.09.035; Ming-Che Shen, Xiangmin Zhao, Gene P. Siegal, Renee Desmond, and Robert W. Hardy, "Dietary Stearic Acid Leads to a Reduction of Visceral Adipose Tissue in Athymic Nude Mice," *PLoS ONE* 9, no. 9 (2014): e104083, https://doi.org/10.1371/journal.pone.0104083.

97. B. J. Meyer, E. J. de Bruin, D. G. Du Plessis, et al., "Some Biochemical Effects of Mainly Fruit Diet in Man," *South African Medical Journal* 45, no. 10 (1971): 253–61.

98. M. Schneeberger et al., "Akkermansia Muciniphila Inversely Correlates with the Onset of Inflammation, Altered Adipose Tissue Metabolism, and Metabolic Disorders during Obesity in Mice," *Science Reports* 5 (2015): 16643, https://doi.org/10.1038/srep16643.

99. S. Samarghandian, T. Farkhondeh, and F. Samini, "Honey and Health: A Review of Recent Clinical Research," *Pharmacognosy Research* 9, no. 2 (2017): 121–27, https://doi.org/10.4103/0974-8490.204647.

100. Mamdouh M. Abdulrhman, Mohamed H. El-Hefnawy, Rasha H. Aly, Rania H. Shatla, Rasha M. Mamdouh, Doaa M. Mahmoud, and Waheed S. Mohamed, "Metabolic Effects of Honey in Type 1 Diabetes Mellitus: A Randomized Crossover Pilot Study," *Journal of Medicinal Food* 16, no. 1 (2013): 66–72, https://doi.org/10.1089/jmf.2012.0108.

101. Reem M. Galal, Hala F. Zaki, Mona M. Seif El-Nasr, and Azza M. Agha, "Potential Protective Effect of Honey against Paracetamol-Induced Hepatotoxicity," *Archives of Iranian Medicine* 15, no. 11 (2012): 674–80, http://www.ncbi.nlm.nih.gov/pubmed/23102243.

102. J. Legault, K. Girard-Lalancette, C. Grenon, C. Dussault, and A. Pichette, "Antioxidant Activity, Inhibition of Nitric Oxide Overproduction, and In Vitro Antiproliferative Effect of Maple Sap and Syrup from Acer Saccharum," *Journal of Medicinal Food* 13, no. 2 (2010): 460–68, https://doi.org/10.1089/jmf.2009.0029; M. M. Abou-Zaid, C. Nozzolillo, A. Tonon, M. D. Coppens, and D. A. Lombardo, "High-Performance Liquid Chromatography Characterization and Identification of Antioxidant Polyphenols in Maple Syrup," *Pharmaceutical Biology* 46 (2008): 117–25, https://cfs.nrcan.gc.ca/publications?id=28297.

103. A. González-Sarrías, L. Li, and N. P. Seeram, "Effects of Maple (Acer) Plant Part Extracts on Proliferation, Apoptosis and Cell Cycle Arrest of Human Tumorigenic and Non-tumorigenic Colon Cells," *Phytotherapy Research* 26, no. 7 (2012): 995–1002, https://doi.org/10.1002/ptr.3677; A. González-Sarrías, H. Ma, M. Edmonds, and N. P. Seeram, "Maple Polyphenols, Ginnalins A-C, Induce S- and G2/M-Cell Cycle Arrest in Colon and Breast Cancer Cells Mediated by Decreasing Cyclins A and D1 Levels," *Food Chemistry* 136, no. 2 (2013): 636–42, https://doi.org/10.1016/j.food chem.2012.08.023.

104. M. T. Montagna, G. Diella, F. Triggiano, et al., "Chocolate, 'Food of the Gods': History, Science, and Human Health," *International Journal of Environmental Research and Public Health* 16, no. 24 (2019): 4960, https://doi.org/10.3390/ijerph 16244960.

105. Bob L. Smith, "Organic Foods vs Supermarket Foods: Element Levels," Journey to Forever, accessed February 24, 2021, http://journeytoforever.org/farm_library /bobsmith.html.

106. K. L. Bassil, C. Vakil, M. Sanborn, et al., "Cancer Health Effects of Pesticides: Systemic Review," *Canadian Family Physician* 53, no. 10 (October 2007): 1704–11.

107. J. R. Robert, C. J. Karr, and Council on Environmental Health, "Pesticide Exposure in Children," *Pediatrics* 130, no. 6 (December 2012): e1765–88, https://doi .org/10.1542/peds.2012-2758. See erratum: J. R. Robert, C. J. Karr, and Council on Environmental Health, "Technical Report: Pesticide Exposure in Children," *Pediatrics* 131, no. 5 (2013): 1013–14, https://doi.org/10.1542/peds.2013-0577.

108. Smith, "Organic Foods vs Supermarket Foods: Element Levels."

109 Yohei Ohashi, Katsuya Yamada, Ikuyo Takemoto, Takaharu Mizutani, and Ken-ichi Saeki, "Inhibition of Human Cytochrome P450 2E1 by Halogenated Anilines, Phenols, and Thiophenols," *Biological and Pharmaceutical Bulletin* 28, no. 7 (2005): 1221–23, https://doi.org/10.1248/bpb.28.1221.

110. M. F. Bouchard, D. C. Bellinger, R. O. Wright, and M. G. Weisskopf, "Attention-Deficit/Hyperactivity Disorder and Urinary Metabolites of Organophosphate Pesticides," *Pediatrics* 125, no. 6 (June 2010): e1270–77, https://doi.org/10.1542 /peds.2009-3058.

111. R. J. Buralli, A. F. Dultra, and H. Ribeiro, "Respiratory and Allergic Effects in Children Exposed to Pesticides: A Systematic Review," *International Journal of Environmental Research and Public Health* 17, no. 8 (2020), https://doi.org/10.3390 /ijerph17082740.

112. M. C. Buser, H. E. Murray, and S. Franco, "Association of Urinary Phenols with Increased Body Weight Measures and Obesity in Children and Adolescents,"

Journal of Pediatrics 165, no. 4 (October 2014): 744–49, https://doi.org/10.1016 /j.jpeds.2014.06.039; E. Jerschow, P. Parikh, A. P. McGinn, S. Jariwala, G. Hudes, and D. Rosenstreich, "Relationship between Urine Dichlorophenol Levels and Asthma Morbidity," *Annals of Allergy, Asthma & Immunology* 112, no. 6 (2014): 511–18, https://doi.org/10.1016/j.anai.2014.03.011; E. Jerschow, A. P. McGinn, G. de Vos, S. Jariwala, G. Hudes, and D. R. Rosenstreich, "Dichlorophenol-Containing Pesticides and Allergies: Results from the US National Health and Nutrition Examination Survey 2005–2006," *Annals of Allergy, Asthma & Immunology* 109, no. 6 (2012): 420–25, https://doi.org/10.1016/j.anai.2012.09.005.

113. Robert, Karr, and Council on Environmental Health, "Pesticide Exposure in Children." See erratum: Robert, Karr, and Council on Environmental Health, "Technical Report: Pesticide Exposure in Children."

114. Rosalind S. Gibson, L. Perlas, and C. Hotz, "Improving the Bioavailability of Nutrients in Plant Foods at the Household Level," *Proceedings of the Nutrition Society* 65, no. 2 (2006): 160–68, https://doi.org/10.1079/pns2006489.

115. Michelle Pietzak, "Celiac Disease, Wheat Allergy, and Gluten Sensitivity," *Journal of Parenteral and Enteral Nutrition* 36, suppl. 1 (2012): 68S–75S, https:// doi.org/10.1177/0148607111426276; A. Fasano, A. Sapone, V. Zevallos, and D. Schuppan, "Nonceliac Gluten Sensitivity," *Gastroenterology* 148, no. 6 (May 2015): 1195–204, https://doi.org/10.1053/j.gastro.2014.12.049; M. R. Barbaro, C. Cremon, G. Caio, U. Volta, V. Stanghellini, and G. Barbara, "247 Zonulin Serum Levels Are Increased in Non-celiac Gluten Sensitivity and Irritable Bowel Syndrome with Diarrhea," *Gastroenterology* 148, no. 4, suppl. 1 (2015), https://doi.org/10.1016 /S0016-5085(15)30192-X.

116. S. E. Byrnes, J. C. Miller, and G. S. Denyer, "Amylopectin Starch Promotes the Development of Insulin Resistance in Rats," *Journal of Nutrition* 125, no. 6 (June 1995): 1430–37, https://doi.org/10.1093/jn/125.6.1430.

117. John S. Punzi, Martha Lamont, Diana Haynes, and Robert L. Epstein, "USDA Pesticide Data Program: Pesticide Residues on Fresh and Processed Fruit and Vegetables, Grains, Meats, Milk, and Drinking Water," *Outlooks on Pest Management* 16, no. 3 (June 2005): 131–37, https://doi.org/10.1564/16jun12.

118. *Diabetologia*, "Child's Gluten Intake during Infancy, Rather Than Mother's during Pregnancy, Linked to Increased Risk of Developing Type 1 Diabetes," *ScienceDaily*, accessed February 22, 2021, https://www.sciencedaily.com/releases/2019 /09/190918184459.htm.

119. C. Andrén Aronsson, H. S. Lee, E. M. Hård Af Segerstad, U. Uusitalo, J. Yang, S. Koletzko, E. Liu, K. Kurppa, P. J. Bingley, J. Toppari, A. G. Ziegler, J. X. She, W. A. Hagopian, M. Rewers, B. Akolkar, J. P. Krischer, S. M. Virtanen, J. M. Norris, and D. Agardh (TEDDY Study Group), "Association of Gluten Intake during the First 5 Years of Life with Incidence of Celiac Disease Autoimmunity and Celiac Disease among Children at Increased Risk," *Journal of the American Medical Association* 322, no. 6 (August 2019): 514–23, https://doi.org/10.1001/jama.2019.10329.

120. K. M. Behall, D. J. Scholfield, I. Yuhaniak, and J. Canary, "Diets Containing High Amylose vs Amylopectin Starch: Effects on Metabolic Variables in Human

Subjects," *American Journal of Clinical Nutrition* 49, no. 2 (1989): 337–44, https://doi .org/10.1093/ajcn/49.2.337.

121. U.S. Department of Agriculture, "Adoption of Genetically Engineered Crops in the U.S.: Recent Trends in GE Adoption," November 3, 2016, https://www.ers .usda.gov/data-products/adoption-of-genetically-engineered-crops-in-the-us.aspx.

122. Q. Sun, D. Spiegelman, R. M. van Dam, et al., "White Rice, Brown Rice, and Risk of Type 2 Diabetes in US Men and Women," *Archives of Internal Medicine* 170, no. 11 (June 2010): 961–69, https://doi.org/10.1001/archinternmed.2010.109; G. F. Deng, X. R. Xu, Y. Zhang, et al., "Phenolic Compounds and Bioactivities of Pigmented Rice," *Critical Reviews in Food Science and Nutrition* 53, no. 3 (2013): 296–306, https://doi.org/10.1080/10408398.2010.529624.

123. Consumer Reports, "Arsenic in Your Food," November 2012, https://www .consumerreports.org/cro/magazine/2012/11/arsenic-in-your-food/index.htm; Consumer Reports, "How Much Arsenic Is in Your Rice?" January 2015, http://www .consumerreports.org/cro/magazine/205/01/how-much-arsenic-is-in-your-rice /index.htm.

124. C. B. Ebbeling, J. F. Swain, H. A. Feldman, et al., "Effects of Dietary Composition on Energy Expenditure during Weight-Loss Maintenance," *Journal of the American Medical Association* 307, no. 24 (June 2012): 2627–34, https://doi.org/10.1001 /jama.2012.6607; D. S. Ludwig, J. A. Majzoub, A. Al-Zahrani, G. E. Dallal, I. Blanco, and S. B. Roberts, "High Glycemic Index Foods, Overeating and Obesity," *Pediatrics* 103, no. 3 (March 1999): E26.

125. Benoit Bérengère, P. Plaisancié, A. Géloën, M. Estienne, C. Debard, E. Meugnier, E. Loizon, et al., "Pasture v. Standard Dairy Cream in High-Fat Diet-Fed Mice: Improved Metabolic Outcomes and Stronger Intestinal Barrier," *British Journal of Nutrition* 112, no. 4 (2014): 520–35, https://doi.org/10.1017/S0007114514001172.

126. Richard A. Forsgård, "Lactose Digestion in Humans: Intestinal Lactase Appears to Be Constitutive Whereas the Colonic Microbiome Is Adaptable," *American Journal of Clinical Nutrition* 110, no. 2 (2019): 273–79, https://doi.org/10.1093/ajcn /nqz104.

127. L. E. Macdonald, J. Brett, D. Kelton, S. E. Majowicz, K. Snedeker, and J. M. Sargeant, "A Systematic Review and Meta-analysis of the Effects of Pasteurization on Milk Vitamins, and Evidence for Raw Milk Consumption and Other Health-Related Outcomes," *Journal of Food Protection* 74, no. 11 (November 2011): 1814–32, https:// doi.org/10.4315/0362-028X.JFP-10-269.

128. F. M. Biro, M. P. Galvez, L. C. Greenspan, P. A. Succop, N. Vangeepuram, S. M. Pinney, S. Teitelbaum, G. C. Windham, L. H. Kushi, and M. S. Wolff, "Pubertal Assessment Method and Baseline Characteristics in a Mixed Longitudinal Study of Girls," *Pediatrics* 126, no. 3 (2010): e583–90, https://doi.org/10.1542 /peds.2009-3079.

129. S. Sanshiroh, T. Sato, H. Harada, and T. Takita, "Transfer of Soy Isoflavone into the Egg Yolk of Chickens," *Bioscience, Biotechnology, and Biochemistry* 65, no. 10 (2001): 2220–25, https://doi.org/10.1271/bbb.65.2220.

130. F. W. Danby, "Acne, Dairy and Cancer: The 5alpha-P Link," *Dermato-Endocrinology* 1, no. 1 (January 2009): 12–16, https://doi.org/10.4161/derm.1.1.7124.

131. H. Hochwallner, U. Schulmeister, I. Swoboda, et al., "Microarray and Allergenic Activity Assessment of Milk Allergens," *Clinical & Experimental Allergy* 40, no. 12 (December 2010): 1809–18, https://doi.org/10.1111/j.1365-2222.2010.03602.x.

132. H. Howchwallner, U. Schulmeister, I. Swoboda, et al., "Cow's Milk Allergy: From Allergens to New Forms of Diagnosis, Therapy and Prevention," *Methods* 66, no. 1 (March 2014): 2–33, https://doi.org/10.1016/j.ymeth.2013.08.00.

133. C. Lill, B. Loader, R. Seemann, et al., "Milk Allergy Is Frequent in Patients with Chronic Sinusitis and Nasal Polyposis," *American Journal of Rhinology & Allergy* 25, no. 6 (November–December 2011): e221–24, https://doi.org/10.2500/ajra.2011.25.3686.

134. J. Harkinson, "You're Drinking the Wrong Kind of Milk," *Mother Jones*, March 12, 2014, https://www.motherjones.com/environment/2014/03/a1-milk-a2-milk-america/.

135. R. Deth, A. Clarke, J. Ni, and M. Trivedi, "Clinical Evaluation of Glutathione Concentration after Consumption of Milk Containing Different Subtypes of B-casein: Results from Randomized, Cross-over Clinical Trial," *Nutrition Journal* 15, no. 1 (September 2016): 82, https://doi.org/10.1186/s12937-016-0201-x.

136. R. B. Elliott, D. P. Harris, J. P. Hill, N. J. Bibby, and H. E. Wasmuth, "Type 1 (Insulin Dependent) Diabetes Mellitus and Cow Milk: Casein Variant Consumption," *Diabetologia* 42, no. 3 (March 1999): 292–96.

137. R. G. Sherman, C. R. Fourtner, and C. D. Drewes, "Invertebrate Nerve-Muscle Systems," *Comparative Biochemistry and Physiology Part A: Physiology* 53, no. 3 (1976): 227–33, https://doi.org/10.1016/s0300-9629(76)80025-4; A. Mukherjee, S. Bandyopadhyay, and P. K. Basu, "Seizures Due to Food Allergy," *Journal of the Association of Physicians of India* 42, no. 8 (1994): 662–63, http://www.ncbi.nlm.nih.gov/pubmed/7868571.

138. B. Grenov, A. Larnkjær, C. Mølgaard, and K. F. Michaelsen, "Role of Milk and Dairy Products in Growth of the Child," *Nestlé Nutrition Institute Workshop Series* 93 (2020): 77–90, https://doi.org/10.1159/000503357.

139. Georg Loss, S. Bitter, J. Wohlgensinger, R. Frei, C. Roduit, J. Genuneit, J. Pekkanen, et al., "Prenatal and Early-Life Exposures Alter Expression of Innate Immunity Genes: The PASTURE Cohort Study," *Journal of Allergy and Clinical Immunology* 130, no. 2 (August 2012): 523–30, https://doi.org/10.1016/j.jaci.2012.05.049.

140. Gaofeng Yuan, C. Xiaoe, and D. Li, "Modulation of Peroxisome Proliferator-Activated Receptor Gamma (PPAR γ) by Conjugated Fatty Acid in Obesity and Inflammatory Bowel Disease," *Journal of Agricultural and Food Chemistry* 63, no. 7 (February 2015): 1883–95, https://doi.org/10.1021/jf505050c; Monica Viladomiu, Raquel Hontecillas, and Josep Bassaganya-Riera, "Modulation of Inflammation and Immunity by Dietary Conjugated Linoleic Acid," *European Journal of Pharmacology* 785 (August 2016): 87–95, https://doi.org/10.1016/j.ejphar.2015.03.095.

141. Ramdas Kanissery, Biwek Gairhe, Davie Kadyampakeni, Ozgur Batuman, and Fernando Alferez, "Glyphosate: Its Environmental Persistence and Impact on Crop Health and Nutrition," *Plants* (Basel) 8, no. 11 (November 2019), https://doi.org/10.3390/plants8110499.

142. Luoping Zhang, Iemaan Rana, Rachel M. Shaffer, Emanuela Tailoli, and Lianne Sheppard, "Exposure to Glyphosate-Based Herbicides and Risk for Non-Hodgkin Lymphoma: A Meta-analysis and Supporting Evidence," *Mutation Research / Reviews in Mutation Research* 781 (July–September 2019): 186–206, https://doi.org/10.1016/j.mrrev.2019.02.001.

143. N. Benachour and G. E. Seralini, "Glyphosate Formulations Induce Apoptosis and Necrosis in Human Umbilical, Embryonic, and Placental Cells," *Chemical Research in Toxicology* 22, no. 1 (January 2009): 97–105, https://doi.org/10.1021/tx800218n.

144. J. Marc et al., "A Glyphosate-Based Pesticide Impinges on Transcription," *Toxicology and Applied Pharmacology* 203, no. 1 (2005): 1–8, https://doi.org/10.1016/j.taap.2004.07.014.

145. R. M. Romano, M. A. Romano, M. M. Bernardi, P. V. Furtado, and C. A. Oliveira, "Prepubertal Exposure to Commercial Formulation of the Herbicide Glyphosate Alters Testosterone Levels and Testicular Morphology," *Archives of Toxicology* 84, no. 4 (April 2010): 309–17, https://doi.org/10.1007/s00204-009-0494-z.

146. Anthony Samsel and Stephanie Seneff, "Glyphosate's Suppression of Cytochrome P450 Enzymes and Amino Acid Biosynthesis by the Gut Microbiome: Pathways to Modern Diseases," *Entropy* 15 (2013), https://doi.org/10.3390/e15041416.

147. D. Huber, "What about Glyphosate-Induced Manganese Deficiency?" *Journal of Fluid Mechanics* 15 (2007): 20–22.

148. Ameena Batada and Michael F. Jacobson, "Prevalence of Artificial Food Colors in Grocery Store Products Marketed to Children," *Clinical Pediatrics*, June 6, 2016, https://pubmed.ncbi.nlm.nih.gov/27270961/.

149. Center for Science in the Public Interest, "Food Dyes: A Rainbow of Risks," June 1, 2010, http://cspinet.org/new/pdf/food-dyes-rainbow-of-risks.pdf.

150. C. J. Lowe, J. B. Morton, and A. C. Reichelt, "Adolescent Obesity and Dietary Decision Making: A Brain-Health Perspective," *Lancet Child & Adolescent Health* 4, no. 5 (May 2020): 388–96, https://doi.org/10.1016/S2352-4642(19)30404-3.

151. F. N. Jacka, C. Rothon, S. Taylor, M. Berk, and S. A. Stansfeld, "Diet Quality and Mental Health Problems in Adolescents from East London: A Prospective Study," *Social Psychiatry and Psychiatry Epidemiology* 48, no. 8 (August 2013): 1297–306, https://doi.org/10.1007/s00127-012-0623-5.

152. Q. P. Wang, Y. Q. Lin, L. Zhang, et al., "Sucralose Promotes Food Intake through NPY and a Neuronal Fasting Response," *Cell Metabolism* 24, no. 1 (July 2016): 75–90; S. E. Swithers and T. L. Davidson, "A Role of Sweet Taste: Calorie Predictive Relations in Energy Regulation by Rats," *Behavioral Neuroscience* 122, no. 1 (February 2008): 161–67, https://doi.org/10.1037/0735-7044.122.1.161.

153. T. J. Maher and R. J. Wurtman, "Possible Neurologic Effects of Aspartame, a Widely Used Food Additive," *Environmental Health Perspectives* 75 (November 1987): 53–57, https://doi.org/10.1289/ehp.877553.

154. I. Simintzi, K. H. Schulpis, P. Angelogianni, C. Liapi, and S. Tsakiris, "1-Cysteine and Glutathione Restore the Modulation of Rat Frontal Cortex Na+, K+-ATPase Activity Induced by Aspartame Metabolites," *Food and Chemical Toxicology* 46, no. 6 (June 2008): 2074–79.

155. K. Toru, T. Mlmura, Y. Takasakl, and M. Ichlmura, "Dietary Aspartame with Protein on Plasma and Brain Amino Acids, Brain Monoamines, and Behavior in Rats," *Physiology Behavior*, no. 36 (1986): 765.

156. J. Suez, T. Korem, D. Zeevi, et al., "Artificial Sweeteners Induce Glucose Intolerance by Altering the Gut Microbiota," *Nature* 514, no. 7521 (2014): 181–86, https://doi.org/10.1038/nature13793.

157. F. J. Ruiz-Ojeda, J. Plaza-Díaz, M. J. Sáez-Lara, and A. Gil, "Effects of Sweeteners on the Gut Microbiota: A Review of Experimental Studies and Clinical Trials," *Advances in Nutrition* 10, suppl. 1 (2019): S31–S48, https://doi.org/10.1093/advances/nmy037.

158. M. Soffritti, F. Belpoggi, M. Manservigi, et al., "Aspartame Administered in Feed, Beginning Prenatally through Life Span, Induces Cancer of the Liver and Lung in Male Swill Mice," *American Journal of Industrial Medicine* 53, no. 12 (2010): 1197–1206, https://doi.org/10.1002/ajim.20896.

159. Jotham Suez, Tal Korem, David Zeevi, Gili Zilberman-Schapira, Christoph A. Thaiss, Ori Maza, David Israeli, Niv Zmora, Shlomit Gilad, Adina Weinberger, Yael Kuperman, Alon Harmelin, Ilana Kolodkin-Gal, Hagit Shapiro, Zamir Halpern, Eran Segal, and Eran Elinav, "Artificial Sweeteners Induce Glucose Intolerance by Altering the Gut Microbiota," *Obstetrical & Gynecological Survey* 70, no. 1 (January 2015): 31–32, https://doi.org/10.1097/01.ogx.0000460711.58331.94.

160. Susan S. Schiffman and Kristina I. Rother, "Sucralose, a Synthetic Organochlorine Sweetener: Overview of Biological Issues," *Journal of Toxicology and Environmental Health*, Part B 16, no. 7 (October 2013): 399–451, https://doi.org/10.1080/10937404.2013.842523.

161. D. McCann, A. Barrett, A. Cooper, D. Crumpler, L. Dalen, K. Grimshaw, E. Kitchin, K. Lok, L. Porteous, and E. Prince, "Food Additives and Hyperactive Behaviour in 3-Year-Old and 8/9-Year-Old Children in the Community: A Randomized, Double-Blinded, Placebo-Controlled Trial," *Lancet* 370, no. 9598 (November 2007): 1560–67, https://doi.org/10.1016/S0140-6736(07)61306-3.

162. David W. Freeman, "Food Dyes Linked to Allergies, ADHD and Cancer: Group Calls on US to Outlaw Their Use," CBS Interactive, June 29, 2010, https://www.cbsnews.com/news/food-dyes-linked-to-allergies-adhd-and-cancer-group-calls-on-us-to-outlaw-their-use/.

163. Sarah Kobylewski and F. J. Michael, "Toxicology of Food Dyes," *International Journal of Occupational and Environmental Health* 18, no. 3 (July–September 2012): 220–46, https://doi.org/10.1179/1077352512Z.00000000034.

164. H. M. El-Wahab and G. S. Moram, "Toxic Effects of Some Synthetic Food Colorants and/or Flavor Additives on Male Rats," *Toxicology and Industrial Health* 29, no. 2 (March 2013): 224–32, https://doi.org/10.1177/0748233711433935.

165. International Agency for Research on Cancer, "Agents Classified by the IARC Monographs, Volumes 1–121," accessed April 19, 2021, https://monographs.iarc.who.int/agents-classified-by-the-iarc/.

166. Jing Ye et al., "Assessment of the Determination of Azodicarbonamide and Its Decomposition Product Semicarbazide: Investigation of Variation in Flour and Flour Products," *Journal of Agricultural and Food Chemistry* 59, no. 17 (2011): 9313–18,

https://doi.org/10.1021/jf201819x; Lisa Lefferts, "FDA Should Ban Azodicarbon-amide, Says CSPI," Center for Science in the Public Interest, February 4, 2014, https://cspinet.org/new/201402041.html.

167. Martha Henriques, "Additive in Breakfast Cereals Could Make the Brain 'Forget' to Stop Eating," *International Business Times*, August 10, 2017, http://www.ib times.co.uk/additive-breakfast-cereals-could-make-brain-forget-stop-eating-1634413.

168. Environmental Working Group, "EWG's Dirty Dozen Guide to Food Additives," accessed April 19, 2021, https://www.ewg.org/research/ewg-s-dirty-dozen -guide-food-additives/generally-recognized-as-safe-but-is-it#.W4hygpNKiRs.

169. S. Dengate and A. Ruben, "Controlled Trial of Cumulative Behavioural Effects of a Common Bread Preservative," *Journal of Paediatrics and Child Health* 38 (202): 373–76, https://doi.org/10.1046/j.1440-1754.2002.00009.x.

170. J. K. Tobacman, "Review of Harmful Gastrointestinal Effects of Carrageenan in Animal Experiments," *Environmental Health Perspectives* 109, no. 10 (2001): 983–94, https://doi.org/10.1289/ehp.01109983.

171. Raphaëlle Santarelli, Fabrice Pierre, and Denis Corpet, "Processed Meat and Colorectal Cancer: A Review of Epidemiologic and Experimental Evidence," *Nutrition and Cancer* 60, no. 2 (March 2008): 131–44, https://doi.org/10.1080 /01635580701684872.

172. Stephen R. Padgette et al., "The Composition of Glyphosate-Tolerant Soybean Seeds Is Equivalent to That of Conventional Soybeans," *Journal of Nutrition* 126, no. 4 (April 1996).

173. Nutrition Source, "Shining the Spotlight on Trans Fats," Harvard School of Public Health, accessed February 25, 2021, https://www.hsph.harvard.edu/nutrition source/what-should-you-eat/fats-and-cholesterol/types-of-fat/transfats/.

174. M. L. Slattery, J. Benson, K.-N. Ma, D. Schaffer, and J. D. Potter, "Trans-Fatty Acids and Colon Cancer," *Nutrition and Cancer* 39, no. 2 (2001): 170–75, https:// doi.org/10.1207/S15327914nc392_2; Véronique Chajès, Anne C. M. Thiébaut, Maxime Rotival, Estelle Gauthier, Virginie Maillard, Marie-Christine Boutron-Ruault, Virginie Joulin, Gilbert M. Lenoir, and Françoise Clavel-Chapelon, "Association between Serum Trans-monounsaturated Fatty Acids and Breast Cancer Risk in the E3N-EPIC Study," *American Journal of Epidemiology* 167, no. 11 (2008): 1312–20, https://doi.org/10.1093/aje/kwn069.

175. Kirsten A. Herrick, Cynthia L. Ogden, Sohyun Park, Heather C. Hamner, and Cheryl D. Fryar, "Added Sugars Intake among US Infants and Toddlers," *Journal of the Academy of Nutrition and Dietetics*, November 19, 2019, https://pubmed.ncbi.nlm .nih.gov/31735600/.

176. D. R. Felix, F. Costenaro, C. B. A. Gottschall, and G. P. Coral, "Non-alcoholic Fatty Liver Disease in Obese Children—Effect of Refined Carbohydrates in Diet," *BMC Pediatrics* 16, no. 1 (November 2016): 187, https://doi.org/10.1186 /s12887-016-0726-3; K. Kavanagh, A. T. Wylie, K. L. Tucker, et al., "Dietary Fructose Induces Endotoxemia and Hepatic Injury in Calorically Controlled Primates," *American Journal of Clinical Nutrition* 98, no. 2 (August 2013): 349–57, https://doi .org/10.3945/ajcn.112.057331.

177. M. Winterdahl, N. Ove, O. Dariusz, A. C. Schacht, S. Jakobsen, A. K. O. Alstrup, A. Gjedde, and A. M. Landau, "Sucrose Intake Lowers μ-Opioid and Dopamine D2/3 Receptor Availability in Porcine Brain," *Scientific Reports* 9, no. 1 (2019), https://www.nature.com/articles/s41598-019-53430-9#Abs1.

178. L. Azadbakht and A. Esmaillzadeh, "Dietary Patterns and Attention Deficit Hyperactivity Disorder among Iranian Children," *Nutrition* 28, no. 3 (March 2012): 242–49, https://doi.org/10.1016/j.nut.2011.05.018.

179. P. K. Olszewski, E. L. Wood, A. Klockars, and A. S. Levine, "Excessive Consumption of Sugar: An Insatiable Drive for Reward," *Current Nutrition Reports* 8 (2019): 120–28, https://doi.org/10.1007/s13668-019-0270-5.

180. A. Chaix, A. Zarrinpar, P. Miu, and S. Panda, "Time-Restricted Feeding Is a Preventative and Therapeutic Intervention against Diverse Nutritional Challenges," *Cell Metabolism* 20, no. 6 (2014): 991–1005, https://doi.org/10.1016/j.cmet.2014.11.001.

181. UT Southwestern Medical Center, "Fasting Kills Cancer Cells of Most Common Type of Childhood Leukemia Study Shows," *ScienceDaily*, accessed February 22, 2021, https://www.sciencedaily.com/releases/2016/12/161212133654.htm.

182. W. W. Au, "Susceptibility of Children to Environmental Toxic Substances," *International Journal of Hygiene and Environmental Health* 205, no. 6 (October 2002): 501–3, https://doi.org/10.1078/1438-4639-00179.

183. P. M. Rodier, "Developing Brain as a Target of Toxicity," *Environmental Health Perspectives* 103, suppl. 6 (September 1995): 73–76, https://doi.org/10.1289/ehp.95103s673; B. P. Lanphear, "The Impact of Toxins on the Developing Brain," *Annual Review of Public Health* 36 (March 2015): 211–30, https://doi.org/10.1146/annurev-publhealth-031912-114413.

184. Environment Working Group, "Body Burden—the Pollution in Newborns: A Benchmark Investigation of Industrial Chemicals, Pollutants and Pesticides in Umbilical Cord Blood," July 14, 2005, https://www.ewg.org/research/body-burden-pollution-newborns.

185. Teresa Valero, "Mitochondrial Biogenesis: Pharmacological Approaches," *Current Pharmaceutical Design* 20, no. 35 (2014): 5507–9, https://doi.org/10.2174/138161282035140911142118.

186. University of Rochester Medical Center, "Environmental Toxins Impair Immune System over Multiple Generations," *ScienceDaily*, accessed February 22, 2021, https://www.sciencedaily.com/releases/2019/10/191002144257.htm.

187. D. C. Jones and G. W. Miller, "The Effects of Environmental Neurotoxicants on the Dopaminergic System: A Possible Role in Drug Addiction," *Biochemical Pharmacology* 76, no. 5 (September 2008): 569–81, https://doi.org/10.1016/j.bcp.2008.05.010.

188. M. Hauptman and A. D. Woolf, "Childhood Ingestions of Environmental Toxins: What Are the Risks?" *Pediatric Annals* 46, no. 12 (2017): e466–71, https://doi.org/10.3928/19382359-20171116-01.

189. Jones and Miller, "The Effects of Environmental Neurotoxicants on the Dopaminergic System."

190. M. S. Jackson-Browne, G. D. Papandonatos, A. Chen, K. Yolton, B. P. Lanphear, and J. M. Braun, "Early-Life Triclosan Exposure and Parent-Reported Behavior Problems in 8-Year-Old Children," *Environment International* 128 (July 2019): 446–56, https://doi.org/10.1016/j.envint.2019.01.021.

191. N. Li, G. D. Papandonatos, A. M. Calafat, K. Yolton, B. P. Lanphear, A. Chen, and J. M. Braun, "Gestational and Childhood Exposure to Phthalates and Child Behavior," *Environment International* 144 (November 2020): 106036, https://doi.org/10.1016/j.envint.2020.106036; J. R. Shoaff, B. Coull, J. Weuve, et al., "Association of Exposure to Endocrine-Disrupting Chemicals during Adolescence with Attention-Deficit/Hyperactivity Disorder–Related Behaviors," *JAMA Network Open* 3, no. 8 (2020): e2015041, https://doi.org/10.1001/jamanetworkopen.2020.15041.

192. Jackson-Browne et al., "Early-Life Triclosan Exposure and Parent-Reported Behavior Problems in 8-Year-Old Children."

193. P. Grandjean and P. J. Landrigan, "Neurobehavioural Effects of Developmental Toxicity," *Lancet Neurology* 13, no. 3 (March 2014): 330–38, https://doi.org/10.1016/S1474-4422(13)70278-3.

194. T. F. Collins, R. L. Sprando, T. N. Black, M. E. Shackelford, N. Olejnik, M. J. Ames, J. I. Rorie, and D. I. Ruggles, "Developmental Toxicity of Sodium Fluoride Measured during Multiple Generations," *Food and Chemical Toxicology* 39, no. 8 (August 2001): 867–76, https://doi.org/10.1016/s0278-6915(01)00033-3.

195. Anna L. Choi, G. Sun, Y. Zhang, and P. Grandjean, "Developmental Fluoride Neurotoxicity: A Systematic Review and Meta-analysis," *Environmental Health Perspectives* 120, no. 10 (October 2012): 1362–68, https://doi.org/10.1289/ehp.1104912.

196. P. Grandjean, "Developmental Fluoride Neurotoxicity: An Updated Review," *Environmental Health* 18 (December 2019): 110, https://doi.org/10.1186/s12940-019-0551-x.

197. V. Mustieles and M. F. Fernández, "Bisphenol A Shapes Children's Brain and Behavior: Towards an Integrated Neurotoxicity Assessment Including Human Data," *Environmental Health* 19, no. 66 (2020), https://doi.org/10.1186/s12940-020-00620-y.

198. M. Fisher, T. E. Arbuckle, C. L. Liang, et al., "Concentrations of Persistent Organic Pollutants in Maternal and Cord Blood from the Maternal–Infant Research on Environmental Chemicals (MIREC) Cohort Study," *Environmental Health* 15, no. 59 (2016), https://doi.org/10.1186/s12940-016-0143-y.

199. S. M. Engel and M. S. Wolff, "Causal Inference Considerations for Endocrine Disruptor Research in Children's Health," *Annual Review of Public Health* 34 (2013): 139–58, https://doi.org/10.1146/annurev-publhealth-031811-124556.

200. Joseph L. Jacobson, Gina Muckle, Pierre Ayotte, Éric Dewailly, and Sandra W. Jacobson, "Relation of Prenatal Methylmercury Exposure from Environmental Sources to Childhood IQ," *Environmental Health Perspectives* 123, no. 8 (August 2015): 827–33, https://doi.org/10.1289/ehp.1408554.

201. K. M. Rice, E. M. Walker, M. Wu, C. Gillette, and E. R. Blough, "Environmental Mercury and Its Toxic Effects," *Journal of Preventive Medicine and Public Health* 47, no. 2 (2014): 74–83, https://doi.org/10.3961/jpmph.2014.47.2.74.

202. P. Grandjean, E. Budtz-Jørgensen, R. F. White, P. J. Jørgensen, P. Weihe, F. Debes, and N. Keiding, "Methylmercury Exposure Biomarkers as Indicators of

Neurotoxicity in Children Aged 7 Years," *American Journal of Epidemiology* 150, no. 3 (August 1999): 301–5, https://doi.org/10.1093/oxfordjournals.aje.a010002.

203. Mariah Blake, "Those BPA-Free Plastics You Thought Were Safe? Think Again," *Mother Jones*, March 3, 2014, https://www.motherjones.com/environment /2014/03/tritan-certichem-eastman-bpa-free-plastic-safe/.

204. Hauptman and Woolf, "Childhood Ingestions of Environmental Toxins: What Are the Risks?"

205. Norwegian University of Science and Technology, "800 Million Children Still Exposed to Lead: Study Documents a Persistent, Dangerous Problem," *ScienceDaily*, accessed February 22, 2021, https://www.sciencedaily.com/releases /2020/10/201001113555.htm.

206. D. K. Marcus, J. J. Fulton, and E. J. Clarke, "Lead and Conduct Problems: A Meta-analysis," *Journal of Clinical Child & Adolescent Psychology* 39, no. 2 (2010): 234–41, https://doi.org/10.1080/15374411003591455.

207. Consumer Reports, "Arsenic in Your Juice," last updated October 3, 2013, http://www.consumerreports.org/cro/magazine/2012/01/arsenic-in-your-juice /index.htm; Consumer Reports, "How Much Arsenic Is in Your Rice?"

208. Yale University, "Cell Phone Use in Pregnancy May Cause Behavioral Disorders in Offspring, Mouse Study Suggests," *ScienceDaily*, accessed February 21, 2021, https://www.sciencedaily.com/releases/2012/03/120315110138.htm; Swiss Tropical and Public Health Institute, "Mobile Phone Radiation May Affect Memory Performance in Adolescents, Study Finds," *ScienceDaily*, accessed February 22, 2021, https:// www.sciencedaily.com/releases/2018/07/180719121803.htm; E. G. Kivrak, K. K. Yurt, A. A. Kaplan, I. Alkan, and G. Altun, "Effects of Electromagnetic Fields Exposure on the Antioxidant Defense System," *Journal of Microscopy and Ultrastructure* 5, no. 4 (October–December 2017): 167–76, https://doi.org/10.1016/j.jmau.2017.07.003.

CHAPTER 4: THE FOUR S'S

1. Naja H. Rod, Jessica Bengtsson, Esben Budtz-Jørgensen, Clara Clipet-Jensen, David Taylor-Robinson, Anne-Marie Nybo Andersen, Nadya Dich, and Andreas Rieckmann, "Trajectories of Childhood Adversity and Mortality in Early Adulthood: A Population-Based Cohort Study," *Lancet* 396, no. 10249 (2020): 489, https://doi .org/10.1016/S0140-6736(20)30621-8.

2. Matthew D. Albaugh, James J. Hudziak, Catherine Orr, Philip A. Spechler, Bader Chaarani, Scott Mackey, Claude Lepage, et al., "Amygdalar Reactivity Is Associated with Prefrontal Cortical Thickness in a Large Population-Based Sample of Adolescents," *PLoS ONE* 14, no. 5 (2019): e216152, https://doi.org/10.1371 /journal.pone.0216152.

3. M. D. De Bellis and A. Zisk, "The Biological Effects of Childhood Trauma," *Child and Adolescent Psychiatric Clinics of North America* 23, no. 2 (2014): 185–222, https://doi.org/10.1016/j.chc.2014.01.002.

4. David Q. Stoye, Manuel Blesa, Gemma Sullivan, Paola Galdi, Gillian J. Lamb, Gill S. Black, Alan J. Quigley, Michael J. Thrippleton, Mark E. Bastin, Rebecca M. Reynolds, and James P. Boardman, "Maternal Cortisol Is Associated with Neonatal Amygdala Microstructure and Connectivity in a Sexually Dimorphic Manner," *eLife* 9 (2020): E60729, https://doi.org/10.7554/eLife.60729.

5. K. L. Humphreys, M. C. Camacho, M. C. Roth, and E. C. Estes, "Prenatal Stress Exposure and Multimodal Assessment of Amygdala-Medial Prefrontal Cortex Connectivity in Infants," *Developmental Cognitive Neuroscience* 46 (December 2020): 100877, https://doi.org/10.1016/j.dcn.2020.100877.

6. Stoye et al., "Maternal Cortisol Is Associated with Neonatal Amygdala Microstructure and Connectivity in a Sexually Dimorphic Manner."

7. Stoye et al., "Maternal Cortisol Is Associated with Neonatal Amygdala Microstructure and Connectivity in a Sexually Dimorphic Manner."

8. A. F. T. Arnsten, "Stress Signaling Pathways That Impair Prefrontal Cortex Structure and Function," *Nature Reviews Neruoscience* 10, no. 6 (June 2009): 410–22, https://doi.org/10.1038/nrn2648.

9. M. D. Teicher, "Wounds That Time Won't Heal: The Neurobiology of Child Abuse," *Cerebrum: The Dana Forum on Brain Science* 2 (2000): 50–67, https://www.researchgate.net/publication/215768752_Wounds_that_time_won't_heal_The_neurobiology_of_child_abuse.

10. Stanford Medicine, "Stanford Study Finds Stronger One-Way Fear Signals in Brains of Anxious Kids," News Center, April 2020, https://med.stanford.edu/news/all-news/2020/04/stanford-study-finds-stronger-one-way-fear-signals-in-brains-of-.html.

11. A. T. Park, J. A. Leonard, P. K. Saxler, A. B. Cyr, J. D. E. Gabrieli, and A. P. Mackey, "Amygdala-Medial Prefrontal Cortex Connectivity Relates to Stress and Mental Health in Early Childhood," *Social Cognitive and Affective Neuroscience* 13, no. 4 (April 2018): 430–39, https://doi.org/10.1093/scan/nsy017.

12. A. Galván and A. Rahdar, "The Neurobiological Effects of Stress on Adolescent Decision Making," *Neuroscience* 249 (September 26, 2013): 223–31, https://doi.org/10.1016/j.neuroscience.2012.09.074.

13. Tim Vanuytsel, Sander van Wanrooy, Hanne Vanheel, Christophe Vanormelingen, Sofie Verschueren, Els Houben, Shadea Salim Rasoel, Joran Toth, Lieselot Holvoet, Ricard Farre, Lukas Van Oudenhove, Guy Boeckxstaens, Kristin Verbeke, and Jan Tack, "Psychological Stress and Corticotropin-Releasing Hormone Increase Intestinal Permeability in Humans by a Mast Cell-Dependent Mechanism," *Gut* 63, no. 8 (August 2014): 1293–99, https://doi.org/10.1136/gutjnl-2013-305690.

14. Rafael Campos-Rodríguez, Marycarmen Godinez-Victoria, Edgar Abarca-Rojano, Judith Pacheo-Yepez, Humberto Reyna-Garfias, Reyna E. Barbosa-Cabrera, and Maria E. Drago-Serrano, "Stress Modulates Intestinal Secretory Immunoglobulin A," *Frontiers in Integrative Neuroscience* 7 (December 2013), https://doi.org/10.3389/fnint.2013.00086.

15. N. Michels, T. Van de Wiele, F. Fouhy, S. O'Mahony, G. Clarke, and J. Keane, "Gut Microbiome Patterns Depending on Children's Psychosocial Stress:

Reports versus Biomarkers," *Brain, Behavior, and Immunity* 80 (August 2019): 751–62, https://doi.org/10.1016/j.bbi.2019.05.024.

16. G. Holtmann, R. Kriebel, and M. V. Singer, "Mental Stress and Gastric Acid Secretion: Do Personality Traits Influence the Response?" *Digestive Diseases and Sciences* 35, no. 8 (1990): 998–1007, https://doi.org/10.1007/BF01537249.

17. Alison C. Bested, Alan C. Logan, and Eva M. Selhub, "Intestinal Microbiota, Probiotics and Mental Health: From Metchnikoff to Modern Advances: Part II—Contemporary Contextual Research," *Gut Pathogens* 5, no. 1 (2013): 3, https://doi.org/10.1186/1757-4749-5-3.

18. K. Schmidt, P. Cowen, C. J. Harmer, G. Tzortzis, and P. W. J. Burnet, "P.1.e.003 Prebiotic Intake Reduces the Waking Cortisol Response and Alters Emotional Bias in Healthy Volunteers," *European Neuropsychopharmacology* 24 (October 2014), https://doi.org/10.1016/s0924-977x (14)70294-9.

19. K. E. Wellen and G. S. Hotamisligil, "Inflammation, Stress, and Diabetes," *Journal of Clinical Investigation* 115, no. 5 (2005): 1111–19, https://doi.org/10.1172/JCI25102.

20. Centers for Disease Control and Prevention, "Preventing Adverse Childhood Experiences," accessed April 6, 2021, https://www.cdc.gov/violenceprevention/aces/fastfact.html.

21. Sara F. Waters, Helena Rose Karnilowicz, Tessa V. West, and Wendy Berry Mendes, "Keep It to Yourself? Parent Emotion Suppression Influences Physiological Linkage and Interaction Behavior," *Journal of Family Psychology* 34, no. 7 (2020): 784–93, https://doi.org/10.1037/fam0000664.

22. Caitlin R. Wagner and Jamie L. Abaied, "Skin Conductance Level Reactivity Moderates the Association between Parental Psychological Control and Relational Aggression in Emerging Adulthood," *Journal of Youth and Adolescence* 45 (2016): 687–700, https://doi.org/10.1007/s10964-016-0422-5.

23. A. Nagano-Saito et al., "Stress-Induced Dopamine Release in Human Medial Prefrontal Cortex—18F-Fallypride/PET Study in Healthy Volunteers," *Synapse* 67, no. 12 (December 2013): 821–30, https://doi.org/10.1002/syn.21700.

24. R. A. Dore, K. M. Purtell, and L. M. Justice, "Media Use among Kindergarteners from Low-Income Households during the COVID-19 Shutdown," *Journal of Developmental and Behavioral Pediatrics*, April 7, 2021, https://doi.org/10.1097/DBP.0000000000000955.

25. K. Tamana Sukhpreet, Victor Ezeugwu, Joyce Chikuma, Diana L. Lefebvre, Meghan B. Azad, Theo J. Moraes, Padmaja Subbarao, Allan B. Becker, Stuart E. Turvey, Malcolm R. Sears, Bruce D. Dick, Valerie Carson, Carmen Rasmussen (CHILD Study Investigators), Jacqueline Pei, and Piush J. Mandhane, "Screen-Time Is Associated with Inattention Problems in Preschoolers: Results from the CHILD Birth Cohort Study," *PLoS ONE* 14, no. 4 (April 2019): e0213995, https://doi.org/10.1371/journal.pone.0213995.

26. Cassandra L. Pattinson, Alicia C. Allan, Sally L. Staton, Karen J. Thorpe, and Simon S. Smith, "Environmental Light Exposure Is Associated with Increased Body Mass in Children," *PLoS ONE* 11, no. 1 (2016): e0143578, https://doi.org/10.1371/journal.pone.0143578.

27. J. M. Twenge, T. E. Joiner, M. L. Rogers, et al., "Increases in Depressive Symptoms, Suicide-Related Outcomes, and Suicide Rates among U.S. Adolescents after 2010 and Links to Increased New Media Screen Time," *Clinical Psychological Science* 6, no. 1 (2017): 3–17, https://doi.org/10.1177/2167702617723376; Norihito Oshima, Atsushi Nishida, Shinji Shimodera, Mamoru Tochigi, Shuntaro Ando, Syudo Yamasaki, Yuji Okazaki, and Tsukasa Sasaki, "The Suicidal Feelings, Self-injury, and Mobile Phone Use after Lights Out in Adolescents," *Journal of Pediatric Psychology* 37, no. 9 (2012): 1023–30, https://doi.org/10.1093/jpepsy/jss072; Neza Stiglic and Russell M. Viner, "Effects of Screen Time on the Health and Well-Being of Children and Adolescents: A Systematic Review of Reviews," *BMJ Open* 9, no. 1 (2019): e023191, https://doi.org/10.1136/bmjopen-2018-023191.

28. Brian A. Primack, Ariel Shensa, Jaime E. Sidani, César G. Escobar-Viera, and Michael J. Fine, "Temporal Associations between Social Media Use and Depression," *American Journal of Preventive Medicine* 60, no. 2 (2021): 179–88, https://doi.org/10.1016/j.amepre.2020.09.014.

29. John S. Hutton, Jonathan Dudley, Tzipi Horowitz-Kraus, Tom DeWitt, and Scott K. Holland, "Associations between Screen-Based Media Use and Brain White Matter Integrity in Preschool-Aged Children," *JAMA Pediatrics* 174, no. 1 (2020): e193869, https://doi.org/10.1001/jamapediatrics.2019.3869.

30. Brandon T. McDaniel and Jenny S. Radesky, "Technoference: Longitudinal Associations between Parent Technology Use, Parenting Stress, and Child Behavior Problems," *Pediatric Research* 84, no. 2 (August 2018): 210–18, https://doi.org/10.1038/s41390-018-0052-6.

31. E. M. White, M. D. DeBoer, and R. J. Scharf, "Associations between Household Chores and Childhood Self-Competency," *Journal of Developmental & Behavioral Pediatrics* 40, no. 3 (April 2019): 176–82, https://doi.org/10.1097/DBP.0000000000000637.

32. K. K. Schmeer and A. J. Yoon, "Home Sweet Home? Home Physical Environment and Inflammation in Children," *Social Science Research* 60 (2016): 236–48, https://doi.org/10.1016/j.ssresearch.2016.04.001.

33. Numerous papers have covered the relationship between exposure to nature and human health. For a recent basic review, see M. A. Repke et al., "How Does Nature Exposure Make People Healthier? Evidence for the Role of Impulsivity and Expanded Space Perception," *PLoS ONE* 13, no. 8 (August 2018): e0202246, https://doi.org/10.1371/journal.pone.0202246.

34. M. Kuo, M. Barnes, and C. Jordan, "Do Experiences with Nature Promote Learning? Converging Evidence of a Cause-and-Effect Relationship," *Frontiers in Psychology* 10 (February 2019): 305, https://doi.org/10.3389/fpsyg.2019.00305.

35. John M. Zelenski, Raelyne L. Dopko, and Colin A. Capaldi, "Cooperation Is in Our Nature: Nature Exposure May Promote Cooperative and Environmentally Sustainable Behavior," *Journal of Environmental Psychology* 42 (June 2015): 24–31, https://doi.org/10.1016/j.jenvp.2015.01.005.

36. S. Strife and L. Downey, "Childhood Development and Access to Nature: A New Direction for Environmental Inequality Research," *Organization & Environment* 22 (2009): 99–122, https://doi.org/10.1177/1086026609333340.

37. Gaétan Chevalier, Stephen T. Sinatra, James L. Oschman, Karol Sokal, and Pawel Sokal, "Earthing: Health Implications of Reconnecting the Human Body to the Earth's Surface Electrons," *Journal of Environmental and Public Health* (2012), http://www.doi.org/10.1155/2012/291541.

38. C. C. C. Bauer, C. Caballero, E. Scherer, M. R. West, M. D. Mrazek, D. T. Phillips, S. Whitfield-Gabrieli, and J. D. E. Gabrieli, "Mindfulness Training Reduces Stress and Amygdala Reactivity to Fearful Faces in Middle-School Children," *Behavioral Neuroscience* 133, no. 6 (December 2019): 569–85, https://doi.org/10.1037/bne0000337.

39. E. M. C. Geronimi, B. Arellano, and J. Woodruff-Borden, "Relating Mindfulness and Executive Function in Children," *Clinical Child Psychology and Psychiatry* 25, no. 2 (2020): 435–45, https://doi.org/10.1177/1359104519833737.

40. C. Crescentini, V. Capurso, S. Furlan, and F. Fabbro, "Mindfulness-Oriented Meditation for Primary School Children: Effects on Attention and Psychological Well-Being," *Frontiers in Psychology* 7 (2016): 805, https://doi.org/10.3389/fpsyg.2016.00805; H. Hamasaki, "Effects of Diaphragmatic Breathing on Health: A Narrative Review," *Medicines* (Basel) 7, no. 10 (2020): 65, https://doi.org/10.3390/medicines7100065.

41. C. Perry-Parrish, N. Copeland-Linder, L. Webb, and E. M. Sibinga, "Mindfulness-Based Approaches for Children and Youth," *Current Problems in Pediatric and Adolescent Health Care* 46, no. 6 (June 2016): 172–78, https://doi.org/10.1016/j.cppeds.2015.12.006.

42. L. Hilton et al., "Mindfulness Meditation for Chronic Pain: Systemic Review and Meta-analysis," *Annals of Behavioral Medicine* 51, no. 2 (April 2017): 199–213, https://doi.org/10.1007/s12160-016-9844-2.

43. Y.-Y. Tang, Q. Lu, H. Feng, R. Tang, and M. I. Posner, "Short-Term Meditation Increases Blood Flow in Anterior Cingulate Cortex and Insula," *Frontiers in Psychology* 6 (2015), https://doi.org/10.3389/fpsyg.2015.00212.

44. M. de Fatima Rosas Marchiori, E. H. Kozasa, R. D. Miranda, A. L. M. Andrade, T. C. Perrotti, and J. R. Leite, "Decrease in Blood Pressure and Improved Psychological Aspects through Meditation Training in Hypertensive Older Adults: A Randomized Control Study," *Geriatrics & Gerontology International* 15, no. 10 (2015): 1158–64, https://doi.org/10.1111/ggi.12414.

45. National Center for Complementary and Integrative Health, "Meditation: In Depth," accessed February 25, 2021, https://nccih.nih.gov/health/meditation/overview.htm.

46. A. A. Taren, J. D. Creswell, and P. J. Gianaros, "Dispositional Mindfulness Covaries with Smaller Amygdala and Caudate Volumes in Community Adults," *PLoS ONE* 8, no. 5 (May 2013): e64574, https://doi.org/10.1371/journal.pone.0064574.

47. Vania Modesto-Lowe, Pantea Farahmand, Margaret Chaplin, and Lauren Sarro, "Does Mindfulness Meditation Improve Attention in Attention Deficit Hyperactivity Disorder?" *World Journal of Psychiatry* 5, no. 4 (2015): 397–403, https://doi.org/10.5498/wjp.v5.i4.397.

48. F. Saatcioglu, "Regulation of Gene Expression by Yoga, Meditation and Related Practices: A Review of Recent Studies," *Asian Journal of Psychiatry* 6, no. 1 (2013): 74–77, https://doi.org/10.1016/j.ajp.2012.10.002.

49. D. S. Black and G. M. Slavich, "Mindfulness Meditation and the Immune System: A Systemic Review of Randomized Controlled Trials," *Annals of the New York Academy of Sciences* 1373, no. 1 (June 2016): 13–24, https://doi.org/10.1111/nyas.12998.

50. Y.-Y. Tang, B. K. Holzel, and M. I. Posner, "The Neuroscience of Mindfulness Meditation," *Nature Reviews Neuroscience* 16, no. 4 (April 2015): 213–25, https://doi.org/10.1038/nrn3954.

51. Hamasaki, "Effects of Diaphragmatic Breathing on Health: A Narrative Review."

52. Neuroscience News, "Laughing Is Good for Your Mind and Your Body, Here's What the Research Shows," November 29, 2020, https://neurosciencenews.com/laughter-physical-mental-psychology-17339.

53. A. Marques, D. A. Santos, C. H. Hillman, and L. B. Sardinha, "How Does Academic Achievement Relate to Cardiorespiratory Fitness, Self-reported Physical Activity and Objectively Reported Physical Activity: A Systematic Review in Children and Adolescents Aged 6–18 Years," *British Journal of Sports Medicine* 52 (2018): 1039, https://doi.org/10.1136/bjsports-2016-097361.

54. Z. Gao, S. Chen, H. Sun, X. Wen, and P. Xiang, "Physical Activity in Children's Health and Cognition," *BioMed Research International* 2018 (2018): 8542403, https://doi.org/10.1155/2018/8542403.

55. R. M. Taylor, S. M. Fealy, A. Bisquera, R. Smith, C. E. Collins, T. J. Evans, and A. J. Hure, "Effects of Nutritional Interventions during Pregnancy on Infant and Child Cognitive Outcomes: A Systematic Review and Meta-analysis," *Nutrients* 9 (2017): 1265, https://doi.org/10.3390/nu9111265.

56. Centers for Disease Control and Prevention, "Do Your Children Get Enough Sleep?" accessed April 21, 2021, https://www.cdc.gov/chronicdisease/resources/infographic/children-sleep.htm.

57. "Blue Light Has a Dark Side," *Harvard Health*, July 7, 2020, https://www.health.harvard.edu/staying-healthy/blue-light-has-a-dark-side.

58. Common Sense Media, "The Common Sense Census: Media Use by Kids Age Zero to Eight, 2020," accessed April 21, 2021, https://www.commonsensemedia.org/research/the-common-sense-census-media-use-by-kids-age-zero-to-eight-2020.

59. Salome Kurth, Douglas C. Dean, Peter Achermann, Jonathan O'Muircheartaigh, Reto Huber, Sean C. L. Deoni, and Monique K. LeBourgeois, "Increased Sleep Depth in Developing Neural Networks: New Insights from Sleep Restriction in Children," *Frontiers in Human Neuroscience* 10 (2016), https://doi.org/10.3389/fnhum.2016.00456.

60. University of South Australia, "Sleep Keeps Teens on Track for Good Mental Health," *ScienceDaily*, accessed February 22, 2021, https://www.sciencedaily.com/releases/2021/02/210210091215.htm.

61. A. Cremone, D. M. de Jong, L. B. F. Kurdziel, P. Desrochers, A. Sayer, M. K. LeBourgeois, R. M. C. Spencer, and J. M. McDermott, "Sleep Tight, Act

Right: Negative Affect, Sleep and Behavior Problems during Early Childhood," *Child Development* 89 (2018): e42–e59, https://doi.org/10.1111/cdev.12717.

62. R. E. Dahl, "Sleep and the Developing Brain," *Sleep* 30, no. 9 (2007): 1079–80, https://doi.org/10.1093/sleep/30.9.1079.

63. Michael Murack, Rajini Chandrasegaram, Kevin B. Smith, Emily G. Ah-Yen, Étienne Rheaume, Étienne Malette-Guyon, Nanji Zahra, Seana N. Semchishen, Olivia Latus, Claude Messier, and Nafissa Ismail, "Chronic Sleep Disruption Induces Depression-Like Behavior in Adolescent Male and Female Mice and Sensitization of the Hypothalamic-Pituitary-Adrenal Axis in Adolescent Female Mice," *Behavioural Brain Research* 399 (2020): 113001, https://doi.org/10.1016/j.bbr.2020.113001.

64. K. P. Maski and S. V. Kothare, "Sleep Deprivation and Neurobehavioral Functioning in Children," *International Journal of Psychophysiology* 89, no. 2 (August 2013): 259–64, https://doi.org/10.1016/j.ijpsycho.2013.06.019.

65. K. Turnbull, G. J. Reid, and J. B. Morton, "Behavioral Sleep Problems and Their Potential Impact on Developing Executive Function in Children," *Sleep* 36, no. 7 (2013): 1077–84, https://doi.org/10.5665/sleep.2814.

66. L. Xiu, M. Ekstedt, M. Hagströmer, O. Bruni, L. Bergqvist-Norén, and C. Marcus, "Sleep and Adiposity in Children from 2 to 6 Years of Age," *Pediatrics* 145, no. 3 (March 2020): e20191420, https://doi.org/10.1542/peds.2019-1420.

67. Simon L. Evans and Ray Norbury, "Associations between Diurnal Preference, Impulsivity and Substance Use in a Young-Adult Student Sample," *Chronobiology International* 1 (2020), https://doi.org/10.1080/07420528.2020.1810063.

68. A. Miles, "PubMed Health," *Journal of the Medical Library Association* 99, no. 3 (2011): 265–66, https://doi.org/10.3163/1536-5050.99.3.018.

69. Vanuytsel et al., "Psychological Stress and Corticotropin-Releasing Hormone Increase Intestinal Permeability in Humans by a Mast Cell-Dependent Mechanism."

70. Darcia Narvaez, "Dangers of 'Crying It Out,'" *Psychology Today*, December 11, 2011, https://www.psychologytoday.com/us/blog/moral-landscapes/201112/dangers-crying-it-out.

71. W. T. Greenough, J. E. Black, and C. S. Wallace, "Experience and Brain Development," *Child Development* 58 (1987): 539–59, https://doi.org/10.2307/1130197.

72. Daiki Hiraoka, Shota Nishitani, Koji Shimada, Ryoko Kasaba, Takashi X. Fujisawa, and Akemi Tomoda, "Epigenetic Modification of the Oxytocin Gene Is Associated with Gray Matter Volume and Trait Empathy in Mothers," *Psychoneuroendocrinology* 123 (2021): 105026, https://doi.org/10.1016/j.psyneuen.2020.105026.

73. Hiraoka et al., "Epigenetic Modification of the Oxytocin Gene Is Associated with Gray Matter Volume and Trait Empathy in Mothers."

74. J. Cassidy, "Emotion Regulation: Influences of Attachment Relationships," *Monographs of the Society for Research in Child Development* 59, no. 2–3 (1994): 228–49.

75. A. Lingnau and A. Caramazza, "The Origin and Function of Mirror Neurons: The Missing Link," *Behavioral and Brain Sciences* 37, no. 2 (April 2014): 209–10, https://doi.org/10.1017/S0140525X13002380.

76. Sara Scardera, Léa C. Perret, Isabelle Ouellet-Morin, Geneviève Gariépy, Robert-Paul Juster, Michel Boivin, Gustavo Turecki, Richard E. Tremblay, Sylvana Côté, and Marie-Claude Geoffroy, "Association of Social Support during Adolescence with

Depression, Anxiety, and Suicidal Ideation in Young Adults," *JAMA Network Open* 3, no. 12 (2020): e2027491, https://doi.org/10.1001/jamanetworkopen.2020.27491.

77. S. F. Waters, E. A. Virmani, R. A. Thompson, S. Meyer, H. A. Raikes, and R. Jochem, "Emotion Regulation and Attachment: Unpacking Two Constructs and Their Association," *Journal of Psychopathology and Behavioral Assessment* 32, no. 1 (March 2010): 37–47, https://doi.org/10.1007/s10862-009-9163-z; Y. Dvir, J. D. Ford, M. Hill, and J. A. Frazier, "Childhood Maltreatment, Emotional Dysregulation, and Psychiatric Comorbidities," *Harvard Review of Psychiatry* 22, no. 3 (2014): 149–61, https://doi.org/10.1097/HRP.0000000000000014.

78. Frank C. Verhulst, "Early Life Deprivation: Is the Damage Already Done?" *Lancet* 389, no. 10078 (2017): 1496–97, https://doi.org/10.1016/S0140-6736(17)30541-X.

79. Teicher, "Wounds That Time Won't Heal."

80. C. D. Kouros, M. M. Pruitt, N. V. Ekas, R. Kiriaki, and M. Sunderland, "Helicopter Parenting, Autonomy Support, and College Students' Mental Health and Well-Being: The Moderating Role of Sex and Ethnicity," *Journal of Child and Family Studies* 26 (2017): 939–49, https://doi.org/10.1007/s10826-016-0614-3.

81. Shalini Misra, Lulu Cheng, Jamie Genevie, and Miao Yuan, "The iPhone Effect: The Quality of In-Person Social Interactions in the Presence of Mobile Devices," *Environment and Behavior* 48, no. 2 (2016), https://doi.org/10.1177/0013916514539755.

82. M. G. Hunt et al., "No More FOMO: Limiting Social Media Decreases Loneliness and Depression," *Journal of Social and Clinical Psychology* 37, no. 10 (November 2018): 751–68, https://doi.org/10.1521/jscp.2018.37.10.751; B. A. Primack et al., "Social Media Use and Perceived Social Isolation among Young Adults in the U.S.," *American Journal of Preventive Medicine* 53, no. 1 (July 2017): 1–8, https://doi.org/10.1016/j.amepre.2017.01.010.

83. Y. Xerxa, S. W. Delaney, L. A. Rescorla, M. H. J. Hillegers, T. White, F. C. Verhulst, R. L. Muetzel, and H. Tiemeier, "Association of Poor Family Functioning from Pregnancy Onward with Preadolescent Behavior and Subcortical Brain Development," *JAMA Psychiatry* 78, no. 1 (January 2021): 29–37, https://doi.org/10.1001/jamapsychiatry.2020.2862.

84. C. A. Taylor, J. A. Manganello, S. J. Lee, and J. C. Rice, "Mothers' Spanking of 3-Year-Old Children and Subsequent Risk of Children's Aggressive Behavior," *Pediatrics* 125, no. 5 (2010): e1057–e1065, https://doi.org/10.1542/peds.2009-2678.

85. P. Nieman, S. Shea, Canadian Paediatric Society, and Community Paediatrics Committee, "Effective Discipline for Children," *Paediatrics & Child Health* 9, no. 1 (2004): 37–50, https://doi.org/10.1093/pch/9.1.37.

86. D. Wolke and S. T. Lereya, "Long-Term Effects of Bullying," *Archives of Disease in Childhood* 100, no. 9 (2015): 879–85, https://doi.org/10.1136/archdischild-2014-306667.

87. E. B. Quinlan, E. D. Barker, Q. Luo, et al., "Peer Victimization and Its Impact on Adolescent Brain Development and Psychopathology," *Molecular Psychiatry* 25 (2020): 3066–76, https://doi.org/10.1038/s41380-018-0297-9.

88. Wolke and Lereya, "Long-Term Effects of Bullying."

89. L. K. Eaton, I. Kann, S. Kinchen, et al., "Youth Risk Behavior Surveillance—United States: 2007," *Morbidity and Mortality Weekly Report* 57, no. 4 (2008): 1–131, https://pubmed.ncbi.nlm.nih.gov/18528314/.

90. D. G. Amen, *Change Your Brain, Change Your Life: The Breakthrough Program for Conquering Anxiety, Depression, Obsessiveness, Lack of Focus, Anger, and Memory Problems* (New York: Three Rivers Press, 1998).

91. A. M. Hussong, H. A. Langley, W. A. Rothenberg, et al., "Raising Grateful Children One Day at a Time," *Applied Developmental Science* 23, no. 4 (2019): 371–84, https://doi.org/10.1080/10888691.2018.1441713.

92. Ying Chen, Eric S. Kim, Howard K. Koh, A. Lindsay Frazier, and Tyler J. VanderWeele, "Sense of Mission and Subsequent Health and Well-Being among Young Adults: An Outcome-Wide Analysis," *American Journal of Epidemiology* 188, no. 4 (April 2019): 664–73, https://doi.org/10.1093/aje/kwz009.

CHAPTER 5: HELPING YOUR CHILD'S BODY WITH SICKNESS

1. Albert Einstein College of Medicine, "Millions of U.S. Children Low in Vitamin D," *ScienceDaily*, accessed February 23, 2021, https://www.sciencedaily.com/releases/2009/08/090803083633.htm.

2. Seattle Children's, "Vitamin D Levels during Pregnancy Linked with Child IQ," *ScienceDaily*, accessed February 22, 2021, https://www.sciencedaily.com/releases/2020/11/201102142242.htm.

3. University of Turku, "Vitamin D Deficiency during Pregnancy Connected to Elevated Risk of ADHD," *ScienceDaily*, accessed February 22, 2021, https://www.sciencedaily.com/releases/2020/02/200210104120.htm.

4. University of Michigan, "Low Levels of Vitamin D in Elementary School Could Spell Trouble in Adolescence," *ScienceDaily*, accessed February 23, 2021, https://www.sciencedaily.com/releases/2019/08/190820130917.htm.

5. Feiyong Jia, Bing Wang, Ling Shan, Zhida Xu, and Lin Du, "Core Symptoms of Autism Improved after Vitamin D Supplementation," *Pediatrics*, December 15, 2014, https://pubmed.ncbi.nlm.nih.gov/25511123/.

6. A. Rosanoff, C. M. Weaver, and Robert K. Rude, "Suboptimal Magnesium Status in the United States: Are the Health Consequences Underestimated?" *Nutrition Reviews* 70, no. 3 (2012): 153–64, https://doi.org/10.1111/j.1753-4887.2011.00465.x.

7. L J. Black, K. L. Allen, P. Jacoby, G. S. Trapp, C. M. Gallagher, S. M. Byrne, and W. H. Oddy, "Low Dietary Intake of Magnesium Is Associated with Increased Externalising Behaviours in Adolescents," *Public Health Nutrition* 18, no. 10 (July 2015): 1824–30, https://doi.org/10.1017/S1368980014002432.

8. M. Mousain-Bosc, C. Siatka, and J. P. Bali, "Magnesium, Hyperactivity and Autism in Children," in *Magnesium in the Central Nervous System*, eds. R. Vink and M. Nechifor (Adelaide, Australia: University of Adelaide Press, 2011), https://www.ncbi.nlm.nih.gov/books/NBK507249/.

9. S. J. Newberry, M. Chung, M. Booth, M. A. Maglione, A. M. Tang, C. E. O'Hanlon, D. D. Wang, A. Okunogbe, C. Huang, A. Motala, M. Trimmer, W. Dudley, R. Shanman, T. R. Coker, and P. G. Shekelle, "Omega-3 Fatty Acids and Maternal and Child Health: An Updated Systematic Review," *Evidence Report/ Technology Assessment* (Full Report) 224 (October 2016): 1–826, https://doi .org/10.23970/AHRQEPCERTA224.

10. M. J. Heilskov Rytter, L. B. Andersen, T. Houmann, N. Bilenberg, A. Hvolby, C. Mølgaard, K. F. Michaelsen, and L. Lauritzen, "Diet in the Treatment of ADHD in Children: A Systematic Review of the Literature," *Nordic Journal of Psychiatry* 69, no. 1 (January 2015): 1–18, https://doi.org/10.3109/08039488.2014.921933.

11. F. Horak, D. Doberer, E. Eber, et al., "Diagnosis and Management of Asthma—Statement on the 2015 GINA Guidelines," *Wiener klinische Wochenschrift* 128, no. 15–16 (2016): 541–54, https://doi.org/10.1007/s00508-016-1019-4; H. Yang, P. Xun, and K. He, "Fish and Fish Oil Intake in Relation to Risk of Asthma: A Systematic Review and Meta-analysis," *PLoS ONE* 8, no. 11 (2013): e80048, https://doi.org/10.1371/journal.pone.0080048.

12. M. E. Surette, J. Whelan, K. S. Broughton, and J. E. Kinsella, "Evidence for Mechanisms of the Hypotriglyceridemic Effect of N-3 Polyunsaturated Fatty Acids," *Biochimica et Biophysica Acta—Lipids and Lipid Metabolism* 1126, no. 2 (June 1992): 199–205, https://doi.org/10.1016/0005-2760(92)90291-3.

13. P. Montgomery, J. R. Burton, R. P. Sewell, T. F. Spreckelsen, and A. J. Richardson, "Fatty Acids and Sleep in UK Children: Subjective and Pilot Objective Sleep Results from the DOLAB Study—A Randomized Controlled Trial," *Journal of Sleep Research* 23, no. 4 (August 2014): 364–88, https://doi.org/10.1111/jsr.12135.

14. Carrie Ruxton, "Health Benefits of Omega-3 Fatty Acids," *Nursing Standard* 18, no. 48 (August 2004): 38–42, https://doi.org/10.7748/ns2004.08.18.48.38.c3668.

15. R. K. McNamara, J. Able, R. Jandacek, T. Rider, P. Tso, J. C. Eliassen, D. Alfieri, W. Weber, K. Jarvis, M. P. DelBello, S. M. Strakowski, and C. M. Adler, "Docosahexaenoic Acid Supplementation Increases Prefrontal Cortex Activation during Sustained Attention in Healthy Boys: A Placebo-Controlled, Dose-Ranging, Functional Magnetic Resonance Imaging Study," *American Journal of Clinical Nutrition* 91, no. 4 (April 2010): 1060–67, https://doi.org/10.3945/ajcn.2009.28549.

CHAPTER 6: TESTING AND INTEGRATIVE MODALITIES FOR HEALING

1. N. Rao, H. A. Spiller, N. L. Hodges, T. Chounthirath, M. J. Casavant, A. K. Kamboj, and G. A. Smith, "An Increase in Dietary Supplement Exposures Reported to US Poison Control Centers," *Journal of Medical Toxicology* 13, no. 3 (September 2017): 227–37, https://doi.org/10.1007/s13181-017-0623-7.

2. L. Uzun, T. Dal, M. T. Kalcıoğlu, M. Yürek, Z. C. Açıkgöz, and R. Durmaz, "Antimicrobial Activity of Garlic Derivatives on Common Causative Microorganisms of the External Ear Canal and Chronic Middle Ear Infections," *Turkish Archives*

of Otorhinolaryngol 57, no. 4 (2019): 161–65, https://doi.org/10.5152/tao.2019.4413; E. Michael Sarrell, Avigdor Mandelberg, and Herman Avner Cohen, "Efficacy of Naturopathic Extracts in the Management of Ear Pain Associated with Acute Otitis Media," *Archives of Pediatrics and Adolescent Medicine* 155, no. 7 (2001): 796–99, https://doi.org/10.1001/archpedi.155.7.796.

3. D. Bijno, C. Di Vincenzo, E. Lusenti, A. Martina, and R. Petrelli, "Composition for the Treatment and Prevention of Urinary Tract Infections," U.S. Patent, 2017, US20170232051.

4. P. Yousefichaijan, M. Kahbazi, S. Rasti, M. Rafeie, and M. Sharafkhah, "Vitamin E as Adjuvant Treatment for Urinary Tract Infection in Girls with Acute Pyelonephritis," *Iran Journal of Kidney Disease* 9, no. 2 (March 2015): 97–104, https://pubmed.ncbi.nlm.nih.gov/25851287/.

5. P. Yousefichaijan, M. Naziri, H. Taherahmadi, M. Kahbazi, and A. Tabaei, "Zinc Supplementation in Treatment of Children with Urinary Tract Infection," *Iran Journal of Kidney Disease* 10, no. 4 (July 2016): 213–16, https://pubmed.ncbi.nlm.nih.gov/27514768/.

6. E. Barbi, P. Marzuillo, E. Neri, S. Naviglio, and B. S. Krauss, "Fever in Children: Pearls and Pitfalls," *Children* (Basel) 4, no. 9 (2017): 81, https://doi.org/10.3390/children4090081.

7. J. D. Ogilvie, M. J. Rieder, and R. Lim, "Acetaminophen Overdose in Children," *Canadian Medical Association Journal* 184, no. 13 (2012): 1492–96, https://doi.org/10.1503/cmaj.111338.

8. T. Strengell, M. Uhari, R. Tarkka, J. Uusimaa, R. Alen, P. Lautala, and H. Rantala, "Antipyretic Agents for Preventing Recurrences of Febrile Seizures: Randomized Controlled Trial," *Archives of Pediatrics and Adolescent Medicine* 163, no. 9 (September 2009): 799–804, https://doi.org/10.1001/archpediatrics.2009.137.

9. T. Sakulchit and R. D. Goldman, "Acetaminophen Use and Asthma in Children," *Canadian Family Physician* 63, no. 3 (2017): 211–13, https://www.ncbi.nlm.nih.gov/pmc/articles/PMC5349720/.

10. Y. Ji, R. E. Azuine, Y. Zhang, et al., "Association of Cord Plasma Biomarkers of In Utero Acetaminophen Exposure with Risk of Attention-Deficit/Hyperactivity Disorder and Autism Spectrum Disorder in Childhood," *JAMA Psychiatry* 77, no. 2 (2020): 180–89, https://doi.org/10.1001/jamapsychiatry.2019.3259.

Bibliography

INTRODUCTION: FROM MEDICAL DOCTOR TO HOLISTICMOM, MD

Aspril, Joshua, and Johns Hopkins Bloomberg School of Public Health. "U.S. Autism Rates Up 10 Percent in New CDC Report." Johns Hopkins Bloomberg School of Public Health, March 26, 2020. https://www.jhsph.edu/news/news-releases/2020 /us-autism-rates-up-10-percent-in-new-cdc-report.html.

Morin, Amy. "The Truth about Troubled Teens." *Verywell Mind*, March 26, 2020. https://www.verywellmind.com/what-is-happening-to-our-children-2606269.

Ray, Gillian. "Mental and Behavioral Health in Children: A Crisis Made Worse by the Pandemic." Children's Hospital Association, February 24, 2021. https://www .childrenshospitals.org/Newsroom/Press-Releases/2021/Mental-and-Behavioral -Health-Crisis-in-Children.

Weintraub, Karen. "The Prevalence Puzzle: Autism Counts." *Nature* 479, no. 7371 (2011): 22–24. https://doi.org/10.1038/479022a.

World Health Organization. "Obesity and Overweight." Accessed February 24, 2021. https://www.who.int/news-room/fact-sheets/detail/obesity-and-overweight.

CHAPTER 1: TODAY'S DILEMMA: IS OUR CHANGING WORLD THREATENING OUR FUTURE?

Anderson, Pauline. "Inflammatory Dietary Pattern Linked to Brain Aging." *Medscape*, July 19, 2017. https://www.medscape.com/viewarticle/883038.

Appleton, Allison A., Stephen L. Buka, Marie C. McCormick, et al. "Emotional Functioning at Age 7 Years Is Associated with C-Reactive Protein in Middle Adulthood." *Psychosomatic Medicine* 73, no. 4 (2011): 295–303. https://doi.org/10.1097 /psy.0b013e31821534f6.

Arkin, Daniel. "Covid Stress Taking a Toll on Children's Mental Health, CDC Finds." NBCNews.com, November 12, 2020. https://www.nbcnews.com/health /kids-health/covid-stress-taking-toll-children-s-mental-health-cdc-finds-n1247540.

Arnsten, A. F. T. "Stress Signalling Pathways That Impair Prefrontal Cortex Structure and Function." *Nature Reviews Neuroscience* 10, no. 6 (June 2009): 410–22.

Breus, Michael J. "Lack of Sleep Disrupts Our Genes." *Psychology Today*, March 21, 2013. https://www.psychologytoday.com/us/blog/sleep-newzzz/201303/lack -sleep-disrupts-our-genes.

Bushnell, Greta A., Stephen Crystal, and Mark Olfson. "Trends in Antipsychotic Medication Use in Young Privately Insured Children." *Journal of the American Academy of Child & Adolescent Psychiatry*, October 19, 2020. https://doi.org/10.1016 /j.jaac.2020.09.023.

Centers for Disease Control and Prevention. "About the Center." January 19, 2021. https://www.cdc.gov/chronicdisease/center/index.htm.

———. "Children Eating More Fruit, but Fruit and Vegetable Intake Still Too Low." Press release, August 5, 2014. https://www.cdc.gov/media/releases/2014/p0805 -fruits-vegetables.html.

———. "Do Your Children Get Enough Sleep?" March 2, 2020. https://www.cdc .gov/chronicdisease/resources/infographic/children-sleep.htm.

———. "FastStats—Asthma." January 25, 2021. https://www.cdc.gov/nchs/fastats /asthma.htm.

———. "Heart Disease Facts." September 8, 2020. https://www.cdc.gov/heartdisease /facts.htm.

Cosier, Susan. "The World Needs Topsoil to Grow 95% of Its Food—but It's Rapidly Disappearing." *Guardian*, May 30, 2019. https://www.theguardian.com/us-news /2019/may/30/topsoil-farming-agriculture-food-toxic-america.

C. S. Mott Children's Hospital. "Mott Poll Report: Healthy Eating for Children: Parents Not Following the Recipe." National Poll on Children's Health, February 20, 2017. https://mottpoll.org/reports-surveys/healthy-eating-children-parents -not-following-recipe.

Curtin, Sally C., and Melonie Heron. "Death Rates Due to Suicide and Homicide among Persons Aged 10–24: United States, 2000–2017." NCHS Data Brief, October 2019. https://www.cdc.gov/nchs/data/databriefs/db352-h.pdf.

Dantzer, R., Jason C. O'Connor, M. A. Lawson, and K. W. Kelley. "Inflammation-Associated Depression: From Serotonin to Kynurenine." *Psychoneuroendocrinology* 36, no. 3 (2011): 426–36. https://doi.org/10.1016/j.psyneuen.2010.09.012.

David-Ferdon, Corinne, Jeffery E. Hall, Khiya J. Marshall, Linda L. Dahlberg, and Alana M. Vivolo-Kantor. "A Comprehensive Technical Package for the Prevention of Youth Violence and Associated Risk Behaviors." National Center for Injury Prevention and Control, Division of Violence Prevention. Centers for Disease Control and Prevention, 2016. https://www.cdc.gov/violenceprevention/pdf /yv-technicalpackage.pdf.

Denizet-Lewis, Benoit. "Why Are More American Teenagers Than Ever Suffering from Severe Anxiety?" *New York Times Magazine*, October 11, 2017. https://www

.nytimes.com/2017/10/11/magazine/why-are-more-american-teenagers-than
-ever-suffering-from-severe-anxiety.html.

DeVille, Danielle C. "Suicidal Ideation, Suicide Attempts, and Self-Injury in Children Aged 9 to 10 Years." *JAMA Network Open*, February 7, 2020. https://doi.org /10.1001/jamanetworkopen.2019.20956.

Digitale, Erin. "Stanford Study Finds Stronger One-Way Fear Signals in Brains of Anxious Kids." Stanford Medicine News Center, April 21, 2020. https://med .stanford.edu/news/all-news/2020/04/stanford-study-finds-stronger-one-way -fear-signals-in-brains-of-.html.

Dvir, Y., J. D. Ford, M. Hill, and J. A. Frazier. "Childhood Maltreatment, Emotional Dysregulation, and Psychiatric Comorbidities." *Harvard Review of Psychiatry* 22, no. 3 (2014): 149–61. https://doi.org/10.1097/HRP.0000000000000014.

Ericsson. "Ericsson Mobility Report: 70 Percent of World's Population Using Smartphones by 2020." Press release, June 3, 2015. https://www.ericsson.com/en /press-releases/2015/6/ericsson-mobility-report-70-percent-of-worlds-population -using-smartphones-by-2020.

Flood, S. M., and K. R. Genadek. "Time for Each Other: Work and Family Constraints among Couples." *Journal of Marriage and Family* 78, no. 1 (2016): 142–64. https://doi.org/10.1111/jomf.12255.

Food and Agriculture Organization. "Fertilizer Use to Surpass 200 Million Tonnes in 2018." February 16, 2015. http://www.fao.org/news/story/en/item/277488 /icode/.

———. "What Is Happening to Agrobiodiversity?" Accessed February 24, 2021. http://www.fao.org/3/y5609e/y5609e02.htm.

Gevezova, M., V. Sarafian, G. Anderson, and M. Maes. "Inflammation and Mitochondrial Dysfunction in Autism Spectrum Disorder." *CNS & Neurological Disorders—Drug Targets* 19, no. 5 (2020): 320–33. https://doi.org/10.2174/187152 7319666200628015039.

Giollabhui, N. M., et al. "Executive Dysfunction in Depression in Adolescence: The Role of Inflammation and Higher Body Mass." *Psychological Medicine* (March 2019): 1–9. https://www.cambridge.org/core/journals/psychological-medicine/article /abs/executive-dysfunction-in-depression-in-adolescence-the-role-of-inflamma tion-and-higher-body-mass/70A07BF9EE0E8E204792E4C36230E1C5.

Graham, A. M., J. M. Rasmussen, M. D. Rudolph, C. M. Heim, J. H. Gilmore, M. Styner, S. G. Potkin, S. Entringer, P. D. Wadhwa, C. Buss, and D. A. Fair. "Maternal Systemic Interleukin-6 during Pregnancy Is Associated with Newborn Amygdala Phenotypes and Subsequent Behavior at 2 Years of Age." *Biological Psychiatry* 83, no. 2 (2018): 109–19. https://doi.org/10.1016/j.biopsych.2017.05.027.

Gramlich, J. "5 Facts about Crime in the U.S." Pew Research Center, January 3, 2019. http://www.pewresearch.org/fact-tank/2019/01/03/5-facts-about-crime -in-the-u-s/.

Guardian. "Poor Diets May Lower Children's IQ." February 7, 2011. https://www .theguardian.com/science/2011/feb/07/diet-children-iq.

Hanswijk, S. I., M. Spoelder, L. Shan, et al. "Gestational Factors throughout Fetal Neurodevelopment: The Serotonin Link." *International Journal of Molecular Sciences* 21, no. 16 (2020): 5850. https://doi.org/10.3390/ijms21165850.

Harvard School of Public Health. "More Than Half of U.S. Children Will Have Obesity as Adults If Current Trends Continue." June 22, 2018. https://www.hsph .harvard.edu/news/press-releases/childhood-obesity-risk-as-adults/.

Howard, Jenny. "Dead Zones, Facts and Information." *National Geographic Environment*, July 31, 2019. https://www.nationalgeographic.com/environment/article /dead-zones.

Hunt, M. G., et al. "No More FOMO: Limiting Social Media Decreases Loneliness and Depression." *Journal of Social and Clinical Psychology* 37, no. 10 (November 2018): 751–68. https://doi.org/10.1521/jscp.2018.37.10.751.

Inagaki, Tristen K., Keely A. Muscatell, Michael R. Irwin, Steve W. Cole, and Naomi I. Eisenberger. "Inflammation Selectively Enhances Amygdala Activity to Socially Threatening Images." *NeuroImage* 59, no. 4 (2012): 3222–26. https://doi .org/10.1016/j.neuroimage.2011.10.090.

Kirchheimer, Sid. "Year 2000 Babies High Risk for Diabetes." WebMD, October 7, 2003. https://www.webmd.com/diabetes/news/20031007/year-2000-babies -high-risk-for-diabetes.

Kolmychkova, K. I., A. V. Zhelankin, V. P. Karagodin, and A. N. Orekhov. "Mitochondria and Inflammation." *Patologicheskaia Fiziologiia I Eksperimental'naia Terapiia* 60, no. 4 (2016): 114–21.

Lancet. "Worldwide Trends in Body-Mass Index, Underweight, Overweight, and Obesity from 1975 to 2016: A Pooled Analysis of 2416 Population-Based Measurement Studies in 128.9 Million Children, Adolescents, and Adults." December 16, 2017. https://www.thelancet.com/journals/lancet/article/PIIS0140 -6736(17)32129-3/fulltext.

Lanphear, B. P. "The Impact of Toxins on the Developing Brain." *Annual Review of Public Health* 36 (March 2015): 211–30. https://doi.org/10.1146/annurev-publ health-031912-114413.

Lanphear, B. P., C. V. Vorhees, and D. C. Bellinger. "Protecting Children from Environmental Toxins." *PLoS Medicine* 2, no. 3 (2005): e61. https://doi.org/10.1371 /journal.pmed.0020061/.

Lau, J. T. F., et al. "Incidence and Predictive Factors of Internet Addiction among Chinese Secondary School Students in Hong Kong: A Longitudinal Study." *Social Psychiatry and Psychiatric Epidemiology* 52, no. 6 (June 2017): 657–67. https://doi .org/10.3390/ijerph17228547.

Lee, S. H., G. Paz-Filho, C. Mastronardi, J. Licinio, and M-L Wong. "Is Increased Antidepressant Exposure a Contributory Factor to the Obesity Pandemic?" *Translational Psychiatry* 6, no. 3 (2016). https://doi.org/10.1038/tp.2016.25.

Leone, Marica, Ralph Kuja-Halkola, Amy Leva, Brian M. D'Onofrio, Henrick Larsson, Paul Lichtenstein, and Sarah E. Bergen. "Association of Youth Depression with Subsequent Somatic Diseases and Premature Death." *JAMA Psychiatry*, December 9, 2020. https://doi.org/10.1001/jamapsychiatry.2020.3786.

Liu, J., and G. Lewis. "Environmental Toxicity and Poor Cognitive Outcomes in Children and Adults." *Journal of Environmental Health* 76, no. 6 (January–February 2014): 130–38. https://www.ncbi.nlm.nih.gov/pmc/articles/PMC4247328/.

Manzel, Arndt, Dominik N. Muller, David A. Hafler, Susan E. Erdman, Ralf A. Linker, and Markus Kleinewietfeld. "Role of 'Western Diet' in Inflammatory Autoimmune Diseases." *Current Allergy and Asthma Reports* 14, no. 1 (January 2014). http://www.doi.org/10.1007/s11882-013-0404-6.

Massachusetts General Hospital. "Childhood Psychiatric Symptom Risk Strongly Linked to Adverse Exposures during Gestation." *ScienceDaily*, accessed April 28, 2021. https://www.sciencedaily.com/releases/2021/04/210428140901.htm.

MedlinePlus. "What Is Noncoding DNA?" Accessed February 24, 2021. https://ghr.nlm.nih.gov/primer/basics/noncodingdna.

Mehta, Neeti D., Ebrahim Haroon, Xiaodan Xu, Bobbi J. Woolwine, Zhihao Li, and Jennifer C. Felger. "Inflammation Negatively Correlates with Amygdala-Ventromedial Prefrontal Functional Connectivity in Association with Anxiety in Patients with Depression: Preliminary Results." *Brain, Behavior, and Immunity* 73 (October 2018): 725–30. https://doi.org/10.1016/j.bbi.2018.07.026.

Morin, Amy. "The Truth about Troubled Teens." *Verywell Mind*, March 26, 2020. https://www.verywellmind.com/what-is-happening-to-our-children-2606269.

Nagano-Saito, A., et al. "Stress-Induced Dopamine Release in Human Medial Prefrontal Cortex—18F-Fallypride/PET Study in Healthy Volunteers." *Synapse* 67, no. 12 (December 2013): 821–30. https://doi.org/10.1002/syn.21700.

O'Connor, M-F, and M. R. Irwin. "What Is Inflammation? And Why Does It Matter for Child Development?" Center on the Developing Child at Harvard University, November 13, 2020. https://developingchild.harvard.edu/resources/what-is-inflammation-and-why-does-it-matter-for-child-development/.

Popkin, B., and C. Hawks. "The Sweetening of the Global Diet, Particularly Beverages: Patterns, Trends and Policy Responses for Diabetes Prevention." *Lancet Diabetes & Endocrinology* 4, no. 2 (February 2016): 174–86. https://doi.org/10.1016/S2213-8587(15)00419-2.

Posner, J., J. Cha, A. K. Roy, B. S. Peterson, R. Bansal, H. C. Gustafsson, E. Raffanello, J. Gingrich, and C. Monk. "Alterations in Amygdala–Prefrontal Circuits in Infants Exposed to Prenatal Maternal Depression." *Translational Psychiatry* 6, no. 11 (November 2016): e935. https://doi.org/10.1038/tp.2016.146.

"Preventing Bullying | Violence Prevention | Injury Center | CDC." Centers for Disease Control and Prevention, October 21, 2020. https://www.cdc.gov/violenceprevention/youthviolence/bullyingresearch/fastfact.html.

Primack, B. A., et al. "Social Media Use and Perceived Social Isolation among Young Adults in the U.S." *American Journal of Preventive Medicine* 53, no. 1 (July 2017): 1–8. https://doi.org/10.1016/j.amepre.2017.01.010.

Rodier, P. M. "Developing Brain as a Target of Toxicity." *Environmental Health Perspectives* 103, suppl. 6 (September 1995): 73–76. https://doi.org/10.1289/ehp.95103s673.

Rodriguez, Tori. "Impact of the COVID-19 Pandemic on Adolescent Mental Health." *Psychiatry Advisor*, April 30, 2021. https://www.psychiatryadvisor.com

/home/topics/child-adolescent-psychiatry/adolescent-mental-health-issues-are -further-exacerbated-by-the-covid-19-pandemic/.

Rosenkranz, J. A., E. R. Venheim, and M. Padival. "Chronic Stress Causes Amygdala Hyperexcitability in Rodents." *Biological Psychiatry* 67, no. 12 (June 2010): 1128–36.

Rudolph, M. D., A. M. Graham, E. Feczko, O. Miranda-Dominguez, J. M. Rasmus-sen, R. Nardos, S. Entringer, P. D. Wadhwa, C. Buss, and D. A. Fair. "Maternal IL-6 during Pregnancy Can Be Estimated from Newborn Brain Connectivity and Predicts Future Working Memory in Offspring." *Nature Neuroscience* 21, no. 5 (2018): 765–72. https://doi.org/10.1038/s41593-018-0128-y.

Sandoval, Kelsie. "Kids in the U.S. Are Eating More Fast Food, the CDC Reports." NBCNews.com, August 14, 2020. https://www.nbcnews.com/health/kids-health /kids-u-s-are-eating-more-fast-food-cdc-reports-n1236756.

Scholastic. "Classroom Behavior Problems Increasing, Teachers Say." Accessed May 17, 2021. https://www.scholastic.com/teachers/articles/teaching-content/classroom -behavior-problems-increasing-teachers-say/.

Secinti, Ekin, Ellen J. Thompson, Marcus Richards, and Darya Gaysina. "Research Review: Childhood Chronic Physical Illness and Adult Emotional Health—A Sys-tematic Review and Meta-Analysis." *Journal of Child Psychology and Psychiatry* 58, no. 7 (2017): 753–59. https://doi.org/10.1111/jcpp.12727.

Shafiei, Fateme, Asma Salari-Moghaddam, Bagher Larijani, and Ahmad Esmaillzadeh. "Adherence to the Mediterranean Diet and Risk of Depression: A Systematic Re-view and Updated Meta-Analysis of Observational Studies." *Nutrition Reviews* 77, no. 4 (2019): 230–39. https://doi.org/10.1093/nutrit/nuy070.

Stein, Rob. "Sperm Counts Plummet in Western Men, Study Finds." NPR, July 31, 2017. https://www.npr.org/2017/07/31/539517210/sperm-counts-plummet-in -western-men-study-finds.

Stolte, Daniel. "One-Third of Plant and Animal Species Could Be Gone in 50 Years." University of Arizona News, February 12, 2020. https://news.arizona.edu/story /onethird-plant-and-animal-species-could-be-gone-50-years.

Sun, R. C., and D. T. L. Shek. "Student Classroom Misbehavior: An Exploratory Study Based on Teachers' Perceptions." *Scientific World Journal* (2012). https://doi .org/10.1100/2012/208907.

Szabo, A. "Negative Psychological Effects of Watching the News in the Television: Relaxation or Another Intervention May Be Needed to Buffer Them!" *International Journal of Behavioral Medicine* 14, no. 2 (2007): 57–62. https://doi.org/10.1007 /BF03004169.

United Nations. "24 Billion Tons of Fertile Land Lost Every Year, Warns UN Chief on World Day to Combat Desertification." UN News, June 16, 2019. https:// news.un.org/en/story/2019/06/1040561.

United States Department of Justice. "102. Juvenile Crime Facts." January 22, 2020. https://www.justice.gov/archives/jm/criminal-resource-manual-102-juvenile -crime-facts.

University College London. "New Mothers Twice as Likely to Have Post-natal De-pression in Lockdown, Study Finds." *ScienceDaily*, accessed May 11, 2021. https:// www.sciencedaily.com/releases/2021/05/210511123619.htm.

University of Birmingham. "Childhood Cognitive Problems Could Lead to Mental Health Issues in Later Life." *ScienceDaily*, accessed April 7, 2021. https://www.sciencedaily.com/releases/2021/04/210407110411.htm.

Van Cleave, J., S. L. Gortmaker, and J. M. Perrin. "Dynamics of Obesity and Chronic Health Conditions among Children and Youth." *Journal of the American Medical Association* 303, no. 7 (2011): 623–30. https://doi.org/10.1001/jama.2010.104.

Van de Loo, K. F. E., J. A. E. Custers, S. Koene, et al. "Psychological Functioning in Children Suspected for Mitochondrial Disease: The Need for Care." *Orphanet Journal of Rare Diseases* 15, no. 1 (2020): 76. https://doi.org/10.1186/s13023-020-1342-8.

Volkow, Nora D. "Prevalence of Substance Use among Young People in the US." *JAMA Pediatrics*, March 29, 2021. https://doi.org/10.1001/jamapediatrics.2020.6981.

Waters, S. F., E. A. Virmani, R. A. Thompson, S. Meyer, H. A. Raikes, and R. Jochem. "Emotion Regulation and Attachment: Unpacking Two Constructs and Their Association." *Journal of Psychopathology and Behavioral Assessment* 32 (2010): 37–47. https://doi.org/10.1007/s10862-009-9163-z.

Weintraub, K. "The Prevalence Puzzle: Autism Counts." *Nature* 479, no. 7371 (2011): 22–24. https://doi.org/10.1038/479022a.

World Health Organization. "Suicide: One Person Dies Every 40 Seconds." Accessed February 24, 2021. https://www.who.int/news/item/09-09-2019-suicide-one-person-dies-every-40-seconds.

Wright, T. M., and C. A. Feghali. "Cytokines in Acute and Chronic Inflammation." *Frontiers in Bioscience: A Journal and Virtual Library* 2 (January 1997): 12–26. https://doi.org/10.2741/a171.

CHAPTER 2: THE SCIENCE OF HOLISTIC PARENTING

Centers for Disease Control and Prevention. "Early Brain Development and Health." Accessed February 22, 2021. https://www.cdc.gov/ncbddd/childdevelopment/early-brain-development.html.

Cusick, S. E., and M. K. Georgieff. "The Role of Nutrition in Brain Development: The Golden Opportunity of the 'First 1000 Days.'" *Journal of Pediatrics* 175 (2016): 16–21. https://doi.org/10.1016/j.jpeds.2016.05.013.

Feinstein, J. S., et al. "The Human Amygdala and the Induction and Experience of Fear." *Current Biology* 21, no. 1 (2011): 34–38. https://doi.org/10.1016/j.cub.2010.11.042.

Greenough, W. T., J. E. Black, and C. S. Wallace. "Experience and Brain Development." *Child Development* 58 (1987): 539–59. https://doi.org/10.2307/1130197.

Hassevoort, K. M., N. A. Khan, C. H. Hillman, and N. J. Cohen. "Childhood Markers of Health Behavior Relate to Hippocampal Health, Memory, and Academic Performance." *Mind, Brain, and Education* 10 (2016): 162–70. https://doi.org/10.1111/mbe.12108.

Hodel, A. S. "Rapid Infant Prefrontal Cortex Development and Sensitivity to Early Environmental Experience." *Developmental Review* 48 (2018): 113–44. https://doi.org/10.1016/j.dr.2018.02.003.

Jirout, J., J. LoCasale-Crouch, K. Turnbull, et al. "How Lifestyle Factors Affect Cognitive and Executive Function and the Ability to Learn in Children." *Nutrients* 11, no. 8 (2019): 1953. https://doi.org/10.3390/nu11081953.

Kelley, N. J., et al. "Stimulating Self-Regulation: A Review of Non-invasive Brain Stimulation Studies of Goal-Directed Behavior." *Frontiers in Behavioral Neuroscience* 12 (January 2019). https://doi.org/10.3389/fnbeh.2018.00337.

Kolb, B. "Brain and Behavioral Plasticity in the Developing Brain: Neuroscience and Public Policy." *Paediatrics & Child Health* 14, no. 10 (2009): 651–52. https://doi.org/10.1093/pch/14.10.651.

Kuppens, S., and E. Ceulemans. "Parenting Styles: A Closer Look at a Well-Known Concept." *Journal of Child and Family Studies* 28, no. 1 (2019): 168–81. https://doi.org/10.1007/s10826-018-1242-x.

Moreau, D., L. J. Kirk, and K. E. Waldie. "High-Intensity Training Enhances Executive Function in Children in a Randomized, Placebo-Controlled Trial." *Elife* 6 (August 2017). https://elifesciences.org/articles/25062.

Neal, D. T., W. Wood, and J. M. Quinn. "Habits—a Repeat Performance." *Current Directions in Psychological Science* 15, no. 4 (2006): 198–202. https://psycnet.apa.org/record/2006-12374-010.

Newman, J. D., and J. C. Harris. "The Scientific Contributions of Paul D. MacLean (1913–2007)." *Journal of Nervous and Mental Disease* 197, no. 1 (January 2009): 3–5. https://doi.org/10.1097/NMD.0b013e31818ec5d9.

Rotshtein, Pia, Mark P. Richardson, Joel S. Winston, Stefan J. Kiebel, Patrik Vuilleumier, Martin Eimer, Jon Driver, and Raymond J. Dolan. "Amygdala Damage Affects Event-Related Potentials for Fearful Faces at Specific Time Windows." *Human Brain Mapping* 31, no. 7 (2009): 1089–1105. https://doi.org/10.1002/hbm.20921.

Shonkoff, J. P., and P. A. Fisher. "Rethinking Evidence-Based Practice and Two-Generation Programs to Create the Future of Early Childhood Policy." *Development and Psychopathology* 25 (2013): 1635–53. https://doi.org/10.1017/S0954579413000813.

Sukhpreet, K., et al. "Bacteroides-Dominant Gut Microbiome of Late Infancy Is Associated with Enhanced Neurodevelopment." *Gut Microbes* 13, no. 1 (2021). https://doi.org/10.1080/19490976.2021.1930875.

CHAPTER 3: DIGESTIVE HEALTH
AND DETOXIFICATION

Abdulrhman, Mamdouh M., Mohamed H. El-Hefnawy, Rasha H. Aly, Rania H. Shatla, Rasha M. Mamdouh, Doaa M. Mahmoud, and Waheed S. Mohamed. "Metabolic Effects of Honey in Type 1 Diabetes Mellitus: A Randomized Cross-over Pilot Study." *Journal of Medicinal Food* 16, no. 1 (2013): 66–72. https://doi .org/10.1089/jmf.2012.0108.

Abou-Zaid, M. M., C. Nozzolillo, A. Tonon, M. D. Coppens, and D. A. Lombardo. "High-Performance Liquid Chromatography Characterization and Identification of Antioxidant Polyphenols in Maple Syrup." *Pharmaceutical Biology* 46 (2008): 117–25. https://cfs.nrcan.gc.ca/publications?id=28297.

Achanta, L. B., B. D. Rowlands, D. S. Thomas, G. D. Housley, and C. D. Rae. "Beta-Hydroxybutyrate Boosts Mitochondrial and Neuronal Metabolism but Is Not Preferred over Glucose under Activated Conditions." *Neurochemical Research* 42 (2017): 1710–23. https://doi.org/10.1007/s11064-017-2228-6.

Ahmad, M., M. N. Ansari, A. Alam, and T. H. Khan. "Oral Dose of Citrus Peel Extracts Promotes Wound Repair in Diabetic Rats." *Pakistan Journal of Biological Sciences* 16, no. 20 (2013): 1086–94. https://doi.org/10.3923/pjbs.2013.1086.1094.

Andrén Aronsson, C., H. S. Lee, E. M. Hård Af Segerstad, U. Uusitalo, J. Yang, S. Koletzko, E. Liu, K. Kurppa, P. J. Bingley, J. Toppari, A. G. Ziegler, J. X. She, W. A. Hagopian, M. Rewers, B. Akolkar, J. P. Krischer, S. M. Virtanen, J. M. Norris, and D. Agardh (TEDDY Study Group). "Association of Gluten Intake during the First 5 Years of Life with Incidence of Celiac Disease Autoimmunity and Celiac Disease among Children at Increased Risk." *Journal of the American Medical Association* 322, no. 6 (August 2019): 514–23. https://doi.org/10.1001/jama.2019.10329.

Arrieta, M. C., L. Bistritz, and J. B. Meddings. "Alterations in Intestinal Permeability." *Gut* 55, no. 10 (2006): 1512–20. https://doi.org/10.1136/gut.2005.085373.

Au, W. W. "Susceptibility of Children to Environmental Toxic Substances." *International Journal of Hygiene and Environmental Health* 205, no. 6 (October 2002): 501–3. https://doi.org/10.1078/1438-4639-00179.

Azadbakht, L., and A. Esmaillzadeh. "Dietary Patterns and Attention Deficit Hyperactivity Disorder among Iranian Children." *Nutrition* 28, no. 3 (March 2012): 242–49. https://doi.org/10.1016/j.nut.2011.05.018.

Baraldi, L.G., S. E. Martinez, D. S. Cannella, and C. A. Monteiro. "Consumption of Ultra-processed Foods and Associated Sociodemographic Factors in the USA between 2007 and 2012: Evidence from a Nationally Representative Cross-sectional Study." *BMJ Open* 8, no. 3 (2018): e020574.

Barbaro, M. R., C. Cremon, G. Caio, U. Volta, V. Stanghellini, and G. Barbara. "247 Zonulin Serum Levels Are Increased in Non-celiac Gluten Sensitivity and Irritable Bowel Syndrome with Diarrhea." *Gastroenterology* 148, no. 4, suppl. 1 (2015). https://doi.org/10.1016/S0016-5085(15)30192-X.

Barile, D., and R. A. Rastall. "Human Milk and Related Oligosaccharides as Prebiotics." *Current Opinion in Biotechnology* 24, no. 2 (February 2013): 214–19. https:// doi.org/10.1016/j.copbio.2013.01.008.

Bassil, K. L., C. Vakil, M. Sanborn, et al. "Cancer Health Effects of Pesticides: Systemic Review." *Canadian Family Physician* 53, no. 10 (October 2007): 1704–11.

Batada, Ameena, and Michael F. Jacobson. "Prevalence of Artificial Food Colors in Grocery Store Products Marketed to Children." *Clinical Pediatrics*, June 6, 2016. https://pubmed.ncbi.nlm.nih.gov/27270961/.

Batchelor, Nina, Jennifer Kelly, Hyun Choi, and Brona Geary. "Towards Evidence-Based Emergency Medicine: Best BETs from the Manchester Royal Infirmary. BET 2: Probiotics and Crying Time in Babies with Infantile Colic." *Emergency Medicine Journal* 32, no. 7 (July 2015): 575–76. https://doi.org/10.1136 /emermed-2015-204984.2.

Baym, C. L., N. A. Khan, J. M. Monti, L. B. Raine, E. S. Drollette, R. D. Moore, M. R. Scudder, A. F. Kramer, C. H. Hillman, and N. J. Cohen. "Dietary Lipids Are Differentially Associated with Hippocampal-Dependent Relational Memory in Prepubescent Children." *American Journal of Clinical Nutrition* 99, no. 5 (2014): 1026–32. https://doi.org/10.3945/ajcn.113.079624.

Behall, K. M., D. J. Scholfield, I. Yuhaniak, and J. Canary. "Diets Containing High Amylose vs Amylopectin Starch: Effects on Metabolic Variables in Human Subjects." *American Journal of Clinical Nutrition* 49, no. 2 (1989): 337–44. https://doi .org/10.1093/ajcn/49.2.337.

Bellisle, F. "Effects of Diet on Behaviour and Cognition in Children." *British Journal of Nutrition* 92, suppl. 2 (2004): S227–S232. https://doi.org/10.1079/BJN20041171.

Benachour, N., and G. E. Seralini. "Glyphosate Formulations Induce Apoptosis and Necrosis in Human Umbilical, Embryonic, and Placental Cells." *Chemical Research in Toxicology* 22, no. 1 (January 2009): 97–105. https://doi.org/10.1021/tx800218n.

Benton, D. "The Impact of Diet on Anti-social, Violent and Criminal Behaviour." *Neuroscience and Biobehavioral Reviews* 31, no. 5 (2007): 752–74. https://doi.org /10.1016/j.neubiorev.2007.02.002.

Bérengère, Benoit, P. Plaisancié, A. Géloën, M. Estienne, C. Debard, E. Meugnier, E. Loizon, et al. "Pasture v. Standard Dairy Cream in High-Fat Diet-Fed Mice: Improved Metabolic Outcomes and Stronger Intestinal Barrier." *British Journal of Nutrition* 112, no. 4 (2014): 520–35. https://doi.org/10.1017/S0007114514001172.

Bergamo, Paolo, Gianna Palmieri, Ennio Cocca, Ida Ferrandino, Marta Gogliettino, Antonio Monaco, Francesco Maurano, and Mauro Rossi. "Adaptive Response Activated by Dietary Cis9, Trans11 Conjugated Linoleic Acid Prevents Distinct Signs of Gliadin-Induced Enteropathy in Mice." *European Journal of Nutrition* 55, no. 2 (March 2016): 729–40. https://doi.org/10.1007/s00394-015-0893-2.

Biro, F. M., M. P. Galvez, L. C. Greenspan, P. A. Succop, N. Vangeepuram, S. M. Pinney, S. Teitelbaum, G. C. Windham, L. H. Kushi, and M. S. Wolff. "Pubertal Assessment Method and Baseline Characteristics in a Mixed Longitudinal Study of Girls." *Pediatrics* 126, no. 3 (2010): e583–90. https://doi.org/10.1542/peds.2009 -3079.

Birt, D. F., T. Boylston, S. Hendrich, et al. "Resistant Starch: Promise for Improving Human Health." *Advances in Nutrition* 4, no. 6 (November 2013): 587–601. https:// doi.org/10.3945/an.113.004325.

Bischoff, Stephan C., Giovanni Barbara, Wim Buurman, Theo Ockhuizen, Jörg-Dieter Schulzke, Matteo Serino, Herbert Tilg, Alastair Watson, and Jerry M. Wells. "Intestinal Permeability—a New Target for Disease Prevention and Therapy." *BMC Gastroenterology* 14, no. 189 (2014). http://www.ncbi.nlm.nih.gov/pmc /articles/PMC4253991/.

Blake, Mariah. "Those BPA-Free Plastics You Thought Were Safe? Think Again." *Mother Jones*, March 3, 2014. https://www.motherjones.com/environment/2014/03/tritan-certichem-eastman-bpa-free-plastic-safe/.

Bonatto, F., M. Polydoro, M. E. Andrades, M. L. Conte de Fronte Jr., F. Dal-Pizzol, L. N. Rotta, D. O. Souza, M. L. Perry, and J. C. F. Moreira. "Effects of Maternal Protein Malnutrition on Oxidative Markers in the Young Rat Cortex and Cerebellum." *Neuroscience Letters* 406 (2006): 281–84. https://doi.org/10.1016/j.neulet.2006.07.052.

Borrmann, A., and G. B. Mensink; KiGGS Study Group. "Obst- und Gemüsekonsum von Kindern und Jugendlichen in Deutschland, and Ergebnisse der KiGGS-Welle 1" [Fruit and vegetable consumption by children and adolescents in Germany: Results of KiGGS wave 1]. *Bundesgesundheitsblatt Gesundheitsforschung Gesundheitsschutz* 58, no. 9 (September 2015): 1005–14. https://doi.org/10.1007/s00103-015-2208-4.

Bouchard, M. F., D. C. Bellinger, R. O. Wright, and M. G. Weisskopf. "Attention-Deficit/Hyperactivity Disorder and Urinary Metabolites of Organophosphate Pesticides." *Pediatrics* 125, no. 6 (June 2010): e1270–77. https://doi.org/10.1542/peds.2009-3058.

Bouchaud, Gregory, Pascal Gourbeyre, Tiphaine Bihouée, Philippe Aubert, David Lair, Marie-Aude Cheminant, Sandra Denery-Papini, Michel Neunlist, Antoine Magnan, and Marie Bodinier. "Consecutive Food and Respiratory Allergies Amplify Systemic and Gut but Not Lung Outcomes in Mice." *Journal of Agricultural and Food Chemistry* 63, no. 28 (July 2015): 6475–83. https://doi.org/10.1021/acs.jafe.5b02338.

Boyland, E. J., et al. "Food Choice and Overconsumption: Effect of Premium Sports Celebrity Endorser." *Journal of Pediatrics* 163, no. 2 (August 2013): 339–43.

Buralli, R. J., A. F. Dultra, and H. Ribeiro. "Respiratory and Allergic Effects in Children Exposed to Pesticides: A Systematic Review." *International Journal of Environmental Research and Public Health* 17, no. 8 (2020). https://doi.org/10.3390/ijerph17082740.

Buser, M. C., H. E. Murray, and S. Franco. "Association of Urinary Phenols with Increased Body Weight Measures and Obesity in Children and Adolescents." *Journal of Pediatrics* 165, no. 4 (October 2014): 744–49. https://doi.org/10.1016/j.jpeds.2014.06.039.

Byrnes, S. E., J. C. Miller, and G. S. Denyer. "Amylopectin Starch Promotes the Development of Insulin Resistance in Rats." *Journal of Nutrition* 125, no. 6 (June 1995): 1430–37. https://doi.org/10.1093/jn/125.6.1430.

Caballero, B. "The Global Epidemic of Obesity: An Overview." *Epidemiologic Reviews* 29 (2007): 1–5. https://doi.org/10.1093/epirev/mxm012.

Campbell, A. W. "Autoimmunity and the Gut" [Review article]. *Autoimmune Diseases* (2014). https://doi.org/10.1155/2014/152428.

Cantarelli, Maria da Graça, Ana Carolina Tramontina, Marina C. Leite, and Carlos-Alberto Gonçalves. "Potential Neurochemical Links between Cholesterol and Suicidal Behavior." *Psychiatry Research* 220, no. 3 (2014): 745–51. https://doi.org/10.1016/j.psychres.2014.10.017.

Center for Science in the Public Interest. "Food Dyes: A Rainbow of Risks." June 1, 2010. http://cspinet.org/new/pdf/food-dyes-rainbow-of-risks.pdf.

Chaix, A., A. Zarrinpar, P. Miu, and S. Panda. "Time-Restricted Feeding Is a Preventative and Therapeutic Intervention against Diverse Nutritional Challenges." *Cell Metabolism* 20, no. 6 (2014): 991–1005. https://doi.org/10.1016/j.cmet.2014.11.001.

Chajès, Véronique, Anne C. M. Thiébaut, Maxime Rotival, Estelle Gauthier, Virginie Maillard, Marie-Christine Boutron-Ruault, Virginie Joulin, Gilbert M. Lenoir, and Françoise Clavel-Chapelon. "Association between Serum Trans-monounsaturated Fatty Acids and Breast Cancer Risk in the E3N-EPIC Study." *American Journal of Epidemiology* 167, no. 11 (2008): 1312–20. https://doi.org/10.1093/aje/kwn069.

Choi, Anna L., G. Sun, Y. Zhang, and P. Grandjean. "Developmental Fluoride Neurotoxicity: A Systematic Review and Meta-analysis." *Environmental Health Perspectives* 120, no. 10 (October 2012): 1362–68. https://doi.org/10.1289/ehp.1104912.

Chowdhury, R., S. Warnakula, S. Kunutsor, et al. "Association of Dietary, Circulating, and Supplement Fatty Acids with Coronary Risk: A Systemic Review and Meta-analysis." *Annals of Internal Medicine* 160, no. 6 (March 2014): 398–406. https://doi.org/10.7326/M13-1788.

Clarke, D. D., and L. Sokoloff. "Circulation and Energy Metabolism of the Brain." In *Basic Neurochemistry: Molecular, Cellular, and Medical Aspects*, edited by G. Siegel, B. Aranoff, and R. Albers. Philadelphia, PA: Lippincott-Raven, 1999.

Collins, T. F., R. L. Sprando, T. N. Black, M. E. Shackelford, N. Olejnik, M. J. Ames, J. I. Rorie, and D. I. Ruggles. "Developmental Toxicity of Sodium Fluoride Measured during Multiple Generations." *Food and Chemical Toxicology* 39, no. 8 (August 2001): 867–76. https://doi.org/10.1016/s0278-6915(01)00033-3.

Consumer Reports. "Arsenic in Your Food." November 2012. https://www.consumerreports.org/cro/magazine/2012/11/arsenic-in-your-food/index.htm.

———. "Arsenic in Your Juice." Last updated October 3, 2013. http://www.consumerreports.org/cro/magazine/2012/01/arsenic-in-your-juice/index.htm.

———. "How Much Arsenic Is in Your Rice?" January 2015. http://www.consumerreports.org/cro/magazine/205/01/how-much-arsenic-is-in-your-rice/index.htm.

Craig, W. J. "Health Effects of Vegan Diets." *American Journal of Clinical Nutrition* 89, no. 5 (May 2009): 1627S–33S. https://doi.org/10.3945/ajcn.2009.26736N.

Cusick, S. E., and M. K. Georgieff. "The Role of Nutrition in Brain Development: The Golden Opportunity of the 'First 1000 Days.'" *Journal of Pediatrics* 175 (2016): 16–21. https://doi.org/10.1016/j.jpeds.2016.05.013.

Danby, F. W. "Acne, Dairy and Cancer: The 5alpha-P Link." *Dermato-Endocrinology* 1, no. 1 (January 2009): 12–16. https://doi.org/10.4161/derm.1.1.7124.

de Lange, A. G., A. C. S. Bråthen, D. A. Rohani, A. M. Fjell, and K. B. Walhovd. "The Temporal Dynamics of Brain Plasticity in Aging." *Cerebral Cortex* 28, no. 5 (May 2018): 1857–65. https://doi.org/10.1093/cercor/bhy003.

Deng, G. F., X. R. Xu, Y. Zhang, et al. "Phenolic Compounds and Bioactivities of Pigmented Rice." *Critical Reviews in Food Science and Nutrition* 53, no. 3 (2013): 296–306. https://doi.org/10.1080/10408398.2010.529624.

Dengate, S., and A. Ruben. "Controlled Trial of Cumulative Behavioural Effects of a Common Bread Preservative." *Journal of Paediatrics and Child Health* 38 (202): 373–76. https://doi.org/10.1046/j.1440-1754.2002.00009.x.

Deth, R., A. Clarke, J. Ni, and M. Trivedi. "Clinical Evaluation of Glutathione Concentration after Consumption of Milk Containing Different Subtypes of B-casein: Results from Randomized, Cross-over Clinical Trial." *Nutrition Journal* 15, no. 1 (September 2016): 82. https://doi.org/10.1186/s12937-016-0201-x.

Diabetologia. "Child's Gluten Intake during Infancy, Rather Than Mother's during Pregnancy, Linked to Increased Risk of Developing Type 1 Diabetes." *ScienceDaily*, accessed February 22, 2021. https://www.sciencedaily.com/releases/2019/09/190918184459.htm.

Diaz, Brenda, Lizeth Fuentes-Mera, Armando Tovar, Teresa Montiel, Lourdes Massieu, Herminia Guadalupe Martínez-Rodríguez, and Alberto Camacho. "Saturated Lipids Decrease Mitofusin 2 Leading to Endoplasmic Reticulum Stress Activation and Insulin Resistance in Hypothalamic Cells." *Brain Research* 1627 (November 2015): 80–89. https://doi.org/10.1016/j.brainres.2015.09.014.

Diaz Heijtz, R., S. Wang, F. Anuar, Y. Qian, B. Björkholm, A. Samuelsson, M. L. Hibberd, H. Forssberg, and S. Pettersson. "Normal Gut Microbiota Modulates Brain Development and Behavior." *Proceedings of the National Academy of Sciences* 108, no. 7 (2011): 3047–52. https://doi.org/10.1073/pnas.1010529108.

Di Girolamo, A. M., and M. Ramirez-Zea. "Role of Zinc in Maternal and Child Mental Health." *American Journal of Clinical Nutrition* 89 (2009): 940S–45S. https://doi.org/10.3945/ajcn.2008.26692C.

Dominguez-Bello, M. G., E. K. Costello, M. Contreras, M. Magris, G. Hidalgo, N. Fierer, et al. "Delivery Mode Shapes the Acquisition and Structure of the Initial Microbiota across Multiple Body Habitats in Newborns." *Proceedings of the National Academy of Sciences* 107 (2010): 11971–75. https://doi.org/10.1073/pnas.1002601107.

Dulloo, A. G., M. Fathi, N. Mensi, et al. "Twenty-Four-Hour Energy Expenditure and Urinary Catecholamines of Human Consuming Low-to-Moderate Amounts of Medium-Chain Triglycerides: A Dose-Response Study in a Human Respiratory Chamber." *European Journal Clinical Nutrition* 50, no. 3 (March 1996): 152–58.

Ebbeling, C. B., J. F. Swain, H. A. Feldman, et al. "Effects of Dietary Composition on Energy Expenditure during Weight-Loss Maintenance." *Journal of the American Medical Association* 307, no. 24 (June 2012): 2627–34. https://doi.org/10.1001/jama.2012.6607.

Elliott, R. B., D. P. Harris, J. P. Hill, N. J. Bibby, and H. E. Wasmuth. "Type 1 (Insulin Dependent) Diabetes Mellitus and Cow Milk: Casein Variant Consumption." *Diabetologia* 42, no. 3 (March 1999): 292–96.

El-Wahab, H. M., and G. S. Moram. "Toxic Effects of Some Synthetic Food Colorants and/or Flavor Additives on Male Rats." *Toxicology and Industrial Health* 29, no. 2 (March 2013): 224–32. https://doi.org/10.1177/0748233711433935.

Emet, Mucahit, Atakan Yucel, Halil Ozcan, Sultan Tuna Akgol Gur, Murat Saritemur, Nevzat Bulut, and Musa Gumusdere. "Female Attempted Suicide Patients with Low HDL Levels Are at Higher Risk of Suicide Re-attempt within the

Subsequent Year: A Clinical Cohort Study." *Psychiatry Research* 225, no. 1–2 (2015): 202–7. https://doi.org/10.1016/j.psychres.2014.11.026.

Emond, J. A., et al. "Exposure to Child-Directed TV Advertising and Preschoolers' Intake of Advertised Cereal." *American Journal of Preventive Medicine* 56, no. 2 (2019): e35–e43.

Engel, S. M., and M. S. Wolff. "Causal Inference Considerations for Endocrine Disruptor Research in Children's Health." *Annual Review of Public Health* 34 (2013): 139–58. https://doi.org/10.1146/annurev-publhealth-031811-124556.

Environment Working Group. "Body Burden—the Pollution in Newborns: A Benchmark Investigation of Industrial Chemicals, Pollutants and Pesticides in Umbilical Cord Blood." July 14, 2005. https://www.ewg.org/research/body-burden -pollution-newborns.

———. "EWG's Dirty Dozen Guide to Food Additives." Accessed April 19, 2021. https://www.ewg.org/research/ewg-s-dirty-dozen-guide-food-additives/generally -recognized-as-safe-but-is-it#.W4hygpNKiRs.

Fasano, A., A. Sapone, V. Zevallos, and D. Schuppan. "Nonceliac Gluten Sensitivity." *Gastroenterology* 148, no. 6 (May 2015): 1195–204. https://doi.org/10.1053 /j.gastro.2014.12.049.

Felix, D. R., F. Costenaro, C. B. A. Gottschall, and G. P. Coral. "Non-alcoholic Fatty Liver Disease in Obese Children—Effect of Refined Carbohydrates in Diet." *BMC Pediatrics* 16, no. 1 (November 2016): 187. https://doi.org/10.1186/s12887 -016-0726-3.

Fisher, M., T. E. Arbuckle, C. L. Liang, et al. "Concentrations of Persistent Organic Pollutants in Maternal and Cord Blood from the Maternal-Infant Research on Environmental Chemicals (MIREC) Cohort Study." *Environmental Health* 15, no. 59 (2016). https://doi.org/10.1186/s12940-016-0143-y.

Flannery, J. E., K. Stagaman, A. R. Burns, et al. "Gut Feelings Begin in Childhood: The Gut Metagenome Correlates with Early Environment, Caregiving, and Behavior." *mBio* 11, no. 1 (2020): e02780-19. https://doi.org/10.1128/mBio.02780-19.

Forsgård, Richard A. "Lactose Digestion in Humans: Intestinal Lactase Appears to Be Constitutive Whereas the Colonic Microbiome Is Adaptable." *American Journal of Clinical Nutrition* 110, no. 2 (2019): 273–79. https://doi.org/10.1093/ajcn/nqz104.

Fowlie, Greta, Nicholas Cohen, and Xue Ming. "The Perturbance of Microbiome and Gut-Brain Axis in Autism Spectrum Disorders." *International Journal of Molecular Sciences* 19, no. 8 (2018): 2251. https://doi.org/10.3390/ijms19082251.

Freeman, David W. "Food Dyes Linked to Allergies, ADHD and Cancer: Group Calls on US to Outlaw Their Use." CBS Interactive, June 29, 2010. https://www.cbs news.com/news/food-dyes-linked-to-allergies-adhd-and-cancer-group-calls-on -us-to-outlaw-their-use/.

Furness, J. B., W. A. Kunze, and N. Clerc. "Nutrient Tasting and Signaling Mechanisms in the Gut; Part II, The Intestine as a Sensory Organ: Neural, Endocrine, and Immune Responses." *American Journal of Physiology* 277, no. 5 (1999): G922–28. https://doi.org/10.1152/ajpgi.1999.277.5.G922.

Gaidos, S. "The Inconstant Gardener." *Science News*, November 15, 2013. https:// www.sciencenews.org/article/inconstant-gardener?mode=.

Galal, Reem M., Hala F. Zaki, Mona M. Seif El-Nasr, and Azza M. Agha. "Potential Protective Effect of Honey against Paracetamol-Induced Hepatotoxicity." *Archives of Iranian Medicine* 15, no. 11 (2012): 674–80. http://www.ncbi.nlm.nih.gov /pubmed/23102243.

Gardner, Courtney M., Kate Hoffman, Heather M. Stapleton, and Claudia K. Gunsch. "Exposures to Semivolatile Organic Compounds in Indoor Environments and Associations with the Gut Microbiomes of Children." *Environmental Science & Technology Letters* 8, no. 1 (2020): 73–79. https://pubs.acs.org/doi/10.1021/acs .estlett.0c00776.

Garrido, Daniel, David C. Dallas, and David A. Mills. "Consumption of Human Milk Glycoconjugates by Infant-Associated Bifidobacteria: Mechanisms and Implications." *Microbiology* 159, pt. 4 (2013): 649–64. https://doi.org/10.1099/mic .0.064113-0.

GBD 2017 Diet Collaborators. "Health Effects of Dietary Risks in 195 Countries, 1990–2017: A Systemic Analysis for Global Burden of Disease Study 2017." *Lancet* 393, no. 10184 (May 2019): 1958–72.

Gesch, Bernard. "Adolescence: Does Good Nutrition = Good Behaviour?" *Nutrition and Health* 22, no. 1 (January 2013): 55–65. https://doi.org/10.1177/0260106013519552.

Gibson, Rosalind S., L. Perlas, and C. Hotz. "Improving the Bioavailability of Nutrients in Plant Foods at the Household Level." *Proceedings of the Nutrition Society* 65, no. 2 (2006): 160–68. https://doi.org/10.1079/pns2006489.

González-Sarrías, A., L. Li, and N. P. Seeram. "Effects of Maple (Acer) Plant Part Extracts on Proliferation, Apoptosis and Cell Cycle Arrest of Human Tumorigenic and Non-tumorigenic Colon Cells." *Phytotherapy Research* 26, no. 7 (2012): 995–1002. https://doi.org/10.1002/ptr.3677.

González-Sarrías, A., H. Ma, M. Edmonds, and N. P. Seeram. "Maple Polyphenols, Ginnalins A-C, Induce S- and G2/M-Cell Cycle Arrest in Colon and Breast Cancer Cells Mediated by Decreasing Cyclins A and D1 Levels." *Food Chemistry* 136, no. 2 (2013): 636–42. https://doi.org/10.1016/j.foodchem.2012.08.023.

Gopinath, B., V. M. Flood, G. Burlutsky, et al. "Consumption of Nuts and Risk of Total and Cause-Specific Mortality over 15 Years." *Nutrition, Metabolism and Cardiovascular Diseases* 25, no. 12 (December 2015): 1125–31. https://doi.org/10.1016 /j.numecd.2015.09.006.

Graham, Ruby J., et al. "Estimates of the Heritability of Human Longevity Are Substantially Inflated Due to Assortative Mating." *Genetics* 2010, no. 3 (November 1, 2018): 1109–24. https://doi.org/10.1534/genetics.118.301613.

Grandjean, P. "Developmental Fluoride Neurotoxicity: An Updated Review." *Environmental Health* 18 (December 2019): 110. https://doi.org/10.1186/s12940-019 -0551-x.

Grandjean, P., E. Budtz-Jørgensen, R. F. White, P. J. Jørgensen, P. Weihe, F. Debes, and N. Keiding. "Methylmercury Exposure Biomarkers as Indicators of Neurotoxicity in Children Aged 7 Years." *American Journal of Epidemiology* 150, no. 3 (August 1999): 301–5. https://doi.org/10.1093/oxfordjournals.aje.a010002.

Grandjean, P., and P. J. Landrigan. "Neurobehavioural Effects of Developmental Toxicity." *Lancet Neurology* 13, no. 3 (March 2014): 330–38. https://doi.org/10.1016/S1474-4422(13)70278-3.

Grantham-McGregor, S., and H. Baker-Henningham. "Review of the Evidence Linking Protein and Energy to Mental Development." *Public Health Nutrition* 8 (2005): 1191–1201. https://doi.org/10.1079/PHN2005805.

Grenov, B., A. Larnkjær, C. Mølgaard, and K. F. Michaelsen. "Role of Milk and Dairy Products in Growth of the Child." *Nestlé Nutrition Institute Workshop Series* 93 (2020): 77–90. https://doi.org/10.1159/000503357.

Grosso, G., J. Yang, S. Marventano, A. Micek, F. Galvano, and S. N. Kales. "Nut Consumption on All-Cause, Cardiovascular, and Cancer Mortality Risk: A Systematic Review and Meta-analysis of Epidemiologic Studies." *American Journal of Clinical Nutrition* 101, no. 4 (February 2015): 783–93. https://doi.org/10.3945/ajcn.114.099515.

Handeland, K., J. Øyen, S. Skotheim, I. E. Graff, V. Baste, M. Kjellevold, L. Frøyland, Ø. Lie, L. Dahl, and K. M. Stormark. "Fatty Fish Intake and Attention Performance in 14–15-Year-Old Adolescents: FINS-TEENS—a Randomized Controlled Trial." *Nutrition Journal* 16 (2017). https://doi.org/10.1186/s12937-017-0287-9.

Harkinson, J. "You're Drinking the Wrong Kind of Milk." *Mother Jones*, March 12, 2014. https://www.motherjones.com/environment/2014/03/a1-milk-a2-milk-america/.

Harris, J. L., J. A. Bargh, and K. D. Brownell. "Priming Effects of Television Food Advertising on Eating Behavior." *Health Psychology* 28, no. 4 (July 2009): 404–13. https://doi.org/10.1037/a0014399.

Hauptman, M., and A. D. Woolf. "Childhood Ingestions of Environmental Toxins: What Are the Risks?" *Pediatric Annals* 46, no. 12 (2017): e466–71. https://doi.org/10.3928/19382359-20171116-01.

Henriques, Martha. "Additive in Breakfast Cereals Could Make the Brain 'Forget' to Stop Eating." *International Business Times*, August 10, 2017. http://www.ibtimes.co.uk/additive-breakfast-cereals-could-make-brain-forget-stop-eating-1634413.

Herrick, Kirsten A., Cynthia L. Ogden, Sohyun Park, Heather C. Hamner, and Cheryl D. Fryar. "Added Sugars Intake among US Infants and Toddlers." *Journal of the Academy of Nutrition and Dietetics*, November 19, 2019. https://pubmed.ncbi.nlm.nih.gov/31735600/.

Hibbeln, Joseph R., Levi R. G. Nieminen, and William E. M. Lands. "Increasing Homicide Rates and Linoleic Acid Consumption among Five Western Countries, 1961–2000." *Lipids* 39, no. 12 (2004): 1207–13. https://doi.org/10.1007/s11745-004-1349-5.

Hochwallner, H., U. Schulmeister, I. Swoboda, et al. "Microarray and Allergenic Activity Assessment of Milk Allergens." *Clinical & Experimental Allergy* 40, no. 12 (December 2010): 1809–18. https://doi.org/10.1111/j.1365-2222.2010.03602.x.

Holt, E. M., L. M. Steffen, A. Moran, S. Basu, J. Steinberger, J. A. Ross, C.-P. Hong, and A. R. Sinaiko. "Fruit and Vegetable Consumption and Its Relation to Markers of Inflammation and Oxidative Stress in Adolescents." *Journal of the American Dietetic Association* 109, no. 3 (2009): 414–21. https://doi.org/10.1016/j.jada.2008.11.036.

Howchwallner H., U. Schulmeister, I. Swoboda, et al. "Cow's Milk Allergy: From Allergens to New Forms of Diagnosis, Therapy and Prevention." *Methods* 66, no. 1 (March 2014): 2–33. https://doi.org/10.1016/j.ymeth.2013.08.00.

Huber, D. "What about Glyphosate-Induced Manganese Deficiency?" *Journal of Fluid Mechanics* 15 (2007): 20–22.

Huss, M., A. Volp, and M. Stauss-Grabbo. "Supplementation of Polyunsaturated Fatty Acids, Magnesium, and Zinc in Children Seeking Medical Advice for Attention-Deficit/Hyperactivity Problems, an Observational Cohort Study." *Lipids in Health and Disease* 9 (2010): 105. https://doi.org/10.1186/1476-511X-9-105.

Iannotti, L. L., J. M. Tielsch, M. M. Black, and R. E. Black. "Iron Supplementation in Early Childhood: Health Benefits and Risks." *American Journal of Clinical Nutrition* 84 (2006): 1261–76. https://doi.org/10.1093/ajcn/84.6.1261.

International Agency for Research on Cancer. "Agents Classified by the IARC Monographs, Volumes 1–121." Accessed April 19, 2021. https://monographs.iarc.who.int/agents-classified-by-the-iarc/.

Jacka, F. N., C. Rothon, S. Taylor, M. Berk, and S. A. Stansfeld. "Diet Quality and Mental Health Problems in Adolescents from East London: A Prospective Study." *Social Psychiatry and Psychiatry Epidemiology* 48, no. 8 (August 2013): 1297–306. https://doi.org/10.1007/s00127-012-0623-5.

Jackson-Browne, M. S., G. D. Papandonatos, A. Chen, K. Yolton, B. P. Lanphear, and J. M. Braun. "Early-Life Triclosan Exposure and Parent-Reported Behavior Problems in 8-Year-Old Children." *Environment International* 128 (July 2019): 446–56. https://doi.org/10.1016/j.envint.2019.01.021.

Jacobson, Joseph L., Gina Muckle, Pierre Ayotte, Éric Dewailly, and Sandra W. Jacobson. "Relation of Prenatal Methylmercury Exposure from Environmental Sources to Childhood IQ." *Environmental Health Perspectives* 123, no. 8 (August 2015): 827–33. https://doi.org/10.1289/ehp.1408554.

Jakobsson, Hedvig E., Thomas R. Abrahamsson, Maria C. Jenmalm, Keith Harris, Christopher Quince, Cecilia Jernberg, Bengt Björkstén, Lars Engstrand, and Anders F. Andersson. "Decreased Gut Microbiota Diversity, Delayed Bacteroidetes Colonisation and Reduced Th1 Responses in Infants Delivered by Caesarean Section." *Gut* 63, no. 4 (2014): 559–66. https://doi.org/10.1136/gutjnl-2012-303249.

James, W. P. T. "WHO Recognition of the Global Obesity Epidemic." *International Journal of Obesity*, December 2008. https://pubmed.ncbi.nlm.nih.gov/19136980/.

Jašarević, E., C. D. Howard, K. Morrison, A. Misic, T. Weinkopff, P. Scott, C. Hunter, D. Beiting, and T. L. Bale. "The Maternal Vaginal Microbiome Partially Mediates the Effects of Prenatal Stress on Offspring Gut and Hypothalamus." *Nature Neuroscience* 21, no. 8 (August 2018): 1061–71. https://doi.org/10.1038/s41593-018-0182-5.

Jerschow, E., A. P. McGinn, G. de Vos, S. Jariwala, G. Hudes, and D. R. Rosenstreich. "Dichlorophenol-Containing Pesticides and Allergies: Results from the US National Health and Nutrition Examination Survey 2005–2006." *Annals of Allergy, Asthma & Immunology* 109, no. 6 (2012): 420–25. https://doi.org/10.1016/j.anai.2012.09.005.

Jerschow, E., P. Parikh, A. P. McGinn, S. Jariwala, G. Hudes, and D. Rosenstreich. "Relationship between Urine Dichlorophenol Levels and Asthma Morbidity." *Annals of Allergy, Asthma & Immunology* 112, no. 6 (2014): 511–18. https://doi.org/10.1016/j.anai.2014.03.011.

Johnson, C. L., and J. Versalovic. "The Human Microbiome and Its Potential Importance to Pediatrics." *Pediatrics* 129, no. 5 (May 2012): 950–60. https://doi.org/10.1542/peds.2011-2736.

Jones, D. C., and G. W. Miller. "The Effects of Environmental Neurotoxicants on the Dopaminergic System: A Possible Role in Drug Addiction." *Biochemical Pharmacology* 76, no. 5 (September 2008): 569–81. https://doi.org/10.1016/j.bcp.2008.05.010.

Kaczmarczyk, M. M., M. J. Miller, and G. G. Freund. "The Health Benefits of Dietary Fiber: Beyond the Usual Suspects of Type 2 Diabetes Mellitus, Cardiovascular Disease and Colon Cancer." *Metabolism* 61, no. 8 (August 2012): 1058–66. https://doi.org/10.1016/j.metabol.2012.01.017.

Kanissery, Ramdas, Biwek Gairhe, Davie Kadyampakeni, Ozgur Batuman, and Fernando Alferez. "Glyphosate: Its Environmental Persistence and Impact on Crop Health and Nutrition." *Plants* (Basel) 8, no. 11 (November 2019). https://doi.org/10.3390/plants8110499.

Karl, J. P., A. M. Hatch, S. M. Arcidiacono, et al. "Effects of Psychological, Environmental and Physical Stressors on the Gut Microbiota." *Frontiers in Microbiology* 9 (2018): 2013. https://doi.org/10.3389/fmicb.2018.02013.

Kavanagh, K., A. T. Wylie, K. L. Tucker, et al. "Dietary Fructose Induces Endotoxemia and Hepatic Injury in Calorically Controlled Primates." *American Journal of Clinical Nutrition* 98, no 2 (August 2013): 349–57. https://doi.org/10.3945/ajcn.112.057331.

Kivrak, E. G., K. K. Yurt, A. A. Kaplan, I. Alkan, and G. Altun. "Effects of Electromagnetic Fields Exposure on the Antioxidant Defense System." *Journal of Microscopy and Ultrastructure* 5, no. 4 (October–December 2017): 167–76. https://doi.org/10.1016/j.jmau.2017.07.003.

Knuesel, Irene, Laurie Chicha, Markus Britschgi, Scott A. Schobel, Michael Bodmer, Jessica A. Hellings, Stephen Toovey, and Eric P. Prinssen. "Maternal Immune Activation and Abnormal Brain Development across CNS Disorders." *Nature Reviews Neurology* 10 (2014): 643–60. https://doi.org/10.1038/nrneurol.2014.187.

Kobylewski, Sarah, and F. J. Michael. "Toxicology of Food Dyes." *International Journal of Occupational and Environmental Health* 18, no. 3 (July–September 2012): 220–46. https://doi.org/10.1179/1077352512Z.00000000034.

Koenig, J. E., A. Spor, N. Scalfone, A. D. Fricker, J. Stombaugh, R. Knight, et al. "Succession of Microbial Consortia in the Developing Infant Gut Microbiome." *Proceedings of the National Academy of Sciences* 108, suppl. 1 (2011): 4578–85. https://doi.org/10.1073/pnas.1000081107.

Lanphear, B. P. "The Impact of Toxins on the Developing Brain." *Annual Review of Public Health* 36 (March 2015): 211–30. https://doi.org/10.1146/annurev-publhealth-031912-114413.

Learn Genetics. "Your Changing Microbiome." Accessed February 24, 2021. https://learn.genetics.utah.edu/content/microbiome/changing/.

Lee, J. M., D. Appugliese, N. Kaciroti, R. F. Corwyn, R. H. Bradley, and J. C. Lumeng. "Weight Status in Young Girls and the Onset of Puberty." *Pediatrics* 119, no. 3 (March 2007): e624–30. https://doi.org/10.1542/peds.2006-2188.

Lefferts, Lisa. "FDA Should Ban Azodicarbonamide, Says CSPI." Center for Science in the Public Interest, February 4, 2014. https://cspinet.org/new/201402041.html.

Legault, J., K. Girard-Lalancette, C. Grenon, C. Dussault, and A. Pichette. "Antioxidant Activity, Inhibition of Nitric Oxide Overproduction, and In Vitro Antiproliferative Effect of Maple Sap and Syrup from Acer Saccharum." *Journal of Medicinal Food* 13, no. 2 (2010): 460–68. https://doi.org/10.1089/jmf.2009.0029.

Li, N., G. D. Papandonatos, A. M. Calafat, K. Yolton, B. P. Lanphear, A. Chen, and J. M. Braun. "Gestational and Childhood Exposure to Phthalates and Child Behavior." *Environment International* 144 (November 2020): 106036. https://doi.org/10.1016/j.envint.2020.106036.

Li, Wang, Scot E. Dowd, Bobbie Scurlock, Veronica Acosta-Martinez, and Mark Lyte. "Memory and Learning Behavior in Mice Is Temporally Associated with Diet-Induced Alterations in Gut Bacteria." *Physiology & Behavior* 96, no. 4–5 (2009): 557–67. http://www.sciencedirect.com/science/article/pii/S003193840800382X.

Li, Y., Q. Dai, J. C. Jackson, and J. Zhang. "Overweight Is Associated with Decreased Cognitive Functioning among School-Age Children and Adolescents." *Obesity* 16, no. 8 (2008): 1809–15. https://doi.org/10.1038/oby.2008.296.

Lieblein-Boff, J. C., E. J. Johnson, A. D. Kennedy, C. S. Lai, and M. J. Kuchan. "Exploratory Metabolomic Analyses Reveal Compounds Correlated with Lutein Concentration in Frontal Cortex, Hippocampus, and Occipital Cortex of Human Infant Brain." *PLoS ONE* 10 (2015): e0136904. https://doi.org/10.1371/journal.pone.0136904.

Lill, C., B. Loader, R. Seemann, et al. "Milk Allergy Is Frequent in Patients with Chronic Sinusitis and Nasal Polyposis." *American Journal of Rhinology & Allergy* 25, no. 6 (November–December 2011): e221–24. https://doi.org/10.2500/ajra.2011.25.3686.

Lindeberg, Staffan, Eliasson Mats, Lindahl Bernt, and Ahrén Bo. "Low Serum Insulin in Traditional Pacific Islanders—the Kitava Study." *Metabolism* 48, no. 10 (October 1999): 1216–19. https://doi.org/10.1016/s0026-0495(99)90258-5.

Lopez, D. A., J. J. Foxe, Y. Mao, W. K. Thompson, H. J. Martin, and E. G. Freedman. "Breastfeeding Duration Is Associated with Domain-Specific Improvements in Cognitive Performance in 9-10-Year-Old Children." *Frontiers in Public Health*, April 26, 2021. https://doi.org/10.3389/fpubh.2021.657422.

Loss, Georg, S. Bitter, J. Wohlgensinger, R. Frei, C. Roduit, J. Genuneit, J. Pekkanen, et al. "Prenatal and Early-Life Exposures Alter Expression of Innate Immunity Genes: The PASTURE Cohort Study." *Journal of Allergy and Clinical Immunology* 130, no. 2 (August 2012): 523–30. https://doi.org/10.1016/j.jaci.2012.05.049.

Lowe, C. J., J. B. Morton, and A. C. Reichelt. "Adolescent Obesity and Dietary Decision Making: A Brain-Health Perspective." *Lancet Child & Adolescent Health* 4, no. 5 (May 2020): 388–96. https://doi.org/10.1016/S2352-4642(19)30404-3.

Ludwig, D. S., J. A. Majzoub, A. Al-Zahrani, G. E. Dallal, I. Blanco, and S. B. Roberts. "High Glycemic Index Foods, Overeating and Obesity." *Pediatrics* 103, no. 3 (March 1999): E26.

Macdonald, L. E., J. Brett, D. Kelton, S..E. Majowicz, K. Snedeker, and J. M. Sargeant. "A Systematic Review and Meta-analysis of the Effects of Pasteurization on Milk Vitamins, and Evidence for Raw Milk Consumption and Other Health-Related Outcomes." *Journal of Food Protection* 74, no. 11 (November 2011): 1814–32. https://doi.org/10.4315/0362-028X.JFP-10-269.

Mac Giollabhui, N., et al. "Executive Dysfunction in Depression in Adolescence: The Role of Inflammation and Higher Body Mass." *Psychological Medicine* (March 2019): 1–9. https://doi.org/10.1017/S0033291719000564.

Maher, T. J., and R. J. Wurtman. "Possible Neurologic Effects of Aspartame, a Widely Used Food Additive." *Environmental Health Perspectives* 75 (November 1987): 53–57. https://doi.org/10.1289/ehp.877553.

Malaisse, Willy J. "Insulin Release: The Receptor Hypothesis." *Diabetologia* 57, no. 7 (July 2014): 1287–90. https://doi.org/10.1007/s00125-014-3221-0.

Mangels, Ann Reed. "Bone Nutrients for Vegetarians." *American Journal of Clinical Nutrition* 100, suppl. 1 (July 2014): 469S–75S. https://doi.org/10.3945/ajcn.113.071423.

Marc, J., et al. "A Glyphosate-Based Pesticide Impinges on Transcription." *Toxicology and Applied Pharmacology* 203, no. 1 (2005): 1–8. https://doi.org/10.1016/j.taap.2004.07.014.

Marcus, D. K., J. J. Fulton, and E. J. Clarke. "Lead and Conduct Problems: A Meta-analysis." *Journal of Clinical Child & Adolescent Psychology* 39, no. 2 (2010): 234–41. https://doi.org/10.1080/15374411003591455.

Martín, Mauricio G., Frank Pfrieger, and Carlos G. Dotti. "Cholesterol in Brain Disease: Sometimes Determinant and Frequently Implicated." *EMBO Reports* 15, no. 10 (2014): 1036–52. https://doi.org/10.15252/embr.201439225.

McCann, D., A. Barrett, A. Cooper, D. Crumpler, L. Dalen, K. Grimshaw, E. Kitchin, K. Lok, L. Porteous, and E. Prince. "Food Additives and Hyperactive Behaviour in 3-Year-Old and 8/9-Year-Old Children in the Community: A Randomized, Double-Blinded, Placebo-Controlled Trial." *Lancet* 370, no. 9598 (November 2007): 1560–67. https://doi.org/10.1016/S0140-6736(07)61306-3.

Meyer, B. J., E. J. de Bruin, D. G. Du Plessis, et al. "Some Biochemical Effects of Mainly Fruit Diet in Man." *South African Medical Journal* 45, no. 10 (1971): 253–61.

Michels, N., T. Van de Wiele, F. Fouhy, S. O'Mahony, G. Clarke, and J. Keane. "Gut Microbiome Patterns Depending on Children's Psychosocial Stress: Reports versus Biomarkers." *Brain, Behavior, and Immunity* 80 (August 2019): 751–62. https://doi.org/10.1016/j.bbi.2019.05.024.

Montagna, M. T., G. Diella, F. Triggiano, et al. "Chocolate, 'Food of the Gods': History, Science, and Human Health." *International Journal of Environmental Research and Public Health* 16, no. 24 (2019): 4960. https://doi.org/10.3390/ijerph16244960.

Mozaffarian, D., et al. "Plasma Phospholipids Long-Chain w-3 Fatty Acids and Total and Cause-Specific Mortality in Older Adults: A Cohort Study." *Annals of Internal*

Medicine 158, no. 7 (2013): 515–25. https://doi.org/10.7326/0003-4819-158-7 -201304020-00003.

Mukherjee, A., S. Bandyopadhyay, and P. K. Basu. "Seizures Due to Food Allergy." *Journal of the Association of Physicians of India* 42, no. 8 (1994): 662–63. http://www .ncbi.nlm.nih.gov/pubmed/7868571.

Mustieles, V., and M. F. Fernández. "Bisphenol A Shapes Children's Brain and Behavior: Towards an Integrated Neurotoxicity Assessment Including Human Data." *Environmental Health* 19, no. 66 (2020). https://doi.org/10.1186/s12940-020-00620-y.

Nagakura, T., S. Matsuda, K. Shichijyo, H. Sugimoto, and K. Hata. "Dietary Supplementation with Fish Oil Rich in Omega-3 Polyunsaturated Fatty Acids in Children with Bronchial Asthma." *European Respiratory Journal* 16, no. 5 (November 2000): 861–65.

National Institutes of Health. "Human Microbiome Project Defines Normal Bacterial Makeup of the Body." Accessed February 24, 2021. https://www.nih.gov/news -events/news-releases/nih-human-microbiome-project-defines-normal-bacterial -makeup-body.

National Library of Medicine. http://www.ncbi.nlm.nih.gov/rn/pubmed/26109549/.

Niu, J., L. Xu, Y. Qian, et al. "Evolution of the Gut Microbiome in Early Childhood: A Cross-sectional Study of Chinese Children." *Frontiers in Microbiology* 11 (2020): 439. https://doi.org/10.3389/fmicb.2020.00439.

Norwegian University of Science and Technology. "800 Million Children Still Exposed to Lead: Study Documents a Persistent, Dangerous Problem." *ScienceDaily*, accessed February 22, 2021. https://www.sciencedaily.com/releases/2020 /10/201001113555.htm.

Nutrition Source. "Shining the Spotlight on Trans Fats." Harvard School of Public Health, accessed February 25, 2021. https://www.hsph.harvard.edu/nutritionsource /what-should-you-eat/fats-and-cholesterol/types-of-fat/transfats/.

Ohashi, Yohei, Katsuya Yamada, Ikuyo Takemoto, Takaharu Mizutani, and Ken-ichi Saeki. "Inhibition of Human Cytochrome P450 2E1 by Halogenated Anilines, Phenols, and Thiophenols." *Biological and Pharmaceutical Bulletin* 28, no. 7 (2005): 1221–23. https://doi.org/10.1248/bpb.28.1221.

Olszewski, P. K., E. L. Wood, A. Klockars, and A. S. Levine. "Excessive Consumption of Sugar: An Insatiable Drive for Reward." *Current Nutrition Reports* 8 (2019): 120–28. https://doi.org/10.1007/s13668-019-0270-5.

Osborne, M. T., et al. "Amygdalar Activity Predicts Future Incident Diabetes Independently of Adiposity." *Psychoneuroendocrinology* 100 (February 2019): 32–40. https://doi.org/10.1016/j.psyneuen.2018.09.024.

Özyurt, Gonca, Yusuf Öztürk, Yeliz Çağan Appak, Fatma Demet Arslan, Maşallah Baran, İnanç Karakoyun, Ali Evren Tufan, and Aynur Akay Pekcanlar. "Increased Zonulin Is Associated with Hyperactivity and Social Dysfunctions in Children with Attention Deficit Hyperactivity Disorder." *Comprehensive Psychiatry* 87 (November 2018): 138–42. https://doi.org/10.1016/j.comppsych.2018.10.006.

Padgette, Stephen R., et al. "The Composition of Glyphosate-Tolerant Soybean Seeds Is Equivalent to That of Conventional Soybeans." *Journal of Nutrition* 126, no. 4 (April 1996).

Pandey, K. B., and S. I. Rizvi. "Plant Polyphenols as Dietary Antioxidants in Human Health and Disease." *Oxidative Medicine and Cellular Longevity* 2, no. 5 (November–December 2009): 270–78.

Paus, T., M. Keshavan, and J. N. Giedd. "Why Do Many Psychiatric Disorders Emerge during Adolescence?" *Nature Reviews Neuroscience* 9 (2008): 947–57. https://doi.org/10.1038/nrn2513.

Pesonen, M., A. Ranki, M. A. Siimes, and M. J. T. Kallio. "Serum Cholesterol Level in Infancy Is Inversely Associated with Subsequent Allergy in Children and Adolescents: A 20-Year Follow-Up Study." *Clinical & Experimental Allergy* 38, no. 1 (January 2008): 178–84. https://doi.org/10.1111/j.1365-2222.2007.02875.x.

Pietzak, Michelle. "Celiac Disease, Wheat Allergy, and Gluten Sensitivity." *Journal of Parenteral and Enteral Nutrition* 36, suppl. 1 (2012): 68S–75S. https://doi.org/10.1177/0148607111426276.

Pratt, Lorelei, Li Ni, Nicholas M. Ponzio, and G. Miller Jonakait. "Maternal Inflammation Promotes Fetal Microglial Activation and Increased Cholinergic Expression in the Fetal Basal Forebrain: Role of Interleukin-6." *Pediatric Research* 74, no. 4 (2013): 393–401. https://doi.org/10.1038/pr.2013.126.

Punzi, John S., Martha Lamont, Diana Haynes, and Robert L. Epstein. "USDA Pesticide Data Program: Pesticide Residues on Fresh and Processed Fruit and Vegetables, Grains, Meats, Milk, and Drinking Water." *Outlooks on Pest Management* 16, no. 3 (June 2005): 131–37. https://doi.org/10.1564/16jun12.

Rice, K. M., E. M. Walker, M. Wu, C. Gillette, and E. R. Blough. "Environmental Mercury and Its Toxic Effects." *Journal of Preventive Medicine and Public Health* 47, no. 2 (2014): 74–83. https://doi.org/10.3961/jpmph.2014.47.2.74.

Robert, J. R., C. J. Karr, and Council on Environmental Health. "Pesticide Exposure in Children." *Pediatrics* 130, no. 6 (December 2012): e1765–88. https://doi.org/10.1542/peds.2012-2758.

———. "Erratum: 'Technical Report: Pesticide Exposure in Children.'" *Pediatrics* 131, no. 5 (2013): 1013–14. https://doi.org/10.1542/peds.2013-0577.

Roberto, Christina, and Mary Gorski. "Public Health Policies to Encourage Healthy Eating Habits: Recent Perspectives." *Journal of Healthcare Leadership* 7 (2015): 81–90. https://doi.org/10.2147/JHL.S69188.

Rodier, P. M. "Developing Brain as a Target of Toxicity." *Environmental Health Perspectives* 103, suppl. 6 (September 1995): 73–76. https://doi.org/10.1289/ehp.95103s673.

Romano, R. M., M. A. Romano, M. M. Bernardi, P. V. Furtado, and C. A. Oliveira. "Prepubertal Exposure to Commercial Formulation of the Herbicide Glyphosate Alters Testosterone Levels and Testicular Morphology." *Archives of Toxicology* 84, no. 4 (April 2010): 309–17. https://doi.org/10.1007/s00204-009-0494-z.

Ruiz-Ojeda, F. J., J. Plaza-Díaz, M. J. Sáez-Lara, and A. Gil. "Effects of Sweeteners on the Gut Microbiota: A Review of Experimental Studies and Clinical Trials." *Advances in Nutrition* 10, suppl. 1 (2019): S31–S48. https://doi.org/10.1093/advances/nmy037.

Russo, Gian Luigi. "Dietary N–6 and N–3 Polyunsaturated Fatty Acids: From Biochemistry to Clinical Implications in Cardiovascular Prevention." *Biochemi-*

cal Pharmacology 77, no. 6 (March 2009): 937–46. https://doi.org/10.1016/j.bcp.2008.10.020.

Saint, S. E., L. M. Renzi-Hammond, N. A. Khan, C. H. Hillman, J. E. Frick, and B. R. Hammond. "The Macular Carotenoids Are Associated with Cognitive Function in Preadolescent Children." *Nutrients* 10 (2018): 193. https://doi.org/10.3390/nu10020193.

Samarghandian, S., T. Farkhondeh, and F. Samini. "Honey and Health: A Review of Recent Clinical Research." *Pharmacognosy Research* 9, no. 2 (2017): 121–27. https://doi.org/10.4103/0974-8490.204647.

Samsel, Anthony, and Stephanie Seneff. "Glyphosate's Suppression of Cytochrome P450 Enzymes and Amino Acid Biosynthesis by the Gut Microbiome: Pathways to Modern Diseases." *Entropy* 15 (2013). https://doi.org/10.3390/e15041416.

Sanshiroh, S., T. Sato, H. Harada, and T. Takita, "Transfer of Soy Isoflavone into the Egg Yolk of Chickens." *Bioscience, Biotechnology, and Biochemistry* 65, no. 10 (2001): 2220–25. https://doi.org/10.1271/bbb.65.2220.

Santarelli, Raphaëlle, Fabrice Pierre, and Denis Corpet. "Processed Meat and Colorectal Cancer: A Review of Epidemiologic and Experimental Evidence." *Nutrition and Cancer* 60, no. 2 (March 2008): 131–44. https://doi.org/10.1080/01635580701684872.

Sarris, J., D. Mischoulon, and I. Schweitzer. "Omega-3 for Bipolar Disorder: Meta-analyses of Use in Mania and Bipolar." *Journal of Clinical Psychiatry* 73, no. 1 (August 2011): 81–86. https://doi.org/10.4088/JCP.10r06710.

Schiffman, Susan S., and Kristina I. Rother. "Sucralose, a Synthetic Organochlorine Sweetener: Overview of Biological Issues." *Journal of Toxicology and Environmental Health*, Part B 16, no. 7 (October 2013): 399–451. https://doi.org/10.1080/10937404.2013.842523.

Schnabel, L., E. Kesse-Guyot, B. Allès, M. Touvier, B. Srour, S. Hercberg, C. Buscail, and C. Julia. "Association between Ultraprocessed Food Consumption and Risk of Mortality among Middle-Aged Adults in France." *JAMA Internal Medicine* 179, no. 4 (2019): 490–98. https://doi.org/10.1001/jamainternmed.2018.7289.

Schneeberger, M., et al. "Akkermansia Muciniphila Inversely Correlates with the Onset of Inflammation, Altered Adipose Tissue Metabolism, and Metabolic Disorders during Obesity in Mice." *Science Reports* 5 (2015): 16643. https://doi.org/10.1038/srep16643.

Schoenthaler, S., S. Amos, and W. Doraz. "The Effect of Randomized Vitamin-Mineral Supplementation on Violent and Non-violent Antisocial Behavior among Incarcerated Juveniles." *Journal of Nutritional & Environmental Medicine* 7, no. 4 (1997). https://doi.org/10.1080/13590849762475.

Shen, Ming-Che, Xiangmin Zhao, Gene P. Siegal, Renee Desmond, and Robert W. Hardy. "Dietary Stearic Acid Leads to a Reduction of Visceral Adipose Tissue in Athymic Nude Mice." *PLoS ONE* 9, no. 9 (2014): e104083. https://doi.org/10.1371/journal.pone.0104083.

Sherman, R. G., C. R. Fourtner, and C. D. Drewes. "Invertebrate Nerve-Muscle Systems." *Comparative Biochemistry and Physiology Part A: Physiology* 53, no. 3 (1976): 227–33. https://doi.org/10.1016/s0300-9629(76)80025-4.

Shoaff, J. R., B. Coull, J. Weuve, et al. "Association of Exposure to Endocrine-Disrupting Chemicals during Adolescence with Attention-Deficit/Hyperactivity Disorder–Related Behaviors." *JAMA Network Open* 3, no. 8 (2020): e2015041. https://doi.org/10.1001/jamanetworkopen.2020.15041.

Silbernagel, Susan M., David O. Carpenter, Steven G. Gilbert, Michael Gochfeld, Edward Groth, Jane M. Hightower, and Frederick M. Schiavone. "Recognizing and Preventing Overexposure to Methylmercury from Fish and Seafood Consumption: Information for Physicians." *Journal of Toxicology* 2011 (July 2011). https://doi.org/10.1155/2011/983072.

Simintzi, I., K. H. Schulpis, P. Angelogianni, C. Liapi, and S. Tsakiris. "1-Cysteine and Glutathione Restore the Modulation of Rat Frontal Cortex Na+, K+-ATPase Activity Induced by Aspartame Metabolites." *Food and Chemical Toxicology* 46, no. 6 (June 2008): 2074–79.

Simopoulos, Artemis P. "Omega-3 Fatty Acids in Inflammation and Autoimmune Diseases." *Journal of the American College of Nutrition* 21, no. 6 (December 2002): 495–505. https://doi.org/10.1080/07315724.2002.10719248.

Slattery, M. L., J. Benson, K.-N. Ma, D. Schaffer, and J. D. Potter. "Trans-Fatty Acids and Colon Cancer." *Nutrition and Cancer* 39, no. 2 (2001): 170–75. https://doi.org/10.1207/S15327914nc392_2.

Smith, Bob L. "Organic Foods vs Supermarket Foods: Element Levels." Journey to Forever, accessed February 24, 2021. http://journeytoforever.org/farm_library/bobsmith.html.

Soffritti, M., F. Belpoggi, M. Manservigi, et al. "Aspartame Administered in Feed, Beginning Prenatally through Life Span, Induces Cancer of the Liver and Lung in Male Swill Mice." *American Journal of Industrial Medicine* 53, no. 12 (December 2010): 1197–1206. https://doi.org/10.1002/ajim.20896.

Soliman, A. T., M. Yasin, and A. Kassem. "Leptin in Pediatrics: A Hormone from Adipocyte That Wheels Several Functions in Children." *Indian Journal of Endocrinology and Metabolism* 16, suppl. 3 (2012): S577–S587. https://doi.org/10.4103/2230-8210.105575.

Suez, J., T. Korem, D. Zeevi, et al. "Artificial Sweeteners Induce Glucose Intolerance by Altering the Gut Microbiota." *Nature* 514, no. 7521 (2014): 181–86. https://doi.org/10.1038/nature13793.

Suez, Jotham, Tal Korem, David Zeevi, Gili Zilberman-Schapira, Christoph A. Thaiss, Ori Maza, David Israeli, Niv Zmora, Shlomit Gilad, Adina Weinberger, Yael Kuperman, Alon Harmelin, Ilana Kolodkin-Gal, Hagit Shapiro, Zamir Halpern, Eran Segal, and Eran Elinav. "Artificial Sweeteners Induce Glucose Intolerance by Altering the Gut Microbiota." *Obstetrical & Gynecological Survey* 70, no. 1 (January 2015): 31–32. https://doi.org/10.1097/01.ogx.0000460711.58331.94.

Sun, Q., D. Spiegelman, R. M. van Dam, et al. "White Rice, Brown Rice, and Risk of Type 2 Diabetes in US Men and Women." *Archives of Internal Medicine* 170, no. 11 (June 2010): 961–69. https://doi.org/10.1001/archinternmed.2010.109.

Swiss Tropical and Public Health Institute. "Mobile Phone Radiation May Affect Memory Performance in Adolescents, Study Finds." *ScienceDaily*, accessed February 22, 2021. https://www.sciencedaily.com/releases/2018/07/180719121803.htm.

Swithers, S. E., and T. L. Davidson. "A Role of Sweet Taste: Calorie Predictive Relations in Energy Regulation by Rats." *Behavioral Neuroscience* 122, no. 1 (February 2008): 161–67. https://doi.org/10.1037/0735-7044.122.1.161.

Tobacman, J. K. "Review of Harmful Gastrointestinal Effects of Carrageenan in Animal Experiments." *Environmental Health Perspectives* 109, no. 10 (2001): 983–94. https://doi.org/10.1289/ehp.01109983.

Toru, K., T. Mlmura, Y. Takasakl, and M. Ichlmura. "Dietary Aspartame with Protein on Plasma and Brain Amino Acids, Brain Monoamines, and Behavior in Rats." *Physiology Behavior,* no. 36 (1986): 765.

Underwood, Mark A., J. Bruce German, Carlito B. Lebrilla, and David A. Mills. "Bifidobacterium Longum Subspecies Infantis: Champion Colonizer of the Infant Gut." *Pediatric Research* 77 (2015): 229–35. https://doi.org/10.1038/pr.2014.156.

University of Rochester Medical Center. "Environmental Toxins Impair Immune System over Multiple Generations." *ScienceDaily,* accessed February 22, 2021. https://www.sciencedaily.com/releases/2019/10/191002144257.htm.

U.S. Department of Agriculture. "Adoption of Genetically Engineered Crops in the U.S.: Recent Trends in GE Adoption." November 3, 2016. https://www.ers.usda.gov/data-products/adoption-of-genetically-engineered-crops-in-the-us.aspx.

UT Southwestern Medical Center. "Fasting Kills Cancer Cells of Most Common Type of Childhood Leukemia Study Shows." *ScienceDaily,* accessed February 22, 2021. https://www.sciencedaily.com/releases/2016/12/161212133654.htm.

Valero, Teresa. "Mitochondrial Biogenesis: Pharmacological Approaches." *Current Pharmaceutical Design* 20, no. 35 (2014): 5507–9. https://doi.org/10.2174/1381612 82035140911142118.

van Vliet, S., N. A. Burd, and L. J. C. van Loon. "The Skeletal Muscle Anabolic Response to Plant- versus Animal-Based Protein Consumption." *Journal of Nutrition* 145, no. 9 (September 2015): 1981–91. https://doi.org/10.3945/jn.114.204305.

Viladomiu, Monica, Raquel Hontecillas, and Josep Bassaganya-Riera. "Modulation of Inflammation and Immunity by Dietary Conjugated Linoleic Acid." *European Journal of Pharmacology* 785 (August 2016): 87–95. https://doi.org/10.1016 /j.ejphar.2015.03.095.

Visser, Jeroen, Jan Rozing, Anna Sapone, Karen Lammers, and Alessio Fasano. "Tight Junctions, Intestinal Permeability, and Autoimmunity." *Annals of the New York Academy of Sciences* 1165, no. 1 (May 2009): 195–205. https://doi.org/10.1111/j.1749-6632 .2009.04037.x.

Vuong, H. E., J. M. Yano, T. C. Fung, and E. Y. Hsiao. "The Microbiome and Host Behavior." *Annual Review of Neuroscience* 25, no. 40 (July 2017): 21–49. https://doi.org /10.1146/annurev-neuro-072116-031347.

Wang, Hansen. "Lipid Rafts: A Signaling Platform Linking Cholesterol Metabolism to Synaptic Deficits in Autism Spectrum Disorders." *Frontiers in Behavioral Neuroscience* 8 (March 2014). https://doi.org/10.3389/fnbeh.2014.00104.

Wang, Q. P., Y. Q. Lin, L. Zhang, et al. "Sucralose Promotes Food Intake through NPY and a Neuronal Fasting Response." *Cell Metabolism* 24, no. 1 (July 2016): 75–90.

Whelan, Jay. "The Health Implications of Changing Linoleic Acid Intakes." *Prostaglandins Leukotrienes & Essential Fatty Acids* 79, no. 3–5 (September–November 2008): 165–67. https://doi.org/10.1016/j.plefa.2008.09.013.

Winterdahl, M., N. Ove, O. Dariusz, A. C. Schacht, S. Jakobsen, A. K. O. Alstrup, A. Gjedde, and A. M. Landau. "Sucrose Intake Lowers µ-Opioid and Dopamine D2/3 Receptor Availability in Porcine Brain." *Scientific Reports* 9, no. 1 (2019). https://www.nature.com/articles/s41598-019-53430-9#Abs1.

Work Group on Breastfeeding. "Breastfeeding and Use of Human Milk." *Pediatrics* 129, no. 3 (2012): e827–41. Revised from *Pediatrics* 100, no. 6 (December 1997): 1035–39. https://doi.org/10.1542/peds.100.6.1035.

Yale University. "Cell Phone Use in Pregnancy May Cause Behavioral Disorders in Offspring, Mouse Study Suggests." *ScienceDaily*, accessed February 21, 2021. https://www.sciencedaily.com/releases/2012/03/120315110138.htm.

Yang, I., E. J. Corwin, P. A. Brennan, S. Jordan, J. R. Murphy, and A. Dunlop. "The Infant Microbiome: Implications for Infant Health and Neurocognitive Development." *Nursing Research* 65, no. 1 (2016): 76–88. https://doi.org/10.1097/NNR.0000000000000133.

Yatsunenko, T., F. E. Rey, M. J. Manary, I. Trehan, M. G. Dominguez-Bello, M. Contreras, et al. "Human Gut Microbiome Viewed across Age and Geography." *Nature* 486 (2012): 222–27. https://doi.org/10.1038/nature11053.

Ye, Jing, et al. "Assessment of the Determination of Azodicarbonamide and Its Decomposition Product Semicarbazide: Investigation of Variation in Flour and Flour Products." *Journal of Agricultural and Food Chemistry* 59, no. 17 (2011): 9313–18. https://doi.org/10.1021/jf201819x.

Yore, Mark M., Ismail Syed, Pedro M. Moraes-Vieira, Tejia Zhang, Mark A. Herman, Edwin A. Homan, Rajesh T. Patel, et al. "Discovery of a Class of Endogenous Mammalian Lipids with Anti-diabetic and Anti-inflammatory Effects." *Cell* 159, no. 2 (2014): 318–32. https://doi.org/10.1016/j.cell.2014.09.035.

Yuan, Gaofeng, C. Xiaoe, and D. Li. "Modulation of Peroxisome Proliferator-Activated Receptor Gamma (PPAR γ) by Conjugated Fatty Acid in Obesity and Inflammatory Bowel Disease." *Journal of Agricultural and Food Chemistry* 63, no. 7 (February 2015): 1883–95. https://doi.org/10.1021/jf505050c.

Zahedi, H., R. Kelishadi, R. Heshmat, M. E. Motlagh, S. H. Ranjbar, G. Ardalan, M. Payab, M. Chinian, H. Asayesh, B. Larijani, and M. Qorbani. "Association between Junk Food Consumption and Mental Health in a National Sample of Iranian Children and Adolescents: The CASPIAN-IV Study." *Nutrition* 30, no. 11–12 (November–December 2014): 1391–97. https://doi.org/10.1016/j.nut.2014.04.014.

Zhang, Luoping, Iemaan Rana, Rachel M. Shaffer, Emanuela Taioli, and Lianne Sheppard. "Exposure to Glyphosate-Based Herbicides and Risk for Non-Hodgkin Lymphoma: A Meta-analysis and Supporting Evidence." *Mutation Research/Reviews in Mutation Research* 781 (July–September 2019): 186–206. https://doi.org/10.1016/j.mrrev.2019.02.001.

CHAPTER 4: THE FOUR S'S

Albaugh, Matthew D., James J. Hudziak, Catherine Orr, Philip A. Spechler, Bader Chaarani, Scott Mackey, Claude Lepage, et al. "Amygdalar Reactivity Is Associated with Prefrontal Cortical Thickness in a Large Population-Based Sample of Adolescents." *PLoS ONE* 14, no. 5 (2019): e216152. https://doi.org/10.1371/journal.pone.0216152.

Amen, D. G. *Change Your Brain, Change Your Life: The Breakthrough Program for Conquering Anxiety, Depression, Obsessiveness, Lack of Focus, Anger, and Memory Problems.* New York: Three Rivers Press, 1998.

Arnsten, A. F. T. "Stress Signaling Pathways That Impair Prefrontal Cortex Structure and Function." *Nature Reviews Neruoscience* 10, no. 6 (June 2009): 410–22. https://doi.org/10.1038/nrn2648.

Bauer, C. C. C., C. Caballero, E. Scherer, M. R. West, M. D. Mrazek, D. T. Phillips, S. Whitfield-Gabrieli, and J. D. E. Gabrieli. "Mindfulness Training Reduces Stress and Amygdala Reactivity to Fearful Faces in Middle-School Children." *Behavioral Neuroscience* 133, no. 6 (December 2019): 569–85. https://doi.org/10.1037/bne0000337.

Bested, Alison C., Alan C. Logan, and Eva M. Selhub. "Intestinal Microbiota, Probiotics and Mental Health: From Metchnikoff to Modern Advances: Part II—Contemporary Contextual Research." *Gut Pathogens* 5, no. 1 (2013): 3. https://doi.org/10.1186/1757-4749-5-3.

Black, D. S., and G. M. Slavich. "Mindfulness Meditation and the Immune System: A Systemic Review of Randomized Controlled Trials." *Annals of the New York Academy of Sciences* 1373, no. 1 (June 2016): 13–24. https://doi.org/10.1111/nyas.12998.

"Blue Light Has a Dark Side." *Harvard Health*, July 7, 2020. https://www.health.harvard.edu/staying-healthy/blue-light-has-a-dark-side.

Campos-Rodríguez, Rafael, Marycarmen Godinez-Victoria, Edgar Abarca-Rojano, Judith Pacheo-Yepez, Humberto Reyna-Garfias, Reyna E. Barbosa-Cabrera, and Maria E. Drago-Serrano. "Stress Modulates Intestinal Secretory Immunoglobulin A." *Frontiers in Integrative Neuroscience* 7 (December 2013). https://doi.org/10.3389/fnint.2013.00086.

Cassidy, J. "Emotion Regulation: Influences of Attachment Relationships." *Monographs of the Society for Research in Child Development* 59, no. 2–3 (1994): 228–49.

Centers for Disease Control and Prevention. "Do Your Children Get Enough Sleep?" Accessed April 21, 2021. https://www.cdc.gov/chronicdisease/resources/info graphic/children-sleep.htm.

———. "Preventing Adverse Childhood Experiences." Accessed April 6, 2021. https://www.cdc.gov/violenceprevention/aces/fastfact.html.

Chen, Ying, Eric S. Kim, Howard K. Koh, A. Lindsay Frazier, and Tyler J. VanderWeele. "Sense of Mission and Subsequent Health and Well-Being among Young Adults: An Outcome-Wide Analysis." *American Journal of Epidemiology* 188, no. 4 (April 2019): 664–73. https://doi.org/10.1093/aje/kwz009.

Chevalier, Gaétan, Stephen T. Sinatra, James L. Oschman, Karol Sokal, and Pawel Sokal. "Earthing: Health Implications of Reconnecting the Human Body to the Earth's Surface Electrons." *Journal of Environmental and Public Health* (2012). http://www.doi.org/10.1155/2012/291541.

Common Sense Media. "The Common Sense Census: Media Use by Kids Age Zero to Eight, 2020." Accessed April 21, 2021. https://www.commonsensemedia.org/research/the-common-sense-census-media-use-by-kids-age-zero-to-eight-2020.

Cremone, A., D. M. de Jong, L. B. F. Kurdziel, P. Desrochers, A. Sayer, M. K. LeBourgeois, R. M. C. Spencer, and J. M. McDermott. "Sleep Tight, Act Right: Negative Affect, Sleep and Behavior Problems during Early Childhood." *Child Development* 89 (2018): e42–e59. https://doi.org/10.1111/cdev.12717.

Crescentini, C., V. Capurso, S. Furlan, and F. Fabbro. "Mindfulness-Oriented Meditation for Primary School Children: Effects on Attention and Psychological Well-Being." *Frontiers in Psychology* 7 (2016): 805. https://doi.org/10.3389/fpsyg.2016.00805.

Dahl, R. E. "Sleep and the Developing Brain." *Sleep* 30, no. 9 (2007): 1079–80. https://doi.org/10.1093/sleep/30.9.1079.

De Bellis, M. D., and A. Zisk. "The Biological Effects of Childhood Trauma." *Child and Adolescent Psychiatric Clinics of North America* 23, no. 2 (2014): 185–222. https://doi.org/10.1016/j.chc.2014.01.002.

Dore, R. A., K. M. Purtell, and L. M. Justice. "Media Use among Kindergarteners from Low-Income Households during the COVID-19 Shutdown." *Journal of Developmental and Behavioral Pediatrics*, April 7, 2021. https://doi.org/10.1097/DBP.0000000000000955.

Dvir, Y., J. D. Ford, M. Hill, and J. A. Frazier. "Childhood Maltreatment, Emotional Dysregulation, and Psychiatric Comorbidities." *Harvard Review of Psychiatry* 22, no. 3 (2014): 149–61. https://doi.org/10.1097/HRP.0000000000000014.

Eaton, L. K., I. Kann, S. Kinchen, et al. "Youth Risk Behavior Surveillance—United States: 2007." *Morbidity and Mortality Weekly Report* 57, no. 4 (2008): 1–131. https://pubmed.ncbi.nlm.nih.gov/18528314/.

Evans, Simon L., and Ray Norbury. "Associations between Diurnal Preference, Impulsivity and Substance Use in a Young-Adult Student Sample." *Chronobiology International* 1 (2020). https://doi.org/10.1080/07420528.2020.1810063.

Fatima Rosas Marchiori, M. de, E. H. Kozasa, R. D. Miranda, A. L. M. Andrade, T. C. Perrotti, and J. R. Leite. "Decrease in Blood Pressure and Improved Psychological Aspects through Meditation Training in Hypertensive Older Adults: A Randomized Control Study." *Geriatrics & Gerontology International* 15, no. 10 (2015): 1158–64. https://doi.org/10.1111/ggi.12414.

Galván, A., and A. Rahdar. "The Neurobiological Effects of Stress on Adolescent Decision Making." *Neuroscience* 249 (September 26, 2013): 223–31. https://doi.org/10.1016/j.neuroscience.2012.09.074.

Gao, Z., S. Chen, H. Sun, X. Wen, and P. Xiang. "Physical Activity in Children's Health and Cognition." *BioMed Research International* (2018): 8542403. https://doi.org/10.1155/2018/8542403.

Geronimi, E. M. C., B. Arellano, and J. Woodruff-Borden. "Relating Mindfulness and Executive Function in Children." *Clinical Child Psychology and Psychiatry* 25, no. 2 (2020): 435–45. https://doi.org/10.1177/1359104519833737.

Greenough, W. T., J. E. Black, and C. S. Wallace. "Experience and Brain Development." *Child Development* 58 (1987): 539–59. https://doi.org/10.2307/1130197.

Hamasaki, H. "Effects of Diaphragmatic Breathing on Health: A Narrative Review." *Medicines* (Basel) 7, no. 10 (2020): 65. https://doi.org/10.3390/medicines7100065.

Hilton, L., et al. "Mindfulness Meditation for Chronic Pain: Systemic Review and Meta-analysis." *Annals of Behavioral Medicine* 51, no. 2 (April 2017): 199–213. https://doi.org/10.1007/s12160-016-9844-2.

Hiraoka, Daiki, Shota Nishitani, Koji Shimada, Ryoko Kasaba, Takashi X. Fujisawa, and Akemi Tomoda. "Epigenetic Modification of the Oxytocin Gene Is Associated with Gray Matter Volume and Trait Empathy in Mothers." *Psychoneuroendocrinology* 123 (2021): 105026. https://doi.org/10.1016/j.psyneuen.2020.105026.

Holtmann, G., R. Kriebel, and M. V. Singer. "Mental Stress and Gastric Acid Secretion: Do Personality Traits Influence the Response?" *Digestive Diseases and Sciences* 35, no. 8 (1990): 998–1007. https://doi.org/10.1007/BF01537249.

Humphreys, K. L., M. C. Camacho, M. C. Roth, and E. C. Estes. "Prenatal Stress Exposure and Multimodal Assessment of Amygdala-Medial Prefrontal Cortex Connectivity in Infants." *Developmental Cognitive Neuroscience* 46 (December 2020): 100877. https://doi.org/10.1016/j.dcn.2020.100877.

Hunt, M. G., et al. "No More FOMO: Limiting Social Media Decreases Loneliness and Depression." *Journal of Social and Clinical Psychology* 37, no. 10 (November 2018): 751–68. https://doi.org/10.1521/jscp.2018.37.10.751.

Hussong, A. M., H. A. Langley, W. A. Rothenberg, et al. "Raising Grateful Children One Day at a Time." *Applied Developmental Science* 23, no. 4 (2019): 371–84. https://doi.org/10.1080/10888691.2018.1441713.

Hutton, John S., Jonathan Dudley, Tzipi Horowitz-Kraus, Tom DeWitt, and Scott K. Holland. "Associations between Screen-Based Media Use and Brain White Matter Integrity in Preschool-Aged Children." *JAMA Pediatrics* 174, no. 1 (2020): e193869. https://doi.org/10.1001/jamapediatrics.2019.3869.

Kouros, C. D., M. M. Pruitt, N. V. Ekas, R. Kiriaki, and M. Sunderland. "Helicopter Parenting, Autonomy Support, and College Students' Mental Health and Well-Being: The Moderating Role of Sex and Ethnicity." *Journal of Child and Family Studies* 26 (2017): 939–49. https://doi.org/10.1007/s10826-016-0614-3.

Kuo, M., M. Barnes, and C. Jordan. "Do Experiences with Nature Promote Learning? Converging Evidence of a Cause-and-Effect Relationship." *Frontiers in Psychology* 10 (February 2019): 305. https://doi.org/10.3389/fpsyg.2019.00305.

Kurth, Salome, Douglas C. Dean, Peter Achermann, Jonathan O'Muircheartaigh, Reto Huber, Sean C. L. Deoni, and Monique K. LeBourgeois. "Increased Sleep Depth in Developing Neural Networks: New Insights from Sleep Restriction in Children." *Frontiers in Human Neuroscience* 10 (2016). https://doi.org/10.3389/fnhum.2016.00456.

Lingnau, A., and A. Caramazza. "The Origin and Function of Mirror Neurons: The Missing Link." *Behavioral and Brain Sciences* 37, no. 2 (April 2014): 209–10. https://doi.org/10.1017/S0140525X13002380.

Marques, A., D. A. Santos, C. H. Hillman, and L. B. Sardinha. "How Does Academic Achievement Relate to Cardiorespiratory Fitness, Self-reported Physical Activity and Objectively Reported Physical Activity: A Systematic Review in Children and Adolescents Aged 6–18 Years." *British Journal of Sports Medicine* 52 (2018): 1039. https://doi.org/10.1136/bjsports-2016-097361.

Maski, K. P., and S. V. Kothare. "Sleep Deprivation and Neurobehavioral Functioning in Children." *International Journal of Psychophysiology* 89, no. 2 (August 2013): 259–64. https://doi.org/10.1016/j.ijpsycho.2013.06.019.

McDaniel, Brandon T., and Jenny S. Radesky. "Technoference: Longitudinal Associations between Parent Technology Use, Parenting Stress, and Child Behavior Problems." *Pediatric Research* 84, no. 2 (August 2018): 210–18. https://doi.org/10.1038/s41390-018-0052-6.

Michels, N., T. Van de Wiele, F. Fouhy, S. O'Mahony, G. Clarke, and J. Keane. "Gut Microbiome Patterns Depending on Children's Psychosocial Stress: Reports versus Biomarkers." *Brain, Behavior, and Immunity* 80 (August 2019): 751–62. https://doi.org/10.1016/j.bbi.2019.05.024.

Miles, A. "PubMed Health." *Journal of the Medical Library Association* 99, no. 3 (2011): 265–66. https://doi.org/10.3163/1536-5050.99.3.018.

Misra, Shalini, Lulu Cheng, Jamie Genevie, and Miao Yuan. "The iPhone Effect: The Quality of In-Person Social Interactions in the Presence of Mobile Devices." *Environment and Behavior* 48, no. 2 (2016). https://doi.org/10.1177/0013916514539755.

Modesto-Lowe, Vania, Pantea Farahmand, Margaret Chaplin, and Lauren Sarro. "Does Mindfulness Meditation Improve Attention in Attention Deficit Hyperactivity Disorder?" *World Journal of Psychiatry* 5, no. 4 (2015): 397–403. https://doi.org/10.5498/wjp.v5.i4.397.

Murack, Michael, Rajini Chandrasegaram, Kevin B. Smith, Emily G. Ah-Yen, Étienne Rheaume, Étienne Malette-Guyon, Nanji Zahra, Seana N. Semchishen, Olivia Latus, Claude Messier, and Nafissa Ismail. "Chronic Sleep Disruption Induces Depression-Like Behavior in Adolescent Male and Female Mice and Sensitization of the Hypothalamic-Pituitary-Adrenal Axis in Adolescent Female Mice." *Behavioural Brain Research* 399 (2020): 113001. https://doi.org/10.1016/j.bbr.2020.113001.

Nagano-Saito, A., et al. "Stress-Induced Dopamine Release in Human Medial Prefrontal Cortex—18F-Fallypride/PET Study in Healthy Volunteers." *Synapse* 67, no. 12 (December 2013): 821–30. https://doi.org/10.1002/syn.21700.

Narvaez, Darcia. "Dangers of 'Crying It Out.'" *Psychology Today*, December 11, 2011. https://www.psychologytoday.com/us/blog/moral-landscapes/201112/dangers-crying-it-out.

National Center for Complementary and Integrative Health. "Meditation: In Depth." Accessed February 25, 2021. https://nccih.nih.gov/health/meditation/overview.htm.

Neuroscience News. "Laughing Is Good for Your Mind and Your Body, Here's What the Research Shows." November 29, 2020. https://neurosciencenews.com /laughter-physical-mental-psychology-17339.

Nieman, P., S. Shea, Canadian Paediatric Society, and Community Paediatrics Committee. "Effective Discipline for Children." *Paediatrics & Child Health* 9, no. 1 (2004): 37–50. https://doi.org/10.1093/pch/9.1.37.

Oshima, Norihito, Atsushi Nishida, Shinji Shimodera, Mamoru Tochigi, Shuntaro Ando, Syudo Yamasaki, Yuji Okazaki, and Tsukasa Sasaki. "The Suicidal Feelings, Self-injury, and Mobile Phone Use after Lights Out in Adolescents." *Journal of Pediatric Psychology* 37, no. 9 (2012): 1023–30. https://doi.org/10.1093/jpepsy/jss072.

Park, A. T., J. A. Leonard, P. K. Saxler, A. B. Cyr, J. D. E. Gabrieli, and A. P. Mackey. "Amygdala-Medial Prefrontal Cortex Connectivity Relates to Stress and Mental Health in Early Childhood." *Social Cognitive and Affective Neuroscience* 13, no. 4 (April 2018): 430–39. https://doi.org/10.1093/scan/nsy017.

Pattinson, Cassandra L., Alicia C. Allan, Sally L. Staton, Karen J. Thorpe, and Simon S. Smith. "Environmental Light Exposure Is Associated with Increased Body Mass in Children." *PLoS ONE* 11, no. 1 (2016): e0143578. https://doi.org/10.1371 /journal.pone.0143578.

Perry-Parrish, C., N. Copeland-Linder, L. Webb, and E. M. Sibinga. "Mindfulness-Based Approaches for Children and Youth." *Current Problems in Pediatric and Adolescent Health Care* 46, no. 6 (June 2016): 172–78. https://doi.org/10.1016 /j.cppeds.2015.12.006.

Primack, B. A., et al. "Social Media Use and Perceived Social Isolation among Young Adults in the U.S." *American Journal of Preventive Medicine* 53, no. 1 (July 2017): 1–8. https://doi.org/10.1016/j.amepre.2017.01.010.

Primack, Brian A., Ariel Shensa, Jaime E. Sidani, César G. Escobar-Viera, and Michael J. Fine. "Temporal Associations between Social Media Use and Depression." *American Journal of Preventive Medicine* 60, no. 2 (2021): 179–88. https://doi .org/10.1016/j.amepre.2020.09.014.

Quinlan, E. B., E. D. Barker, Q. Luo, et al. "Peer Victimization and Its Impact on Adolescent Brain Development and Psychopathology." *Molecular Psychiatry* 25 (2020): 3066–76. https://doi.org/10.1038/s41380-018-0297-9.

Repke, M. A., et al. "How Does Nature Exposure Make People Healthier? Evidence for the Role of Impulsivity and Expanded Space Perception." *PLoS ONE* 13, no. 8 (August 2018): e0202246. https://doi.org/10.1371/journal.pone.0202246.

Rod, Naja H., Jessica Bengtsson, Esben Budtz-Jørgensen, Clara Clipet-Jensen, David Taylor-Robinson, Anne-Marie Nybo Andersen, Nadya Dich, and Andreas Rieckmann. "Trajectories of Childhood Adversity and Mortality in Early Adulthood: A Population-Based Cohort Study." *Lancet* 396, no. 10249 (2020): 489. https://doi .org/10.1016/S0140-6736(20)30621-8.

Saatcioglu, F. "Regulation of Gene Expression by Yoga, Meditation and Related Practices: A Review of Recent Studies." *Asian Journal of Psychiatry* 6, no. 1 (2013): 74–77. https://doi.org/10.1016/j.ajp.2012.10.002.

Scardera, Sara, Léa C. Perret, Isabelle Ouellet-Morin, Geneviève Gariépy, Robert-Paul Juster, Michel Boivin, Gustavo Turecki, Richard E. Tremblay, Sylvana

Côté, and Marie-Claude Geoffroy. "Association of Social Support during Adolescence with Depression, Anxiety, and Suicidal Ideation in Young Adults." *JAMA Network Open* 3, no. 12 (2020): e2027491. https://doi.org/10.1001/jamanetworkopen.2020.27491.

Schmeer, K. K., and A. J. Yoon. "Home Sweet Home? Home Physical Environment and Inflammation in Children." *Social Science Research* 60 (2016): 236–48. https://doi.org/10.1016/j.ssresearch.2016.04.001.

Schmidt, K., P. Cowen, C. J. Harmer, G. Tzortzis, and P. W. J. Burnet. "P.1.e.003 Prebiotic Intake Reduces the Waking Cortisol Response and Alters Emotional Bias in Healthy Volunteers." *European Neuropsychopharmacology* 24 (October 2014). https://doi.org/10.1016/s0924-977x (14)70294-9.

Stanford Medicine. "Stanford Study Finds Stronger One-Way Fear Signals in Brains of Anxious Kids." News Center, April 2020. https://med.stanford.edu/news/all-news/2020/04/stanford-study-finds-stronger-one-way-fear-signals-in-brains-of-.html.

Stiglic, Neza, and Russell M. Viner. "Effects of Screen Time on the Health and Well-Being of Children and Adolescents: A Systematic Review of Reviews." *BMJ Open* 9, no. 1 (2019): e023191. https://doi.org/10.1136/bmjopen-2018-023191.

Stoye, David Q., Manuel Blesa, Gemma Sullivan, Paola Galdi, Gillian J. Lamb, Gill S. Black, Alan J. Quigley, Michael J. Thrippleton, Mark E. Bastin, Rebecca M. Reynolds, and James P. Boardman. "Maternal Cortisol Is Associated with Neonatal Amygdala Microstructure and Connectivity in a Sexually Dimorphic Manner." *eLife* 9 (2020). E60729. https://doi.org/10.7554/eLife.60729.

Strife, S., and L. Downey. "Childhood Development and Access to Nature: A New Direction for Environmental Inequality Research." *Organization & Environment* 22 (2009): 99–122. https://doi.org/10.1177/1086026609333340.

Sukhpreet, K. Tamana, Victor Ezeugwu, Joyce Chikuma, Diana L. Lefebvre, Meghan B. Azad, Theo J. Moraes, Padmaja Subbarao, Allan B. Becker, Stuart E. Turvey, Malcolm R. Sears, Bruce D. Dick, Valerie Carson, Carmen Rasmussen (CHILD Study Investigators), Jacqueline Pei, and Piush J. Mandhane. "Screen-Time Is Associated with Inattention Problems in Preschoolers: Results from the CHILD Birth Cohort Study." *PLoS ONE* 14, no. 4 (April 2019): e0213995. https://doi.org/10.1371/journal.pone.0213995.

Tang, Y.-Y., B. K. Holzel, and M. I. Posner. "The Neuroscience of Mindfulness Meditation." *Nature Reviews Neuroscience* 16, no. 4 (April 2015): 213–25. https://doi.org/10.1038/nrn3954.

Tang, Y.-Y., Q. Lu, H. Feng, R. Tang, and M. I. Posner. "Short-Term Meditation Increases Blood Flow in Anterior Cingulate Cortex and Insula." *Frontiers in Psychology* 6 (2015). https://doi.org/10.3389/fpsyg.2015.00212.

Taren, A. A., J. D. Creswell, and P. J. Gianaros. "Dispositional Mindfulness Co-varies with Smaller Amygdala and Caudate Volumes in Community Adults." *PLoS ONE* 8, no. 5 (May 2013): e64574. https://doi.org/10.1371/journal.pone.0064574.

Taylor, C. A., J. A. Manganello, S. J. Lee, and J. C. Rice. "Mothers' Spanking of 3-Year-Old Children and Subsequent Risk of Children's Aggressive Behavior." *Pediatrics* 125, no. 5 (2010): e1057–e1065. https://doi.org/10.1542/peds.2009-2678.

Taylor, R. M., S. M. Fealy, A. Bisquera, R. Smith, C. E. Collins, T. J. Evans, and A. J. Hure. "Effects of Nutritional Interventions during Pregnancy on Infant and Child Cognitive Outcomes: A Systematic Review and Meta-analysis." *Nutrients* 9 (2017): 1265. https://doi.org/10.3390/nu9111265.

Teicher, M. D. "Wounds That Time Won't Heal: The Neurobiology of Child Abuse." *Cerebrum: The Dana Forum on Brain Science* 2 (2000): 50–67. https://www.researchgate.net/publication/215768752_Wounds_that_time_won't_heal_The_neurobiology_of_child_abuse.

Turnbull, K., G. J. Reid, and J. B. Morton. "Behavioral Sleep Problems and Their Potential Impact on Developing Executive Function in Children." *Sleep* 36, no. 7 (2013): 1077–84. https://doi.org/10.5665/sleep.2814.

Twenge, J. M., T. E. Joiner, M. L. Rogers, et al. "Increases in Depressive Symptoms, Suicide-Related Outcomes, and Suicide Rates among U.S. Adolescents after 2010 and Links to Increased New Media Screen Time." *Clinical Psychological Science* 6, no. 1 (2017): 3–17. https://doi.org/10.1177/2167702617723376.

University of South Australia. "Sleep Keeps Teens on Track for Good Mental Health." *ScienceDaily*, accessed February 22, 2021. https://www.sciencedaily.com/releases/2021/02/210210091215.htm.

Vanuytsel, Tim, Sander van Wanrooy, Hanne Vanheel, Christophe Vanormelingen, Sofie Verschueren, Els Houben, Shadea Salim Rasoel, Joran Toth, Lieselot Holvoet, Ricard Farre, Lukas Van Oudenhove, Guy Boeckxstaens, Kristin Verbeke, and Jan Tack. "Psychological Stress and Corticotropin-Releasing Hormone Increase Intestinal Permeability in Humans by a Mast Cell-Dependent Mechanism." *Gut* 63, no. 8 (August 2014): 1293–99. https://doi.org/10.1136/gutjnl-2013-305690.

Verhulst, Frank C. "Early Life Deprivation: Is the Damage Already Done?" *Lancet* 389, no. 10078 (2017): 1496–97. https://doi.org/10.1016/S0140-6736(17)30541-X.

Wagner, Caitlin R., and Jamie L. Abaied. "Skin Conductance Level Reactivity Moderates the Association between Parental Psychological Control and Relational Aggression in Emerging Adulthood." *Journal of Youth and Adolescence* 45 (2016): 687–700. https://doi.org/10.1007/s10964-016-0422-5.

Waters, Sara F., Helena Rose Karnilowicz, Tessa V. West, and Wendy Berry Mendes. "Keep It to Yourself? Parent Emotion Suppression Influences Physiological Linkage and Interaction Behavior." *Journal of Family Psychology* 34, no. 7 (2020): 784–93. https://doi.org/10.1037/fam0000664.

Waters, S. F., E. A. Virmani, R. A. Thompson, S. Meyer, H. A. Raikes, and R. Jochem. "Emotion Regulation and Attachment: Unpacking Two Constructs and Their Association." *Journal of Psychopathology and Behavioral Assessment* 32, no. 1 (March 2010): 37–47. https://doi.org/10.1007/s10862-009-9163-z.

Wellen, K. E., and G. S. Hotamisligil. "Inflammation, Stress, and Diabetes." *Journal of Clinical Investigation* 115, no. 5 (2005): 1111–19. https://doi.org/10.1172/JCI25102.

White, E. M., M. D. DeBoer, and R. J. Scharf. "Associations between Household Chores and Childhood Self-Competency." *Journal of Developmental & Behavioral Pediatrics* 40, no. 3 (April 2019): 176–82. https://doi.org/10.1097/DBP.0000000000000637.

Wolke, D., and S. T. Lereya. "Long-Term Effects of Bullying." *Archives of Disease in Childhood* 100, no. 9 (2015): 879–85. https://doi.org/10.1136/archdischild -2014-306667.

Xerxa, Y., S. W. Delaney, L. A. Rescorla, M. H. J. Hillegers, T. White, F. C. Verhulst, R. L. Muetzel, and H. Tiemeier. "Association of Poor Family Functioning from Pregnancy Onward with Preadolescent Behavior and Subcortical Brain Development." *JAMA Psychiatry* 78, no. 1 (January 2021): 29–37. https://doi .org/10.1001/jamapsychiatry.2020.2862.

Xiu, L., M. Ekstedt, M. Hagströmer, O. Bruni, L. Bergqvist-Norén, and C. Marcus. "Sleep and Adiposity in Children from 2 to 6 Years of Age." *Pediatrics* 145, no. 3 (March 2020): e20191420. https://doi.org/10.1542/peds.2019-1420.

Zelenski, John M., Raelyne L. Dopko, and Colin A. Capaldi. "Cooperation Is in Our Nature: Nature Exposure May Promote Cooperative and Environmentally Sustainable Behavior." *Journal of Environmental Psychology* 42 (June 2015): 24–31. https:// doi.org/10.1016/j.jenvp.2015.01.005.

CHAPTER 5: HELPING YOUR CHILD'S BODY WITH SICKNESS

Albert Einstein College of Medicine. "Millions of U.S. Children Low in Vitamin D." *ScienceDaily*, accessed February 23, 2021. https://www.sciencedaily.com/releases /2009/08/090803083633.htm.

Black, L. J., K. L. Allen, P. Jacoby, G. S. Trapp, C. M. Gallagher, S. M. Byrne, and W. H. Oddy. "Low Dietary Intake of Magnesium Is Associated with Increased Externalising Behaviours in Adolescents." *Public Health Nutrition* 18, no. 10 (July 2015): 1824–30. https://doi.org/10.1017/S1368980014002432.

Heilskov Rytter, M. J., L. B. Andersen, T. Houmann, N. Bilenberg, A. Hvolby, C. Mølgaard, K. F. Michaelsen, and L. Lauritzen. "Diet in the Treatment of ADHD in Children: A Systematic Review of the Literature." *Nordic Journal of Psychiatry* 69, no. 1 (January 2015): 1–18. https://doi.org/10.3109/08039488.2014.921933.

Horak, F., D. Doberer, E. Eber, et al. "Diagnosis and Management of Asthma— Statement on the 2015 GINA Guidelines." *Wiener klinische Wochenschrift* 128, no. 15–16 (2016): 541–54. https://doi.org/10.1007/s00508-016-1019-4.

Jia, Feiyong, Bing Wang, Ling Shan, Zhida Xu, and Lin Du. "Core Symptoms of Autism Improved after Vitamin D Supplementation." *Pediatrics*, December 15, 2014. https://pubmed.ncbi.nlm.nih.gov/25511123/.

McNamara, R. K., J. Able, R. Jandacek, T. Rider, P. Tso, J. C. Eliassen, D. Alfieri, W. Weber, K. Jarvis, M. P. DelBello, S. M. Strakowski, and C. M. Adler. "Docosahexaenoic Acid Supplementation Increases Prefrontal Cortex Activation during Sustained Attention in Healthy Boys: A Placebo-Controlled, Dose-Ranging, Functional Magnetic Resonance Imaging Study." *American Journal of Clinical Nutrition* 91, no. 4 (April 2010): 1060–67. https://doi.org/10.3945/ajcn.2009.28549.

Montgomery, P., J. R. Burton, R. P. Sewell, T. F. Spreckelsen, and A. J. Richardson. "Fatty Acids and Sleep in UK Children: Subjective and Pilot Objective Sleep Results from the DOLAB Study—a Randomized Controlled Trial." *Journal of Sleep Research* 23, no. 4 (August 2014): 364–88. https://doi.org/10.1111/jsr.12135.

Mousain-Bosc, M., C. Siatka, and J. P. Bali. "Magnesium, Hyperactivity and Autism in Children." In *Magnesium in the Central Nervous System*, edited by R. Vink and M. Nechifor. Adelaide, Australia: University of Adelaide Press, 2011. https://www.ncbi.nlm.nih.gov/books/NBK507249/.

Newberry, S. J., M. Chung, M. Booth, M. A. Maglione, A. M. Tang, C. E. O'Hanlon, D. D. Wang, A. Okunogbe, C. Huang, A. Motala, M. Trimmer, W. Dudley, R. Shanman, T. R. Coker, and P. G. Shekelle. "Omega-3 Fatty Acids and Maternal and Child Health: An Updated Systematic Review." *Evidence Report/Technology Assessment* (Full Report) 224 (October 2016): 1–826. https://doi.org/10.23970/AHRQEPCERTA224.

Rosanoff, A., C. M. Weaver, and Robert K. Rude. "Suboptimal Magnesium Status in the United States: Are the Health Consequences Underestimated?" *Nutrition Reviews* 70, no. 3 (2012): 153–64. https://doi.org/10.1111/j.1753-4887.2011.00465.x.

Ruxton, Carrie. "Health Benefits of Omega-3 Fatty Acids." *Nursing Standard* 18, no. 48 (August 2004): 38–42. https://doi.org/10.7748/ns2004.08.18.48.38.c3668.

Seattle Children's. "Vitamin D Levels during Pregnancy Linked with Child IQ." *ScienceDaily*, accessed February 22, 2021. https://www.sciencedaily.com/releases/2020/11/201102142242.htm.

Surette, M. E., J. Whelan, K. S. Broughton, and J. E. Kinsella. "Evidence for Mechanisms of the Hypotriglyceridemic Effect of N-3 Polyunsaturated Fatty Acids." *Biochimica et Biophysica Acta—Lipids and Lipid Metabolism* 1126, no. 2 (June 1992): 199–205. https://doi.org/10.1016/0005-2760(92)90291-3.

University of Michigan. "Low Levels of Vitamin D in Elementary School Could Spell Trouble in Adolescence." *ScienceDaily*, accessed February 23, 2021. https://www.sciencedaily.com/releases/2019/08/190820130917.htm.

University of Turku. "Vitamin D Deficiency during Pregnancy Connected to Elevated Risk of ADHD." *ScienceDaily*, accessed February 22, 2021. https://www.sciencedaily.com/releases/2020/02/200210104120.htm.

Yang, H., P. Xun, and K. He. "Fish and Fish Oil Intake in Relation to Risk of Asthma: A Systematic Review and Meta-analysis." *PLoS ONE* 8, no. 11 (2013): e80048. https://doi.org/10.1371/journal.pone.0080048.

CHAPTER 6: TESTING AND INTEGRATIVE MODALITIES FOR HEALING

Barbi, E., P. Marzuillo, E. Neri, S. Naviglio, and B. S. Krauss. "Fever in Children: Pearls and Pitfalls." *Children* (Basel) 4, no. 9 (2017): 81. https://doi.org/10.3390/children4090081.

Bijno, D., C. Di Vincenzo, E. Lusenti, A. Martina, and R. Petrelli. "Composition for the Treatment and Prevention of Urinary Tract Infections." U.S. Patent, 2017. US20170232051.

Ji, Y., R. E. Azuine, Y. Zhang, et al. "Association of Cord Plasma Biomarkers of In Utero Acetaminophen Exposure with Risk of Attention-Deficit/Hyperactivity Disorder and Autism Spectrum Disorder in Childhood." *JAMA Psychiatry* 77, no. 2 (2020): 180–89. https://doi.org/10.1001/jamapsychiatry.2019.3259.

Ogilvie, J. D., M. J. Rieder, and R. Lim. "Acetaminophen Overdose in Children." *Canadian Medical Association Journal* 184, no. 13 (2012): 1492–96. https://doi.org/10.1503/cmaj.111338.

Rao, N., H. A. Spiller, N. L. Hodges, T. Chounthirath, M. J. Casavant, A. K. Kamboj, and G. A. Smith. "An Increase in Dietary Supplement Exposures Reported to US Poison Control Centers." *Journal of Medical Toxicology* 13, no. 3 (September 2017): 227–37. https://doi.org/10.1007/s13181-017-0623-7.

Sakulchit, T., and R. D. Goldman. "Acetaminophen Use and Asthma in Children." *Canadian Family Physician* 63, no. 3 (2017): 211–13. https://www.ncbi.nlm.nih.gov/pmc/articles/PMC5349720/.

Sarrell, E. Michael, Avigdor Mandelberg, and Herman Avner Cohen. "Efficacy of Naturopathic Extracts in the Management of Ear Pain Associated with Acute Otitis Media." *Archives of Pediatrics and Adolescent Medicine* 155, no. 7 (2001): 796–99. https://doi.org/10.1001/archpedi.155.7.796.

Strengell, T., M. Uhari, R. Tarkka, J. Uusimaa, R. Alen, P. Lautala, and H. Rantala. "Antipyretic Agents for Preventing Recurrences of Febrile Seizures: Randomized Controlled Trial." *Archives of Pediatrics and Adolescent Medicine* 163, no. 9 (September 2009): 799–804. https://doi.org/10.1001/archpediatrics.2009.137.

Uzun, L., T. Dal, M. T. Kalcıoğlu, M. Yürek, Z. C. Açıkgöz, and R. Durmaz. "Antimicrobial Activity of Garlic Derivatives on Common Causative Microorganisms of the External Ear Canal and Chronic Middle Ear Infections." *Turkish Archives of Otorhinolaryngol* 57, no. 4 (2019): 161–65. https://doi.org/10.5152/tao.2019.4413.

Yousefichaijan, P., M. Kahbazi, S. Rasti, M. Rafeie, and M. Sharafkhah. "Vitamin E as Adjuvant Treatment for Urinary Tract Infection in Girls with Acute Pyelonephritis." *Iran Journal of Kidney Disease* 9, no. 2 (March 2015): 97–104. https://pubmed.ncbi.nlm.nih.gov/25851287/.

Yousefichaijan, P., M. Naziri, H. Taherahmadi, M. Kahbazi, and A. Tabaei. "Zinc Supplementation in Treatment of Children with Urinary Tract Infection." *Iran Journal of Kidney Disease* 10, no. 4 (July 2016): 213–16. https://pubmed.ncbi.nlm.nih.gov/27514768/.

Index

ACEs. *See* adverse childhood experiences
acne, 16
acupressure, 160–62, *161*, 165
acute conditions, 156–57
addiction, 27, 100; development of, 39; nutrition impacted by, 52; to processed foods, 52, 66, 102; stress influencing, 44; to sugar, 84; technology and, 104, 114; in teenagers, 14, 121
additives, 82
ADHD. *See* attention-deficit/ hyperactivity disorder
adverse childhood experiences (ACEs), 102
air filtration, 95
Akkermansia muciniphilia, 56, 73
allergic rhinitis, 160
allergies, 160
aluminum additives, 82
amygdala, 45, 100, 106, 107; decisions controlled by, 16–17; inflammation and, 17, 19–20, *42*; in limbic system, 37–38; prefrontal cortex connected with, 16, *38*, 41–42, 103, 118; stress and, 27, 99
anemia, 158

anti-inflammatory omelet (recipe), 202
anxiety, 82, 114, 120; acupressure points for, *161*; aromatherapy for, 162, 165; separation, 181, 182; stress increasing, 101, 102; sugar and, 85; supplements for, 158; technology causing, 29; in teenagers, 113
appreciation, encouragement and, 125
aromatherapy, 162–63, 165
artificial colorings, 82
artificial sweeteners, 82
attachment. *See* unconditional love
attention-deficit/hyperactivity disorder (ADHD): acupressure for, *161*; detoxification and, 75, 89; medications and, 164; mold impacting, 140; parenting with, 6; pesticides and, 75; and pregnancy, 144; sugar impacting, 85; vitamin supplements for, 158
autism: CDC on, 13; dairy linked to, 79; detoxification aiding, 140, 157; environment improving, 140; inflammation influenced by, 21, 59; processed food linked to, 83; supplements regressing, 138, 145, 157
azodicarbonamide, 82–83

About the Author

Madiha Saeed, MD (also known as HolisticMom, MD, on social media), is a practicing board-certified family physician in the United States, health influencer, and international speaker. She is the author of the bestselling book *The Holistic Rx: Your Guide to Healing Chronic Inflammation and Disease* and the children's book series *Adam's Healing Adventures*. Her goal is to empower the world toward healthier living. Dr. Saeed is the director of education for Documenting Hope and KnoWEwell. She sits on multiple medical advisory boards, including Wellness Mama. Dr. Saeed and her children speak internationally at the most prestigious holistic conferences and summits, and she has appeared on radio and podcasts (including *mindbodygreen*) and in newspapers. She is a regular on the international Emmy-winning medical talk show *The Dr. Nandi Show*. Dr. Saeed's children host *The Holistic Kids Show* podcast, where they interview the biggest names in the functional, holistic, and integrative medicine world and help kids empower and educate other kids.